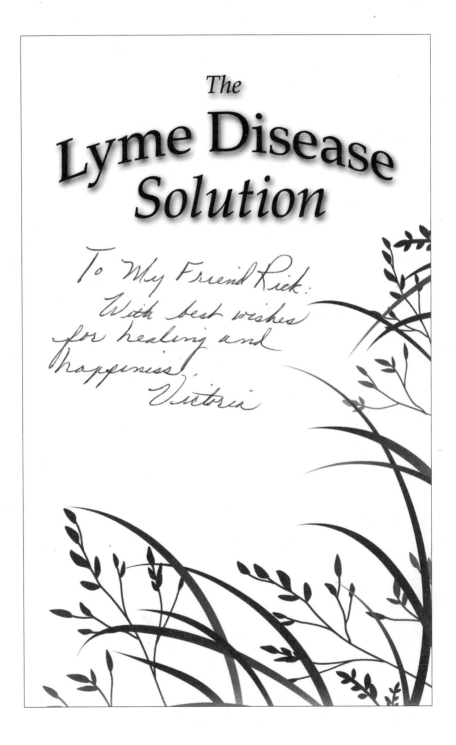

The

Lyme Disease
Solution

To My Friend Rick:
With best wishes
for healing and
happiness,
      Victoria

The

Lyme Disease
Solution

KENNETH B. SINGLETON, M.D., M.P.H.

Foreword by James A. Duke, Ph.D.
Author, *The Green Pharmacy*

BROWN BOOKS 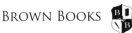 DALLAS, TEXAS

The Lyme Disease Solution™

Manufactured in the United States of America

For information, please contact:

Brown Books Publishing Group
16200 North Dallas Parkway, Suite 170
Dallas, Texas 75248
www.brownbooks.com
972-381-0009

A New Era in Publishing™

ISBN-13: 978-1-934812-00-6
ISBN-10: 1-934812-00-5
LCCN: 2007939144

1 2 3 4 5 6 7 8 9 10

This book is intended for educational purposes only. All information and advice contained herein is based on the author's personal and professional experience. This book exclusively represents the viewpoint and approach of the author, and does not necessarily represent the viewpoint or approach of any other health care practitioner or organization of health care practitioners. Before embarking on any advice given in the book, the reader is advised to consult their health care provider.

Dedication

This book is dedicated to all my Lyme and tick-borne infection patients who have taught me so much over the years. I also dedicate this book to the true pioneers—the two best Lyme doctors that I know—Charles Ray Jones, M.D., and Joseph Burrascano, M.D.—the real heroes of the story.

Page 84
NERVE PAIN

Contents

Acknowledgments

Special Thanks To:

Ursuline Singleton, M.P.H., R.D.

For your patience and diligence in reviewing the manuscript of this book, for your kind and gentle spirit, and for believing in me.

James A. Duke, Ph.D.

For your incredible knowledge and expertise, for your meticulous review and wonderful suggestions, and for being the great teacher that you are.

Mark Garzon, M.D.

For your special contribution to this book in the areas of Endocrinology and Toxicology, for which I am very grateful.

Larry Trivieri, Jr.

For your creativity and your superb writing and editing skills, without which this book would not have been possible.

and

Those Who Took the Time to Review and Offer Excellent Feedback—Dr. Kenneth Liegner, Dr. Binyamin Rothstein, Pastor Kevin McGhee, Mrs. Wendy Goodness.

Special Thanks Also To Others Who Contributed Greatly:

Kathy Norris, Judy Madore, Lori Martell, Marcus Singleton, Myah Singleton, Ursula Beal, Alvin and Gloria Singleton, Marilyn Dimas, Dwight Singleton, Tami Lawyer, Brian Lawyer, Leya Schiller, Pam Andrews, Jean Galbreath, Dr. Brian Heaton, Dr. Mark McClure, and, most importantly, our Creator who makes all things possible.

A Garden Parable

One spring day George decided to plant a garden. He went to the local nursery and bought several beautiful plants. After clearing the land, he put the plants in the ground.

For the first few months, his Garden was magnificent. The colors were spectacular. His neighbors would often slow down as they drove by his home to admire the beautiful Garden that George had created. In fact, George could hardly wait to get home from work every day so he could bask in the lush beauty of his new Garden.

But later in the season, some strange things began to happen in his Garden. He noticed several different varieties of weeds growing where none had ever grown before. He also noted that several of the plants had a peculiar fungus-like material on the leaves and stems. He further observed that some of the trees had insects burrowing under their bark and that the leaves were looking unhealthy.

George nervously ran down to the garden shop where he had bought the plants and bought the best herbicide, fungicide, and insecticide that he could find. Only the best would do for his wonderful Garden. He rushed home and sprayed and sprayed and sprayed.

And for a short time, it seemed that the chemicals worked—the weeds withered, the fungus lightened up, and the insects seemed to go away. But George's elation turned into frustration a few weeks later, when all the problems returned with a vengeance.

In desperation, George asked his neighbor a few doors away for advice. (This neighbor, Kathy, also had a very nice garden, which seemed to be doing well.) Kathy told him that she had had similar problems for the first year of her garden. She had finally gotten advice from an old retired gardener named Frank. And that advice had made all the difference.

George searched and finally was able to contact Frank. He joyfully hopped in his car and drove over to Frank's place a few miles away. There on the front porch sat a quiet old man with weathered skin, Frank.

George introduced himself and asked Frank if he could describe his problems to him and possibly get some advice. Frank said that he would do better than give advice—he wanted to actually take a walk through George's Garden.

They arrived back at the Garden, and Frank carefully examined each of the plants, felt the soil and took a sample, smelled the flowers, analyzed the sun/shade patterns, and observed the wildlife usage of the Garden—the birds, spiders, bees, and so forth.

Frank then spoke to George about the Garden. "George, all the chemicals in the world will not cure the problems of your

Garden. Those give temporary fixes that in the long run might make things worse unless you correct the underlying causes."

George replied, "What underlying causes are you speaking of?"

Frank said, "The Garden is fully capable of healing itself if you obey some very basic rules of gardening."

He went on. "First rule is that you have to prepare the soil and regularly feed the plants. Without proper nutrition, the plants cannot survive in a healthy way; they will always look sick and be more prone to disease.

"Second rule is that proper watering is essential to all vital functions of the Garden. Regular watering whether you think it needs it or not is absolutely critical.

"Next you must make sure that sunlight exposure is appropriate for each of the plants. Some like full sun and others prefer mostly shade. With the wrong amount of sun, the plants will do very poorly. For instance, this azalea is in full sun, and now it is yellowing and drooping. It was intended for shade or indirect light."

Frank went on and on. George frantically took notes as he gave his sage advice.

His final piece of advice was, "So George, put the chemicals away for now. You might need them at some point to help out, but they will never be the whole answer. They are not a substitute for proven rules of gardening from the Creator which when followed strengthen your Garden, enabling it to have health and vitality from the inside out."

George gratefully took all of Frank's advice and obeyed it. His Garden flourished, and he never needed the chemicals again, because the Garden was now equipped to heal itself of all its problems.

Foreword

The Light of the LAMP

by

James A. Duke, Ph.D.

In Dr. Singleton's Garden Parable that opens this book, Frank is an organic gardener, not a chemical gardener. Frank has learned in his gardening experience that harsh chemicals sometimes cause more problems than they solve. Frank knows that in order to grow well, a plant needs the right environment: the right amount of sunshine, the right amount of water, the proper soil and fertility. And Frank's plants grow better and healthier than those of the "inorganic" gardeners in the area.

The "inorganic gardeners" drench any and all diseased plants and weeds with harsh chemicals, harming both the disease agents and ultimately the desired plant itself. Frank has learned in life's school of hard knocks that, when properly nurtured, the plant is much better able to compete with weeds and disease. And, as a result, it will require less and less assistance from potentially dangerous synthetic chemical substances.

Lyme disease is best approached in the same way. Like Frank, I prefer a "Lyme-aware medical practitioner" (or LAMP) who is an organic health practitioner. This kind of practitioner is a beam of light for the observant patient and for the "inorganic" medical practitioners. By inorganic practitioners I am referring to those practitioners who attack every disease symptom only using a plethora of expensive and toxic chemicals—with both beneficial effects and harmful side effects. Sometimes the side effects are worse than the original disease effects.

As with Frank and his plants, the organic LAMP doctor seeks to strengthen his patient, while gently attacking the underlying disease. Given the right nurture, nutrition, exercise, stress reduction, spiritual support, and life style, the patient's immune system grows stronger and healthier. Of course, like the good gardener, the good LAMP knows that not necessarily the same prescription works for each individual patient. The good LAMP enlightens the pathway to health and self-healing. As a result, fewer and fewer potentially harmful chemicals are needed to correct the diminishing symptoms of the healthier patient. The patient is growing happier and healthier in the light of the LAMP.

Living organically, like an organic flower, the patient expands and blossoms in the light. The result is spiritual healing, reflecting the inner strengths that stem from an improved immune system, well cultivated in the temple of the patient. The patient is healed more from inner strengths, without the need of so many synthetic chemical substances.

Life goes on for the patient, and the Lyme is suppressed, sometimes forgotten, thanks to the inner strengths of the organic patient. As sunshine strengthens the plant, the guidance that you will receive from this book can strengthen a cooperating Lyme patient. If you are a Lyme patient and have an open mind, this book will enlighten you on your pathway back to health and wholeness.

Introduction

Do you suffer from health problems that your doctors can't seem to get a handle on? Are you in pain, or tired all the time, or often unable to think straight? Is the quality of your life slipping away despite everything that you and your doctor have tried? If you answered "yes" to any of these questions, it is very possible that you are suffering from a health problem that is often ignored or misdiagnosed—Lyme disease. And you are not alone. Lyme is a problem that has left untold numbers of others suffering with a similar range of debilitating symptoms. To make problems even worse, Lyme disease is often accompanied by other tick-borne infections.

Each year the United States Centers for Disease Control and Prevention (CDC) reports more than 20,000 diagnosed cases of Lyme disease in the United States, but many authorities agree that CDC-reported cases greatly underestimate the number of actual cases. Some estimates place the actual number of cases at 10 times or more higher than reported cases. These staggering statistics indicate that Lyme disease is a major U.S. public health problem. The statistics suggest that Lyme disease is reaching epidemic proportions in the United States. Further, Lyme disease is not confined to the United States and is becoming an increasingly important public health concern in Canada, Europe, and other parts of the world.

Lyme disease is becoming so prevalent in the United States that it has even affected the President of the United States. This fact was revealed on August 8, 2007, by the *Houston Chronicle*, which reported that a year earlier, President Bush was treated for early-stage Lyme disease after developing the "bull's eye" rash associated with Lyme. As this book makes clear, President Bush was fortunate in that in his case Lyme was detected early. For many other people, including myself, Lyme often escapes early detection, making the standard treatment approach that President Bush received (a course of antibiotics) of limited usefulness.

If you have been diagnosed with Lyme disease, you likely know how severe and debilitating its manifestations can be. I know personally about that struggle also. For eight years I had undiagnosed Lyme disease. My symptoms first began in the early 1990s, soon after I helped friends build a mountain log cabin. Shortly afterwards, I developed symptoms of an out-of-season flu. I had not spotted a tick bite nor developed a "bull's eye" rash. Unfortunately, I did not know much about Lyme disease in those days and did not initially suspect it to be the cause of my health problems. (As medicine is an ever-evolving science, at that time very little was known by the medical profession about Lyme disease.)

Over the next few months my symptoms became progressively worse. Because I had no clue as to the cause of these symptoms, I thought it wise to seek help from my medical colleagues. One consultant that I met with was suspicious of Lyme and performed a Lyme blood test. Subsequently, he dismissed Lyme as a possibility for my symptoms because the blood test was normal. Therefore, like many Lyme patients, on the basis of negative lab results and lack of the tell-tale "bull's eye" rash, an accurate Lyme diagnosis was missed.

Over the next seven years, my symptoms continued to worsen—persistent fatigue, foggy thinking, and pain in the joints and muscles. Like many patients I have seen in my practice, I was continuously told by the numerous specialists with whom I consulted that Lyme disease was not a possibility. After all, my blood test for Lyme was normal. I could only guess at the nature of my mysterious illness as I failed to adequately respond to the treatments prescribed by my medical colleagues from whom I sought assistance.

The final diagnosis by the Rheumatology medical specialist was that I had a poorly understood disorder called "fibromyalgia." Whatever relief I experienced from his treatment approach was inconsistent. At this point, I became deliberate in my quest to feel like myself again. I began to research and explore various "alternative" approaches that included acupuncture, nutrition, and herbal therapies. As I incorporated some of these approaches into my treatment regimen, to my surprise, I experienced a significant improvement in my health and discovered a new sense of well-being—something that I had not felt for several years. This improvement in my health led to a new awareness and understanding of how these alternative therapies can complement the conventional treatment therapies that I had been using in my own medical practice. I began to incorporate these techniques into my practice with excellent results. Over time, other "fibromyalgia" patients began to seek me out as I became widely regarded as a physician who was skilled in using alternative, as well as conventional, medical therapies to effectively treat fibromyalgia.

Yet, despite the marked improvements in my health, I still was not completely well. Eight years after the onset of my illness, a fellow physician recommended that I be retested for Lyme disease utilizing a different type of Lyme test—one that was more accurate for detecting Lyme. This time, I tested positive. Within a few months of adding combination antibiotics to my natural therapies regimen, I was well on my way to fully recovering my health. Today, I am helping many other Lyme patients do the same.

If your experience is similar to mine, take heart. In the pages that follow, I will provide you with information that will enable you to develop a powerful, personal action plan for your recovery from Lyme and other tick-borne diseases. In your recovery, you will need the help of knowledgeable Lyme health professionals. In this book, you will learn what to look for in a doctor and how you can locate one that you can work with. In that light, you will also learn about the concept of the "Lyme-aware medical practitioner" (LAMP) that Dr. James Duke referred to in the foreword of this book.

And that's not all. You will also learn about signs, symptoms, and risk factors for Lyme and the other common tick-borne infections. I will discuss with you the reasons that Lyme disease is so difficult to recognize and diagnose. You will get the answer to the question: Why are so many people with Lyme disease incorrectly told they don't have Lyme? Very importantly, you will learn how Lyme doctors reliably and effectively make the diagnosis of Lyme disease and the other tick-borne diseases.

Next, you will learn how the body's natural defense system, the immune system, works to battle Lyme. There are many self-care things that you can do to support your own natural defenses against Lyme. You will further learn how you can have a strong immune system without having an overactive system that causes a problem called "chronic inflammation." I will share with you how to incorporate principles of diet and nutrition to build a healthy immune system that is able to control Lyme and the other tick-borne diseases. You will be introduced to a very effective nutritional approach to healing and balancing your immune system—the Lyme Inflammation Diet.

You will learn about the core natural therapies and about the antibiotics that are used by Lyme doctors like myself to successfully treat Lyme and the other tick-borne disorders. I will discuss the practical ways that you can relay your health information to your Lyme specialist so that your doctor can most effectively help you. You will further learn about methods of dealing with the most common complications of Lyme such as fatigue, chronic pain, inflammation, brain and neurological problems, and many more. I will also deal extensively with the problem of coping with Lyme—from a spiritual and psychological perspective by giving you a road map of mind/body/spirit techniques that I have found to be extremely useful. Finally, you will be provided with a list of the most helpful Lyme disease organizations, as well as a wealth of other helpful resources.

Knowing firsthand the pain and suffering that Lyme disease can cause gives me a unique perspective on Lyme disease. Based on my personal experience and the experiences of my patients, I also know that it is possible that Lyme disease can be reversed. My message to you is simple: There is hope for you, no matter how long you may have suffered with Lyme disease. As with any illness, the key to recovery lies in knowing what you must do in order to get well. If you are ready to make that healing journey, turn the page so that you can discover the Lyme Disease Solution!

PART ONE:

THE LYME DISEASE BASICS

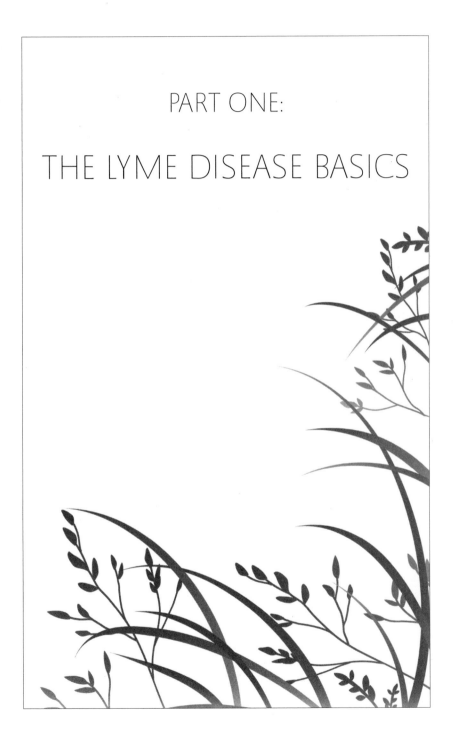

Chapter One

Lyme Disease:
the Facts, Risks, Controversy,
and Prevention

If you are reading this book, most likely you either know or suspect that you or someone you know is suffering from Lyme disease. Unfortunately, many people with Lyme disease are unaware that they are affected by it. This problem is made even worse by the fact that a significant number of Lyme-infected patients are told by their physicians that they don't have Lyme after having a "false negative" blood test for Lyme disease. This means that a true Lyme diagnosis can be missed because the blood test result does not show evidence of the disease despite Lyme being present and active in the body.

As I mentioned in the Introduction, I was one of those patients. I suffered from Lyme disease symptoms for nearly eight years before my condition was accurately diagnosed. Soon after the onset of symptoms, I sought medical help from competent medical professionals. Despite being a physician myself (and consulting with very knowledgeable doctors), I was misdiagnosed as having "fibromyalgia." Lyme disease was considered as a diagnosis but was dismissed because of the false negative result of the conventional ELISA blood test.

Based on my experience in coping with and eventually succeeding in treating my condition, I know firsthand how important a proper diagnosis is in order to effectively treat Lyme disease. For every case of Lyme that is currently detected, there are as many as ten or more cases of Lyme disease that go undetected or misdiagnosed. In this chapter, I will explain why this is so.

What Is Lyme Disease?

Lyme disease is a potentially chronic and debilitating disorder that can manifest with a wide range of possible symptoms. Depending on how it progresses in an individual patient, these symptoms can mimic those of cardiac, neurological, rheumatoid, and many other conditions. At its core, Lyme disease is primarily an infection caused by an invasive spirochetal bacterium known as *Borrelia burgdorferi* (abbreviated *Bb*). The organism was named after Dr. Willy Burgdorfer, who identified the bacterium in 1982. These infectious organisms, which are called spirochetes because of their characteristic cork-screw or spiral shape, are the cause of the disease we call Lyme disease.

The technical name for this disease is actually "Lyme borreliosis." However, for the sake of simplicity, it is commonly known as "Lyme disease" (LD). In the United States, more than 100 strains of *Bb* have been identified so far, while worldwide approximately 300 strains have been found. Although some of these strains are similar, many others are quite distinct from each other.

In addition to having many different strains of Lyme, the bacterium can also exist in three different forms when viewed under a microscope. The most common form is called a "spirochete," which is the cork-screw structure that is transmitted from the tick and causes the infection in humans. Once inside the body, the spirochete can change itself into two alternative structures if it is stressed or threatened (for example, by antibiotics). The first alternative structure is called the "L" form. In this form, the Lyme organism becomes round in shape and its outer coating (called the cell wall) becomes thinned. The second alternative configuration is called the "cyst" form. In this form the Lyme organism becomes thickened, and it ceases its growth and reproductive processes. It goes into hibernation, or dormancy, waiting for a more favorable time and environment in which to grow.

Initially, it was thought that humans only contracted *Borrelia burgdorferi*, or *Bb*, from ticks, a belief that still is commonly accepted by many in the medical field, as well as the public at large. Research strongly suggests that *Bb* can also be transmitted by a variety of other vectors, such as fleas, flies, gnats, mites, and mosquitoes. Evidence also indicates that human-to-human transmission of *Bb* can also occur via the placenta (which accounts for many of the cases of children being born with Lyme disease). It may also occur through blood transfusions. For this reason, the Red Cross now makes it a policy to exclude donors with active Lyme disease, as well as people in whom Lyme disease was active during the previous year. (People with a history of babesiosis, a co-infection, are also not permitted to donate blood.) Some health experts take the position that Lyme disease can be transmitted during sexual intercourse. While this has not been conclusively proven scientifically, it has been documented that Lyme organisms can be present in both semen and vaginal secretions. Animal studies support the contention that Lyme may potentially be transmissible by sexual contact.

A common misconception about Lyme disease is that people who suffer with it develop a specific type of rash soon after they are infected with the *Bb* spirochete. This rash, which has the shape of a "bull's eye," is referred to as "erythema migrans" (EM or ECM). Certainly, it does develop in many cases of Lyme disease as an early warning sign. However, research now shows that less than 50 percent of adults and children with reported cases of Lyme disease exhibit the EM rash. Additionally, other rashes that are not "bull's eye" in appearance often occur with Lyme and are often dismissed by physicians as "not Lyme" because they are not the easily recognized EM rashes.

This lack of appearance of an EM rash is one of the three major reasons why so many cases of Lyme disease escape detection. With no signs of the EM rash, many patients and physicians alike simply assume that Lyme disease is not a factor in the health problems they face.

The second major reason that Lyme escapes detection has to do with the tick bite itself. The deer tick may be extremely small—the size of the period at the end of this sentence. Unless it becomes engorged with blood, it can easily be missed. Therefore, in those cases where no skin reaction or rash occurs, a person may never know that they were bitten.

The third major reason that Lyme goes undetected is the improper use of and dependence on the conventional blood screening tests. So often physicians will perform the test before it has had a chance to become positive (which may take up to six weeks) and dismiss even a classic EM rash because "the Lyme test was negative." Finally, some tests have only been made to detect one strain of Lyme, thereby setting a patient up to fail detection if that patient is not infected with that particular strain.

When Lyme disease is detected soon after a person is exposed to *Bb*, it usually can be treated rather easily. However, if it escapes detection in the very early stages, Lyme disease very commonly passes from an acute, or localized, short-term health problem, to a far more serious and chronic condition. As a result it can disrupt various body systems, including the joints, the immune system (causing autoimmune disorders), the nervous system, and other vital organ structures. When this occurs, effective treatment becomes far more challenging and, often, expensive and time-consuming.

One of the other major reasons that Lyme disease so often escapes detection or is misdiagnosed has to do with the myriad ways in which it can manifest. For this reason, progressive Lyme physicians often refer to it as "The Great Imposter" or "The Great Imitator." These descriptive nicknames are well-earned because of how the symptoms of Lyme disease so often mimic those of other diseases, including chronic fatigue syndrome (CFS/CFIDS), fibromyalgia, Lou Gehrig's disease (amyotrophic lateral sclerosis, or ALS), and multiple sclerosis. In fact, Lyme disease can both cause and mimic heart disease as well as a number of neurological and psychological conditions.

George is a typical example of how Lyme may masquerade as the very common disorder, fibromyalgia syndrome (FMS). As an avid hunter in rural Pennsylvania, it was common for him to pull ticks off of himself. One year, he became sick a few weeks after completion of the hunting season. He recalled a flu-like illness that no one else in the family or at work seemed to catch. There was no rash. Shortly after the main symptoms subsided, he noticed that his knees hurt and even swelled at times. He also noted headaches and that his memory was not as sharp as it had been. He went to his family doctor, who did a Lyme test, which was negative. Anti-inflammatory and antidepressant medications were prescribed, which helped somewhat with his discomfort.

A few months later, he began to notice additional daily symptoms of severe tiredness, lack of motivation, numbness of his feet, ringing in the ears, poor sleep, and muscle and joint pains involving his entire body. Also, he noticed that every three or four weeks all the symptoms would intensify for a few days. After these few days of increased intensity, the symptoms would revert to the previous pattern.

Eventually, his prescribed anti-inflammatory medicines and antidepressants were no longer effective. At this point, he was referred to a rheumatologist. He was evaluated and had extensive testing, including a repeat of the Lyme blood test. The conclusion was that he had fibromyalgia syndrome. Unfortunately, the therapies prescribed for him by the specialist were not effective in reducing his symptoms. Two years later, he was able to locate a doctor who specialized in detecting and treating tick-borne illnesses. Upon further testing, he was found to have Lyme disease. After four months of antibiotic therapy and use of the comprehensive approach described in this book, his symptoms completely resolved.

Based on such experiences in my clinical practice, as well as my own nearly eight-year history of being misdiagnosed, I have learned a considerable amount about chronic "incurable" diseases. I believe that many patients who suffer from chronic health problems that don't abate no matter what is being done to treat them should be thoroughly evaluated for Lyme disease and "co-infections" (other organisms that often infect a person at the same time as Lyme) by a physician who is skilled in evaluating patients for these disorders. In chapter 2, I will discuss the symptoms of Lyme and the co-infections. I will describe the most accurate methods for testing for Lyme and for co-infections in chapter 3.

The Prevalence of Lyme Disease

Another unfortunate reason that Lyme disease is often undiagnosed has to do with the still persistent beliefs that only people in certain geographical regions are at risk for contracting it. Many also believe that Lyme disease is a relatively new health condition. Both of these beliefs are false. Even so, conventional Lyme experts and health institutions, including the Centers for Disease Control and Prevention (CDC), unwittingly continue to perpetuate them. For example, on its Web site, the CDC states: "About 12,000–15,000 cases of Lyme disease are reported each year in the United States, primarily in the Northeast and North Central parts of the country and in parts of California."

Other mainstream sources of health information also primarily relegate Lyme disease to only a handful of states. They report that 95 percent of all cases occur in Connecticut, Delaware, Maryland, Massachusetts, Minnesota, New Hampshire, New Jersey, New York, Pennsylvania, Wisconsin, and Vermont. A major problem with this kind of statistic is that it does not take into account that virtually all Lyme-reporting to CDC is done by practicing doctors and laboratories. However, if doctors are not recognizing Lyme or testing for it, then it goes undetected and thus unreported.

A good example of this is in the state of Virginia. My practice is in Maryland—one of the top ten states for new cases of Lyme according to the CDC. It is generally recognized as one of the "endemic" or hotbed states for Lyme. However, just across the Potomac River is Virginia. That state doesn't seem to have nearly as many cases reported to CDC. Yet many of my new patients are coming from Virginia. The difference is purely due to the fact that Lyme is not yet considered to be a major public health problem there. As a result, many physicians are not yet thinking that Lyme disease could be a serious threat to their patients and are, therefore, not evaluating for it.

This problem of physician unawareness makes it easy for people to wrongly infer that the risk of Lyme disease in other parts of the country is very small and even nonexistent. Nothing could be further from the truth. In actuality, a number of states outside of the Northeast and the upper Central region of the United States, including California, Florida, Illinois, Missouri, North Carolina, Ohio, Texas, and, now even, Virginia, in recent years are reporting substantial increases in the incidence of Lyme disease within their borders. Eventually, all these states will be considered endemic also. And, as of the 2005 CDC statistics, all but one state (Montana) across the nation have reported cases of Lyme disease.

The increasing incidence of Lyme disease is further confirmed by the CDC. According to the CDC: "In 2005, 23,305 cases of Lyme disease were reported, yielding a national average of 7.9 cases for every 100,000 persons. In the ten states where Lyme disease is most common, the average was 31.6 cases for every 100,000 persons." Further, the CDC states that only 5 to 10 percent of Lyme disease cases are actually reported each year by state health officials and physicians. This means that in 2005, there were potentially more than 460,000 new cases of Lyme disease in the United States. And many health experts believe that this number would be much larger if not for the strict reporting criteria recommended by the CDC for Lyme disease. (In chapter 3 we will discuss in detail how Lyme is diagnosed.)

Lyme disease is also a growing problem for countries other than the United States. According to the Canadian equivalent of the CDC, Health Canada's Laboratory Centre for Disease Control, the incidence of Lyme disease is nearing epidemic proportions, and ticks infected with *Bb* are now present in nearly every Canadian province. According to the World Health Organization (WHO), Lyme disease is also present in significant percentages of the populations of most European countries, especially Germany, where it is estimated that up to 15 percent of all Germans are infected. Lyme disease also poses a significant health problem in Great Britain, Australia, China, Japan, New Zealand, and Russia.

A Brief History of Lyme Disease

Lyme disease is commonly thought to be a relatively new disease that originated in and around the town of Lyme, Connecticut (hence its name), in the mid-1970s. Initially, 39 children and 12 adults from within this community were diagnosed with what was first called "Lyme arthritis" by medical researchers from Yale University working in concert with the National Institute of Arthritis and Musculoskeletal and Skin Diseases. Heading up this research was Yale's Dr. Allen Steere, who a few years later (1978) suspected that the symptoms experienced by these patients were related to tick bites. As I mentioned above, in 1982, further investigation by Dr. Willy Burgdorfer led to the discovery that it wasn't the tick bite itself that caused Lyme disease, but rather the presence of the specific *Bb* bacteria that ticks transmitted to humans when bites occurred.

Because it was originally thought that the ticks associated

with Lyme disease were located only in the northeastern United States, for years afterwards, the disease itself was also considered to be a health threat only in that same region. However, the truth is that Lyme disease did not originate in Connecticut, nor is it a condition that has only been around for the last thirty years. In fact, Lyme disease dates back to at least the 1800s, and it was first discovered in Europe, where it has been written about in medical journals since 1883, when German physician Alfred Buchwald first published a description of it. In 1909, another physician, Arvid Afzelius of Sweden, became the first medical physician to present research about the expanding "bull's eye" rash or lesion that is characteristic of some Lyme disease cases in their acute, or early, stage.

In 1921, the first medical report linking joint pain and swelling to what is now known as Lyme disease was published. One year later, further medical research first suggested a link between the erythema migrans (EM) rash and the neurological problems that we now know most definitely can be part of the symptoms caused by Lyme disease. According to Karen Vanderhoof-Forschner, co-founder of the Lyme Disease Foundation, much of what we now know about Lyme disease had already been published in medical journals, "including the variety of skin problems, the common arthritic conditions, and many of the neurological, cardiac, and ophthalmologic problems" that are so often a part of chronic Lyme disease.

It is interesting that now, several decades after the case reported in 1921, the general medical community, along with the public is becoming aware of how widespread Lyme disease is, and how pervasive its symptoms can be. This very long delay is a powerful illustration of the lag that so often occurs between the time in which medical discoveries first occur (and enter the medical literature) and the time in which they first begin to be widely accepted and implemented. As it is, even today there remains a need for a much greater recognition of the problems posed by Lyme disease on the part of physicians and medical researchers. More importantly, there remains a need for more physicians to recognize and implement a comprehensive treatment plan in order to properly treat patients suffering from chronic Lyme disease. My hope, in presenting just such a plan in this book, is that it will be Lyme patients themselves who spur the medical community to move in this direction as quickly as possible and thereby help put an end to the needless suffering and pain experienced by so many Lyme patients and their loved ones.

The Medical Controversy Surrounding Lyme Disease

Physicians and health organizations today are divided into two basic schools of thought when it comes to Lyme disease— those who recognize it as a potentially chronic and debilitating disease that requires a comprehensive treatment approach, and those who continue to regard Lyme disease as a primarily benign illness that can easily be treated with a short course of antibiotic treatment. As a result of this controversy, many people with Lyme disease are unaware that it is the underlying cause of their health symptoms and, therefore, are not being properly treated.

The gravity of the health risks posed by this ongoing controversy is illustrated by the experience of the internationally renowned writer and novelist Amy Tan. On her Web site (www.amytan.net) and in her book, *The Opposite of Fate*, Tan recounts her multiyear struggle to make sense of her health symptoms, which began in 1999. Describing that struggle, she writes that her experience is "in many ways typical," and that, as someone who primarily lives in California, she had little awareness of Lyme disease when she first began to notice her symptoms. Initially, because she had a history of being in good health, she passed off her early symptoms—"a stiff neck, insomnia, a constant headache, and a bad back followed by a frozen shoulder"—as being due to too much air travel. But then she began to experience tingling pains and numbness in her feet, which caused her to recall an odd rash she'd developed months earlier. Beginning as a tiny black dot that she mistakenly assumed was a small blood blister, it turned into "a growing red rash, which, curiously, did not itch, but lasted a month." When she asked her physician if the rash might be related to her symptoms, she was told no.

As her symptoms continued to worsen, Tan was referred to a total of ten health care specialists and had "countless lab tests," including an MRI that revealed lesions on her brain's frontal, temporal, and parietal lobes that her doctors felt were normal for someone her age. Eventually, still without an accurate diagnosis, Tan reached the point where she was unable to leave her house alone, due to extreme fatigue, pain, and mental confusion that she feared were the early signs of Alzheimer's disease. It was only after Tan began researching her symptoms on the Internet that she finally came to realize that she might have Lyme disease. Further online research led her to a physician who specialized in treating Lyme disease, who was able to confirm her diagnosis and begin an effective treatment plan. Today, she reports, she is making steady progress in her journey back to health, but adds, "I know that my late diagnosis means I am in this for years, perhaps even for life. But at least I have my mind back." What makes Tan's experience all the more illustrative of the challenges so many patients with Lyme disease face is the fact that all the doctors she consulted prior to finding her Lyme specialist "were affiliated with major urban hospitals, were tops in their department, well known, well respected." Yet, these very competent medical professionals were unable to properly diagnose her problem, resulting in her condition worsening before she finally began to improve.

Tragically, Tan's experience is all too common, due to the continued lack of understanding of Lyme disease by many in the medical community. But lack of understanding is hardly the only issue involved in the Lyme disease controversy. Far more serious is the ongoing "heated debate" that has arisen between researchers in the academic fields and clinical researchers and physicians who are actually in the trenches, as it were, doing their best to treat Lyme disease effectively. Most of the patients who come to these "doctors in the trenches" are the most difficult cases—those who have failed every other treatment protocol— and very often these cases require lengthy treatments in order to help patients recover their health.

Recently, the Lyme disease controversy became even more pronounced after fourteen members of the Infectious Diseases Society of America (IDSA) issued national guidelines. The unfortunate fact is that these guidelines have received general acceptance in the medical community. However, these guidelines may significantly diminish the ability of physicians who treat and diagnose Lyme disease to properly and effectively treat their patients. I would like to discuss examples of how these guidelines will impact Lyme patients.

Among the recommendations made by the IDSA are that physicians limit their treatment of Lyme disease to ten to twenty-eight days of oral antibiotics, with no more than a month of additional oral antibiotic use for patients with persistent symptoms and then only after a waiting period of time (giving Lyme a chance to further disseminate). The guidelines also recommend that physicians rely solely on two unreliable diagnostic criteria: the characteristic bull's eye or erythema migrans (EM) rash and conventional screening blood tests for Lyme. I've already discussed how one half or more of people who develop Lyme disease never develop the EM rash. The conventional tests recommended by the IDSA for diagnosing Lyme are often of limited value because they only detect 50–60 percent of true Lyme cases. This means one third to one half of Lyme patients will be missed. (We will discuss this diagnostic dilemma in chapter 3.)

Most disturbing of all, the IDSA's guidelines actually deny the existence of chronic or persistent Lyme infection, preferring to call it "Post-Lyme Disease Syndrome" (PLDS). PLDS is viewed as a chronic condition that some patients are left with after the *Bb* bacteria are killed off by the antibiotics. However, studies have shown that Lyme can persist after antibiotic treatment. Culture-confirmed failure of antibiotics was first reported in 1989. Several studies conducted in animals—mice, dogs, monkeys—indicate that *Bb* can persist after treatment is completed. Persistence of Lyme infection after treatment in humans has been confirmed by way of culture or molecular testing in at least twelve different studies.

The IDSA guidelines do not acknowledge that Lyme can

be a chronic and persistent infection nor do they acknowledge the significant role of co-infections in patients with chronic symptoms. When Lyme becomes chronic, or resistant, or if co-infections exist, or if chronic inflammation becomes a problem, it becomes necessary to utilize a multidisciplinary treatment approach that you will learn about in this book.

Fortunately, a number of Lyme advocacy groups, including the International Lyme and Associated Diseases Society (ILADS), have challenged the IDSA's assertions on the following bases:

* They are too restrictive, considering many of the latest published findings about Lyme disease.

* They are likely to stifle new and effective treatments.

* If adopted, they are likely to give insurance companies, which are already resistant to the idea of providing medical coverage for Lyme disease treatments, additional ammunition in the battle to avoid payment for Lyme treatment.

Fortunately, the concerns raised by the ILADS, the Lyme Disease Association (LDA), and other Lyme disease advocacy groups have caught the eye of at least one state's attorney general. In November 2006, Richard Blumenthal, attorney general of Connecticut, announced an investigation into the practices of the IDSA to determine whether it is a "monopolistic organization" attempting to shape the treatment of Lyme disease at the expense of other viable treatment options. In addition, Blumenthal is also investigating whether the IDSA violated antitrust laws due to the way they went about setting their suggested guidelines. "These guidelines were set by a panel that essentially locked out competing points of view," Blumenthal stated at a press conference announcing his investigation.

The outcome of this investigation remains to be seen. For now, it is certain that the controversy that surrounds Lyme disease is ongoing and likely will continue. For this reason, patients with Lyme disease need to do all they can to educate themselves about the legal and political issues concerning their condition, so that they can make the best and most informed choices about their health care. To better assist you in this education process, I've included additional information on this issue in the appendices of this book.

As a result of many years of my personal and professional experience with Lyme disease, my medical preference is to follow the approach to Lyme promoted by ILADS. I will discuss next some of the key points that I believe that you should consider in choosing a doctor to evaluate and treat you for Lyme disease.

The Lyme-Aware Doctors

Given the current state of controversy regarding Lyme disease and its treatment, I feel that it is absolutely essential that people with Lyme be aware of these issues so that they can knowledgeably address them with their physicians. Knowing about these issues can also help patients to be better informed when it comes to selecting the physicians they work with. By being well informed, patients are in a much better position to determine whether or not their physicians have an aware and progressive view of Lyme disease. It is important to work with a physician who recognizes the potential need for comprehensive and possibly ongoing treatment in many cases where Lyme disease has disseminated through the body to become systemic. Working with such physicians can make a profound difference in how well patients recover from Lyme disease.

Dr. James A. Duke mentioned in his foreword a type of Lyme practitioner who is proficient in addressing *both* the conventional medical *and* the natural health aspects of Lyme treatment. Like Dr. Duke, I refer to such physicians as Lyme-Aware Medical Practitioners (LAMPs) or, simply, Lyme-aware doctors. This type of practitioner is also commonly known by the acronym LLMD, which stands for Lyme-Literate Medical Doctor.

In number, they still make up only a small percentage of physicians in the United States. Fortunately, the number of these physicians is continuing to grow. Additionally, some of them, myself included, became members of the Lyme-aware physician group due to personal or family struggles with Lyme disease. This makes us well able to appreciate the challenges and frustrations that Lyme patients can face. What's important is not whether your physician has had Lyme disease; what matters most is that he or she recognizes the multifaceted nature of Lyme disease and is knowledgeable about the comprehensive treatment strategies I will be sharing with you later on in this book. If this is the case, then you are in capable hands.

While it is essential to have the assistance of a competent Lyme doctor to help illuminate your pathway back to health, there is another key component on this journey. It's important for you to realize that the ultimate responsibility for your health rests with you. This is something that many patients don't realize and, in a lot of cases, also don't wish to accept. Too often in our society, we have been taught to place physicians on a pedestal and defer to their judgments. Although some physicians may enjoy such deference, most of my medical colleagues and I find that such an attitude places an undue burden on our profession while simultaneously short-changing the patients who hold it. That is why I like to tell all my new patients that my philosophy of medicine is that a good doctor–patient relationship is a partnership and not a dictatorship.

Certainly, physicians should be respected for their medical expertise. However, as part of this doctor–patient partnership, it is important that you realize that you are your own best expert when it comes to your body and your health. When you agree to take responsibility for your role within this partnership, it means two things. First of all, it means that you agree to work with your physician respecting his or her recommendations. Secondly, you agree to take the time to educate yourself as much as possible about the nature of your condition and the various treatment options that are available to you.

Remember, knowledge is power. You can empower yourself best by learning all you can about your problem and the various therapy choices available to you. The knowledge that you gain will place you in a much better position to ask your doctor appropriate questions.

By taking a proactive stance and seeking out a Lyme-aware physician to work with, you will be in the best possible position from which to reclaim your health. In upcoming sections of this book, you will also learn about many useful self-care tools that can be helpful to you on your journey back to health. And in the resources section of this book, you will find references to organizations you can contact that can refer you to a Lyme-aware physician or an LLMD.

Prevention—The Most Effective Method for Dealing with Lyme Disease

There is one thing about which there is no controversy. Everyone agrees that the best way to handle Lyme disease is to never contract it in the first place. Therefore, efforts to increase public awareness and education concerning Lyme prevention are critical in order to reduce the incidence of this potentially devastating disease. Lyme education and prevention requires a comprehensive approach that focuses on the school systems, the media (print, TV, and radio), and health care providers.

It saddens me when I happen to see children, landscapers, athletes, and everyday people outdoors doing things that I know will place them at a very high risk for contracting Lyme disease. Most people have no idea that they are at such great risk. On the other hand, I don't want people to become paralyzed with fear of contracting Lyme disease to the point that they can't enjoy all the wonders of nature provided to us by our Creator. When it comes to Lyme disease, there needs to be what I call a "common sense balance" of wise caution without paranoia.

There are two wise sayings that address this common sense approach that I advocate: "An ounce of prevention is worth a pound of cure" and "The best time to dig a well is before you are thirsty." Both are especially apt when it comes to Lyme disease. This is because Lyme disease so often escapes early detection and also because it is difficult to treat when detected at a later stage, such as chronic or disseminated Lyme disease. Therefore, preventing Lyme disease is the most important step to protect yourself from the health challenge that many thousands of others have been forced to face because of Lyme.

General Recommendations

Let's begin by listing the Lyme prevention guidelines established by the U.S. Department of Health and Human Services:

- Avoid tick-infested areas.

- When outdoors, wear light-colored clothes so that ticks will be more noticeable. Avoid knit clothing, choosing clothes made of smooth materials such as tightly woven cotton instead, as these are harder for ticks to latch onto.

- Wear long-sleeved shirts, pants, and a hat and closed shoes and socks, and be sure to tuck your shirt into your pants and your pants legs into your socks or shoes. Hats are also advisable if you are going to be hiking through woods or areas of tall vegetation.

- Apply insect repellent to pants, socks, shoes, and exposed skin. (Safe and effective insect repellents, as well as natural alternatives that you can use, are listed below.)

- Avoid walking in overgrown grass and brush. When using hiking trails, stay in the center of the trail.

- When you return indoors after being in tick-infested areas, remove, wash, and dry your clothing. If possible, take a hot shower and use a brush on the skin. (Showering without brushing is ineffective.)

- Inspect your body thoroughly and carefully remove any attached ticks. If you have pets, also check them for ticks. For parents, it is imperative that you inspect your young children from head to toe when they have been outside during high-risk Lyme months.

* If you find a tick, tug gently but firmly with a blunt, fine-point tweezers near the head of the tick until it releases its hold on the skin. Grasp the tick as close to the skin as possible and pull straight out. To reduce the risk of infection, do not crush the tick's body or handle it with bare fingers. Also do not try to dislodge ticks by using heat or chemicals, as this can result in them injecting the *Bb* bacteria and other harmful microorganisms into your skin. (For more information about how to remove ticks, see below.)

* Should you be bitten by a tick, swab the bite area immediately and thoroughly with an antiseptic to help prevent bacterial infection. As a further precaution, consider seeing a Lyme-aware medical practitioner.

These precautions should especially be followed between May through the end of September, particularly in northern regions of the country, as these are the months in which tick infections most frequently occur. However, I have seen tick bites in the mid-Atlantic states as early as March and as late as December.

How to Safely Remove a Tick

If you notice a tick has settled on you, first determine if it has bitten and attached itself to your skin. If not (or if it is only on your clothes), you can flick it aside with your finger, stick, or other tool. Another option would be to apply tape to the tick and then lift the tape away from your body. If the tick is attached to your skin, take the following steps as soon as possible:

- Avoid using your fingers to remove ticks embedded in your skin to avoid infection. Instead, wait until you can use the proper type of tweezers.

- Using blunt-tip, fine-point tweezers, place the tweezers as close as you can to where the tick is biting your skin, grabbing its mouth. Then pull straight back gently yet firmly. (Do not use tweezers with a sharp point, such as eyebrow tweezers, as these can cause pricking, which in turn can lead the tick to transmit infectious fluids into your skin.)

- A novel way to remove a tick taught to me by a patient is to take a cotton ball and place a drop or two of liquid soap on it. Then place the soaked cotton onto the area of the tick and rotate gently but vigorously for about 20 seconds. The tick will usually release immediately.

- Once the tick has been removed, without touching it with exposed fingers, place it into a container or a Ziploc bag, so that it can be later tested for the *Bb* bacteria and other co-infections if necessary. (See chapter 3.) In order for ticks to be properly tested, they should ideally be alive, so try not to kill them before you send them to a lab. It's also best that the head of the tick still be attached to its body. In whatever condition you remove the tick, *save it,* as it might be the only good clue to the cause of illness that might develop later. To find a lab that can test a tick for Lyme disease and other tick-borne infections, contact your local, county, or state health department, or see our resources section at the end of this book.

* If possible, label the container (such as a piece of tape on a Ziploc bag) and include the location and approximate time that you were bitten.

* Swab the bite area of your skin as described above.

* Do not twist, prick, or attempt to crush ticks during the removal process. Twisting ticks can cause them to break apart, leaving parts of them embedded in your skin. Pricking and crushing ticks can cause them to release infectious fluids into the skin.

Additional Prevention Measures

What follows are more extensive precautions I recommend that you take to protect yourself, your loved ones, and your pets from Lyme disease and other tick-borne infections.

Self-Inspection and Tips for Inspecting Your Pets

If you spend a lot of time outdoors, get in the habit of regularly checking yourself for ticks. Most ticks are very small—about the size of a freckle—and can therefore be easily missed, so train yourself to closely inspect your clothing. If you are with others, take turns inspecting each other for a more thorough inspection. In areas that are known to be tick-infested, tick inspections conducted every hour or so are a good idea.

When you return home, strip off your clothes and closely inspect your body for any ticks you might have missed outdoors. Use a mirror for best results, or ask someone to help you. Then be sure to wash and dry your clothes soon after you return home in order to kill any ticks that may still be lodged inside them. Be sure to take these same precautions with your children.

If you have pets, you should also get into the habit of checking them periodically throughout the day, especially during tick season. Use gloves for this purpose, and pay close attention to the areas in and around your pet's ears, eyes, and groin. Consult with your veterinarian about tick collars that your pet can wear, as well as any other recommendations he or she may have for protecting your pets from ticks.

One promising type of collar that has been shown to protect against ticks, along with fleas that can also transmit the *Bb* bacteria, is known as Frontline. To obtain it, however, you will need your vet to provide you with a prescription. As a further precaution against ticks, keep your pets off furniture and bedding, since ticks can easily pass from them onto furniture and beds to later infect family members. It is not a good idea to allow pets access to your sleeping quarters, especially access to your bed.

You should also take care to ensure that your lawn is regularly mowed during tick season. The reason for this is that ticks tend to climb tall grass in order to attach themselves to passing animals and humans, but usually are not found on lawns that are kept trim. Also be sure to thin the underbrush of any shrubbery around your home, as ticks will often take up residence in thick underbrush. Keep areas of leaf litter to a minimum as ticks tend to inhabit these areas also.

The Problem of Mice

Another important point to consider when it comes to protecting yourself and your loved ones from ticks is whether you live in an area that is frequented by field mice. One little known fact about infection-carrying ticks is that nearly all of them spend the early stages of their lives living on the bodies of field mice. Field mice that enter into homes and other buildings can therefore lead to their becoming infested with ticks. According to gardening expert Mike McGrath, one of the most effective ways to deal with tick-infested field mice is to use Daminex tubes. These cardboard tubes are filled with cotton balls that have been soaked with permethrin. Although permethrin is a pesticide, it is synthesized from chrysanthemum flowers, is biodegradable, and relatively safe (except for fish and other aquatic life, so avoid using permethrin products near water). Moreover, since the cotton balls that contain it are enclosed by tubes, there is virtually no risk that you, your family, or your pets will be exposed to it.

Field mice are attracted to Daminex tubes because of the cotton they contain, which they use to line their nests to make bedding. In the process, the permethrin the cotton contains kills any ticks that are living on the mice, but not the mice themselves in most cases. Various garden supply retail outlets carry Daminex tubes. You can also order them directly at www.garden-shops.com.

Lyme disease experts point out that Daminex tubes only protect against tick-bearing field mice for two years or less. They also state that many other small animals also can bear ticks, yet are not attracted to the cotton that the tubes contain. Therefore, for further protection, it is recommended that people who live in areas that are frequented by wildlife also use liquid or granular insecticides. These include permethrin in spray-form, as well as Sevin, both of which are also relatively safe. Spray them in a "fogging" motion, avoiding coarse or concentrated spraying. Areas to be sprayed include shrubbery and underbrush that is close to your home. Also spray any areas of your lawn that border the woods. Spray an area a few feet wide. The best time to apply such products is in late spring and again in early fall.

DEET and Permethrin

DEET is the most common skin-applied tick repellent in use today. It is easily available and inexpensive. While relatively effective as a repellent, I recommend caution when using it because it is a potential neurotoxin, meaning that it can be toxic to the nervous system when absorbed through the skin. In order to work, DEET needs to be applied directly to the skin. If you do happen to use DEET, remember to thoroughly wash the areas where it was applied as soon as possible with soapy water. Alternatives to DEET are discussed in the next section.

Permethrin can also be safely sprayed on your clothing and footwear to protect yourself against ticks while you are outdoors. Permethrin is relatively nontoxic when used in low concentrations. While permethrin is highly effective in killing ticks, properly used it poses no health threats to humans in low doses or to the surrounding environment (except fish, as previously mentioned). Permethrin is **not** intended to be applied directly to your skin or to be taken internally, as it can be neurotoxic if used improperly. When sprayed on clothing and footwear, permethrin does a good job of killing ticks that may land on clothing before they have a chance to bite you. In addition, a single application will protect you against ticks for two to six weeks, even after your clothes have been washed and worn again. Permethrin is available in concentrations of 0.5 percent in aerosol and pump sprays under such brand names as Duranon, Permanone, and Permakill and is usually carried in camping and hunting supply stores. You can also obtain it online by visiting www.permethrin-repellent.com.

Commercial and Natural Tick Repellents

As an alternative to DEET, the product that I most often recommend for topical use is Avon Skin-So-Soft Mosquito, Flea, and Deer Tick Repellent. It is safe and very effective as a tick repellent. It can be used for children and by pregnant women because it is made from natural, non-toxic materials. One of the principal ingredients is citronella, which alone is not a great tick repellent, but when combined with the other components in this product is quite useful. The United States military uses Avon Skin-So-Soft Mosquito, Flea, and Deer Tick Repellent extensively.

Experts in the field of herbal medicine state that "mountain mint" is a plant that works well as a natural tick repellent. However, it has yet to be tested head-to-head with commercially available products. Mountain mint grows as a weed in various sections of the Unites States, such as the piedmont and mountain areas of the Northeast. You can use it by stripping a branch of a few leaves, rubbing them together in your hands, and then applying the crushed leaves directly to your skin. This is perfectly safe if mountain mint is not used in large quantities. Other mint products, such as peppermint oil, may also be helpful as natural tick repellents when diluted and applied directly to the skin.

Eating garlic before you go outdoors may also repel ticks (as well as most other living creatures). Several patients have told me that ticks don't attach to them if garlic has been eaten recently. It is also claimed by some that ingestions of B-complex vitamins may also have some tick-repellent properties.

Prevention Measures for Buildings and Lawns

Another potential risk factor for ticks is recently purchased homes and other buildings, especially if they have been vacant for a while. Vacant properties can be a breeding ground for ticks and other insects. According to McGrath, an easy solution for determining whether such properties have ticks is to set carbon dioxide traps. You can do this by placing dry ice in the middle of each of the suspected building's rooms. (Don't handle dry ice bare-handed; protect yourself by wearing thick, long gloves.) Around the dry ice place a surrounding wide circle of sticky tape. Because ticks are attracted to the carbon dioxide that the dry ice emits as it melts, if they are in the building they will travel towards it and become trapped on the tape. If you find ticks on the tape, then you know the building has a problem and needs to be disinfected. But if no ticks appear within a day of setting the carbon dioxide traps, it's likely that the building is tick-free. Dry ice is commonly available for purchase at many grocery stores, liquor stores, and ice cream parlors.

Another precaution you can take to help protect against ticks is to remove lawn ornaments that attract animals that can carry ticks, such as bird baths and bird feeders. Wood and leaf piles should also be removed. If your property has stone walls, you should also take care not to sit on them and to wear protective clothing if you have to work or garden near them during tick season, as ticks tend to nest in such walls and also to use them as birthing grounds for new generations of ticks.

Two factors that can make your lawn a breeding area for ticks are dense vegetation and humid lawn conditions caused by too little sunlight reaching the ground. Ticks thrive in landscapes that are overgrown with vegetation and have high moisture content due to lack of sunlight. Conversely, ticks do not fare well in dry landscapes where they are susceptible to dehydration. This was proven by research conducted by the Connecticut Agricultural Experiment Station, which showed that dry lawns exposed to sunlight due to sparse overhead vegetation rarely exhibit ticks even when the lawns are close to bordering tick-infested woods.

Another factor that determines how widespread ticks are in lawns and other landscapes is the access that wildlife has to pass through them. Left to themselves, ticks rarely travel more than a dozen feet during their entire lifetime, but by attaching themselves to animals, they can travel much greater distances— up to several miles—should they latch on to creatures like birds or deer.

By taking the following steps you can significantly reduce the likelihood of ticks taking up residence in your lawn:

* Prune any overhanging branches that are near your house. You might even consider cutting down trees in your yard that grow close to your home in order to extend the area of open lawn that is able to receive sunlight.

* Trim or clear away brush and other overgrowth surrounding your house, especially moisture-storing plants such as ivy.

* Keep your lawn free of leaves and fallen branches.

* Mow your lawn weekly.

* Avoid watering your lawn. (Remember, ticks don't like dry conditions.)

* Make sure your garbage is picked up regularly, and keep garbage cans away from your house with their lids securely fastened.

* If you use clotheslines to dry your clothes, make sure that they hang over open lawn areas, away from trees and brush, to prevent ticks from attaching themselves to hanging sheets, towels, and so forth

If you live in an area where deer and other wild animals pass by, consider fencing off your property.

Prevention Tips for Campers, Hikers, and Hunters

Campers, hikers, and hunters need to be especially careful during tick season. One of the worst things people who spend time in the woods can do is sit on the ground with their backs leaning against a tree. This was confirmed by a study that found that people who do this have a high risk of picking up ticks.

In addition to following the relevant guidelines mentioned above, campers should spray their tents and other camping equipment with one of the tick repellents mentioned above. When changing into a new pair of clothes, campers should also place the old clothes in a sealed plastic bag so that ticks do not crawl onto them.

Hunters should follow these same precautions. In addition, they should always wear protective gloves when handling dead animals, to minimize the risk of infection. They should also take care to hang animal game away from their campsite and places of human activity, since ticks are often found on animal carcasses. Hang such game for at least 12 hours, which is usually enough time for ticks to abandon the carcasses. To ensure that ticks don't drop to the ground and crawl away to cause problems later, place game directly above a pail of water to which a solution of concentrated bleach has been added. This will kill ticks as they fall into the water.

These simple precautions can dramatically decrease the likelihood of ticks becoming a problem near your home.

The Use of Antibiotics after a Tick Bite

Appropriate treatment of tick bites with antibiotics can be very beneficial, especially soon after such bites occur. The question that arises concerns the best antibiotic method to employ in order to prevent Lyme after a tick bite. There are two schools of thought.

The first is called the "two Doxy" approach and basically adheres to the following protocol for those at *high risk* for contracting Lyme infection: If a patient resides in an endemic area and is bitten by a deer or lone star tick (with attachment for 36 hours or more), the most effective method to prevent Lyme is to administer one dose of doxycycline (200 mg total) as a preventive measure. This dose needs to be administered within 72 hours of the bite.

This "two Doxy" approach may very well prevent some cases of Lyme. But there are two factors that are of concern. The first concern is that this treatment has the potential to reduce Lyme load slightly while not eradicating the infection. This reduction in Lyme load might in turn have the negative effect of eliminating the earliest signs of the disease (such as EM rash). The second concern is that an individual might be lulled into a false sense of security about "adequate" Lyme preventive coverage. Consequently, if the patient later develops symptoms of Lyme disease, those symptoms will likely be attributed to something other than Lyme.

The second approach for patients at *high risk* of Lyme infection after a tick bite is similar to the "two Doxy" approach, except that it involves keeping the tick for possible future analysis, and it involves a longer course of Doxycycline, namely ten to fourteen days. Both schools of thought agree that doxycycline is the best choice of antibiotics because it will, when administered at this most early stage, adequately cover the *Bb* bacteria that causes Lyme. It has an added benefit in that it will also cover other co-infections such as Rocky Mountain spotted fever, Ehrlichia, Anaplasma, STARI, and possibly even Bartonella. If the patient gets sick—despite treatment with the longer course of doxycycline—the tick is sent to a lab for analysis (being aware that the tick analysis is not perfect). If the tick bite is *low risk* (that is, attached less than 24 hours, not a deer or lone star tick, not from an endemic area, and so forth), the tick is sent for analysis first. Should the tick be positive for any of the infections tested, then antibiotic preventive treatment is begun.

I subscribe to this second approach because, in my experience, I have found that it gives the patient the best chance of clearing nearly all the possible infections that might be present. I am ever aware of the possible unpleasant side effects of antibiotics, but in the case of Lyme disease, with its severity and its complexity, the use of antibiotics is a necessity. Doxycycline (and its entire family of tetracyclines) has a long history of safety as evidenced by its frequent long-term use in treating non life-threatening disorders such as acne.

Meanwhile, the patient needs to be on high alert for the early signs of Lyme disease (and co-infections) and seek treatment as soon as symptoms develop. Always keep in mind that treatment is most effective in the early stages of the illness.

Summing Up

In concluding this chapter, let's review its key points by answering some of the most common questions people have about Lyme disease, its risks, and its prevention.

Isn't Lyme disease a relatively new condition that is limited to certain geographical regions of the United States?

No. Lyme disease is neither new—it was first medically documented by the German physician Alfred Buchwald in 1883—nor is it found only in certain areas of the country. The first modern cases of Lyme disease were detected in and around Lyme, Connecticut, in the mid 1970s, giving the condition its name. Since then, cases of Lyme disease have been reported in every state except Montana, as well as in Washington, D.C. It has also been reported throughout Canada, Great Britain, and many European countries, as well as in Australia, China, Japan, New Zealand, and Russia.

How prevalent is Lyme disease in the United States?

According to the Centers for Disease Control and Prevention (CDC), approximately 23,000 cases of Lyme disease were reported in 2005 (nearly eight cases for every 100,000 people in the United States). However, according to CDC, as many as ten cases are unreported for every case that is reported, indicating that the actual number of annual cases of Lyme disease in the United States may be in the hundreds of thousands.

Are tick bites the only cause of Lyme disease?

While ticks (deer and lone star varieties) are a major source of Lyme disease transmission, via a strain of bacteria known as *Borrelia burgdorferi* (*Bb*) that is passed on to humans at the time that the bites occur, Lyme disease (and other co-infections) can likely also be transmitted via bites from various insects, including fleas, flies (research from Connecticut and Germany), gnats, mites (research from Russia), and mosquitoes. Rocky Mountain spotted fever may be contracted by simply handling an infected tick. Other routes of transmission of *Bb* may also occur via the placenta and through blood transfusions. Animal studies also suggest that Lyme may be transmitted during sex, although this has never been documented scientifically in humans.

Is the characteristic bull's eye rash the only symptom of Lyme disease?

No. This rash, known as erythema migrans, or EM, occurs in less than half of all people infected with Lyme disease. The truth is that if an EM rash is present, this is absolute proof of Lyme disease and no further confirmation for Lyme (such as blood testing) is required for diagnosis. *Keep in mind, however, that Lyme may not be the only problem, and co-infections and other medical disorders may also need to be evaluated.* However, the absence of an EM does not rule out Lyme disease. There are other factors that add to the complexity of diagnosing Lyme disease. One of these factors is the reality that even when a rash does appear, it isn't always in the shape of a bull's eye. Secondly, it can take up to six weeks or longer before blood tests can detect the presence of *Bb* even when the EM rash is present. Remember, there are many other potentially more serious symptoms of Lyme disease beyond the EM rash. These will be discussed in the next chapter.

I thought Lyme disease was a benign condition that is easily treated with a short course of antibiotics?

This is one of the most unfortunate misconceptions about Lyme disease. Although short-course antibiotic treatment often can resolve Lyme disease when it is still in its early, localized stage, once the *Bb* bacteria spreads into other areas of the body, treatment can become far more difficult.

Isn't Lyme disease easily detectable using conventional blood tests?

Once again, the answer is no. The most commonly used blood tests, such as the ELISA/IFA test, often fail to detect the presence of *Bb* even when Lyme disease is in an advanced stage and has spread throughout the body. I can attest to this personally, since I was told I did not have Lyme disease when I was first tested for it. It was nearly eight years later, during which time my condition worsened, that I was finally accurately diagnosed with Lyme disease. To learn about the most effective tests for Lyme disease, see chapter 3.

Why is there so much controversy surrounding Lyme disease?

The truth of the matter is that despite the extensive research that has been done on Lyme disease, there still is no consensus. If the evidence were overwhelmingly clear, we would not have controversy. Obviously, we have much more work to do in order to have a unified approach to diagnosing and treating this very serious illness.

I suspect that I may have Lyme disease. Who can I turn to for help?

Your best choice for getting an accurate diagnosis and beginning an effective treatment program is to seek out what I refer to as a Lyme-aware doctor (also known to many by the acronym LLMD). I discuss such physicians in more detail in chapter 3 and provide a list of organizations that can help you find one in the resources section at the end of this book.

How can I best prevent Lyme disease from occurring to myself and my loved ones?

I cannot overstress how important prevention is when it comes to dealing with Lyme disease. By adopting the guidelines I've shared in this chapter, you can significantly minimize the risk of Lyme disease for you and your loved ones.

If you should still be bitten by a tick despite taking the measures above, don't despair. Instead, seek prompt medical attention, ideally from a Lyme-aware physician who can see to it that you are appropriately and accurately evaluated for Lyme disease. Keep looking until you find someone who understands Lyme disease and can help you get the proper diagnosis and treatment.

Remember, Lyme disease, when caught in its early, localized state, is far more easily treated than it is when it becomes chronic. Therefore, don't wait to see if you develop symptoms if you know or suspect that you've been exposed to ticks and other vectors that carry the *Bb* bacteria and other Lyme-related co-infectious agents. Instead, consult with a physician as soon as possible. This is particularly crucial if you begin to develop flu-like symptoms after you've been bitten by a tick or by insects that can potentially transmit Lyme disease or its co-infections.

In the next chapter, you will learn about symptoms of Lyme disease and symptoms of the most common of the tick-borne co-infections.

Chapter Two

Signs and Symptoms of Lyme Disease and Related Co-infections

✳

Patients and doctors alike face an enormous challenge regarding the diagnosis and treatment of Lyme and other tick-borne illnesses. In this chapter, I want to discuss one very important aspect of this challenge—the recognition of symptoms of Lyme and of the co-infections (other organisms) that may accompany Lyme at the time of Lyme infection.

First of all, let me define two terms. "Symptoms" are subjective feelings as a patient experiences them. For example, knee pain is a symptom of discomfort in the knee as a person experiences it. "Signs" are objective evidences that a doctor examines, observes, or tests for, that allow the doctor to reliably make a diagnosis. For example, a swollen and red knee is a sign of joint inflammation that is called arthritis.

One of the most challenging problems with Lyme disease

is that very often neither a patient's subjective symptoms nor a doctor's objective signs are specific enough to reliably diagnose Lyme or the co-infections. Unfortunately, when a patient comes to a doctor's office, there are very few symptoms that are absolutely specific for Lyme. Likewise, there are very few objective signs that a doctor can examine or test for that are so specific that no one disputes the diagnosis of Lyme disease.

The only indisputable Lyme symptom and sign is the presence of a rash that is diagnosed as the erythema migrans (EM) rash. Therefore, if a person does not have a diagnosed EM rash, there is a good possibility that the Lyme diagnosis will be missed. Consequently, those patients can become chronically ill with Lyme disease.

The symptoms of chronic Lyme are often non-specific symptoms that look like a wide variety of other medical conditions. A good example would be the symptom of chronic fatigue. While fatigue is a universal chronic Lyme disease symptom, it is also a major symptom of literally hundreds of other medical conditions, including depression, cancer, heart disease, hypothyroidism (low thyroid function), and chronic stress to name just a few.

In this chapter, I will discuss the symptom patterns of Lyme disease and the major co-infections that often accompany Lyme. The symptoms presented below should not be considered a complete or exhaustive list. Rather, these symptoms should alert you to the need to seek further care, preferably from a Lyme-aware doctor who can help you get a proper diagnosis and treatment. (I discuss proper diagnostic measures for Lyme disease in chapter 3.) To better help you understand some of the typical symptom patterns of Lyme that are seen clinically, I have included actual clinical case histories. As much as possible, I've also included a brief description of antibiotic therapies that were useful in the treatment of those cases. (Antibiotics will be discussed in detail in chapter 6.)

However, it is important to remember that antibiotics are only part of the answer in a comprehensive approach to treating Lyme disease and the related co-infections. Antibiotic choices change with time; therefore, extensive discussion of antibiotic protocols (including complex combination therapies) for the tick-borne diseases is beyond the scope of this book. For up-to-date information on current antibiotic treatment protocols, I suggest you visit the "Treatment Guidelines" section of the ILADS Web site (www.ilads.org).

Symptoms of Lyme Disease

There are two distinct phases of Lyme disease—acute and chronic. Acute Lyme disease can also be referred to as localized Lyme disease, while chronic Lyme disease can be broken down into two additional classifications—(1) early disseminated (systemic) Lyme disease and (2) late disseminated Lyme disease.

Acute, or localized, Lyme disease refers to the initial stage of the disease, when the only visible symptom, if it exists at all, is the EM rash on or near the site of a tick or insect (flea, fly, etc.) bite. Often no other symptoms are present, but in some cases minor aches and pains, as well as headache and/or fever can also occur.

Remember, however, that in many cases, the EM rash does not appear. This is why localized Lyme disease, which is usually easy to treat with a proper course of antibiotics, so often goes undetected. As a result, the *Bb* bacteria that cause Lyme begin to spread from the localized site of infection to other areas of the body and become "disseminated Lyme disease." Let's take a closer look at the symptom picture of each stage of Lyme disease.

Localized Symptoms (Stage One)

As mentioned, the primary localized symptom of Lyme disease is the EM rash. When it does appear, it is typically, but not always, within a few days following infection with the *Bb* bacteria. However, as you read in chapter 1, the EM rash is not a symptom of many people infected with *Bb*, and in some cases, the rash may not manifest until weeks after infection begins. Usually, if this is the case, the bacteria will have migrated beyond the original infection site to other areas of the body. In addition, persons with darker skin color may not notice the rash if it appears, due to its lightness in color. (In persons with darker complexions, the EM rash may appear as a bruise).

Should the typical EM rash appear, it will usually begin as a small, reddish bump on the skin that then expands into a characteristic bull's eye pattern, with clear skin encircled by a reddish, slightly raised rash. In size, the EM rash can range from as small as one to two inches in diameter to a large red mass that covers a sizeable portion of the torso or extremities, depending on where on the body the infection with the *Bb* bacteria originated. However, not all EM rashes have a bull's eye appearance. They can also be elliptical, oval, or triangular in shape or resemble long, thin, lines. In addition, unlike other types of skin rashes, which typically start to fade away within a few days or less of their appearance, the EM rash can last for a week to several months. In some cases, the rash can also cause blistering, scaling, and, much more rarely, bleeding. The affected area of the skin can also be painful to the touch, feel hot, cold, and numb and/or create burning or mild itching sensations. It is commonly confused with ringworm or with spider bites.

Despite the fact that the EM rash is considered unquestionable evidence of Lyme, some doctors choose not to treat patients presenting with the rash until they receive a blood test that confirms the presence of the *Bb* bacteria. The truth is that if you have the characteristic rash, you have the disease. There are two important reasons why it is an error to wait for blood test confirmation before starting treatment. The first is that it may take up to six weeks after the tick bite for the test to become positive. The second reason is that often the most commonly ordered blood tests fail to detect *Bb* because of poor Lyme blood test accuracy. (I explain this in more detail in chapter 3.) Therefore, waiting for the blood test confirmation dangerously leaves the patient at risk for developing more serious Lyme complications for which treatment may be much more difficult and extensive. Benjamin's case history illustrates this reality.

Benjamin is a veterinarian whom I had successfully treated for Lyme four years ago. Recently, while visiting friends in New Jersey, he noticed a new deer tick bite under his left arm. There was an accompanying six-inch bull's eye rash associated with it. He had no other symptoms. He removed the tick and saved it.

When he got home to Maryland, he called his primary doctor's office immediately for an appointment to get diagnosed and treated. He was told that since he didn't have any other Lyme symptoms, he needed to get a blood test first before seeing the doctor. If that test showed Lyme disease, then the doctor would see him and very likely give him antibiotics. If the test were negative, then the doctor would treat him only if symptoms, like arthritis, later developed.

Benjamin knew better. He called our office and we were able to get him in quickly for an appointment. He had a classic EM rash. We placed him on one month of oral doxycycline. Meanwhile, on his own, he had sent the tick to a lab for analysis. One month later, he returned to the office. The rash had resolved and he had no further symptoms. The tick, incidentally, tested positive for Lyme *Bb*.

As I've already stated, during the localized stage of Lyme disease, headaches, mild aches and pains, fever, and mild flu-like symptoms can also occur, whether or not the EM rash is present. If you experience any of these symptoms, especially following times spent outdoors when you may have been exposed to ticks and disease-carrying insects, seek prompt medical attention so that you can be evaluated for Lyme disease and other arthropod-borne diseases. When accurately diagnosed in time, Lyme disease can usually be easily treated with a course of antibiotics.

Symptoms of Disseminated or Systemic Lyme Disease (Stage Two, or Early Disseminated, and Stage Three, or Late Disseminated)

Once Lyme disease progresses beyond localized infection to migrate to other areas of the body, it can quickly begin to attack various vital organs and body systems. As a result, the symptoms of disseminated Lyme disease can be extremely varied, depending on which body systems are affected, and to what degree. The wide range of Lyme disease symptoms often mimics the symptoms of other diseases. Among these symptoms are: arthritis-like joint pain and swelling (especially migrating joint symptoms), "brain fog" (with poor concentration, focus, and attention), poor sleep, back pain, light sensitivity and/or blurred vision, ear symptoms (hearing loss, ringing in the ears, noise sensitivity), chronic fatigue, facial paralysis (especially Bell's palsy), fibromyalgia, gait and balance problems, headache, impaired muscle coordination, impaired reflexes, memory loss (especially short-term), muscle aches and pains, muscle weakness, and nerve symptoms (described as numbness, tingling, burning, vibrating, or shooting pain). *Two major clues that Lyme is the cause of the above symptoms are: (1) the progressive worsening over time of a multi-system pattern of symptoms and (2) the tendency for these symptoms to wax and wane in a cyclical fashion.* That is, every three to six weeks, it seems that all the symptoms get worse for a few days, after which they resume the previous pattern.

Sarah's case shows how severe Lyme symptoms can become when they are not properly diagnosed. Sarah is a person who loved to hike. One spring while hiking in the Shenandoah National Park she felt something crawling on her leg. Thinking nothing of it, she continued the hike. Later that evening she noticed a black speck in her groin area. She flicked it off using her fingernail and noticed that it was a tick.

When she got back home to Northern Virginia, Sarah observed that the area of the tick bite had become slightly reddish and inflamed. However, a few days later, she felt fine. Two weeks later, she noticed a flu-like illness that was clearly out of season for influenza. When the symptoms persisted for several weeks, she went to her doctor, who did a thorough examination. She informed him that a few weeks ago she had had a tick bite on her leg for a few hours, but developed nothing more than a small area of irritation for a few days after that.

He ordered the usual array of tests to rule out serious illness. A Lyme test was included in that battery of tests. She was reassured and sent home with the diagnosis of "viral infection." His office called a week later to tell her that there was no need to worry about Lyme because the test was negative. And besides, the office stated, Lyme is very rare in the part of Virginia in which she was hiking.

Over the next four months, Sarah noticed increasing amounts of tiredness, anxiety, poor short-term memory, irritability, migrating joint pains, eye "floaters," light sensitivity, heart skipping, and sleep problems. She noticed that her symptoms seemed to be much worse during the week before her menstrual cycle was to begin. A return visit to the doctor's office resulted in a repeat negative Lyme test and further reassurance that this could not possibly be Lyme. She was told that probably stress was the main problem and was told to exercise, to learn relaxation techniques, and to try to avoid stressful situations.

Seven months later, after doing extensive research on the Internet, Sarah became convinced that she did, in fact, have chronic Lyme disease. Once she got an appointment in our office, we were able to confirm her suspicions. This was done with Western Blot testing and PCR testing (both of which will be discussed in chapter 3). Because she had chronic disseminated Lyme, we chose to place her on two antibiotics—amoxicillin and azithromycin—along with the comprehensive therapies you will learn about in the second and third parts of this book.

In the initial stage of her treatment, Sarah experienced what is known as a "Jarish-Herxheimer reaction." I will discuss this reaction in detail in chapter 6. Briefly, this reaction is caused as *Bb* bacteria "die-off" as a result of the antibiotic treatment. The symptoms one can experience when this happens are actually due to the immune system's inflammatory response to the presence of dead Lyme debris circulating in the body. Soon after the reaction ran its course, Sarah began to notice gradual improvement in her symptoms. After three months of antibiotic therapy, her symptoms were totally resolved and the antibiotics were discontinued.

Lyme and Neurological Disease: Lyme disease is also frequently the cause or a significant contributing co-factor in a number of chronic degenerative and neurological diseases, such as Parkinson's, Lou Gehrig's disease (ALS), Alzheimer's disease, and multiple sclerosis (MS). In addition, these same conditions can also be misdiagnosed as a result of Lyme disease, meaning that physicians can fail to detect that Lyme is the underlying cause.

Susan's case illustrates what can result when this happens.

Susan came to our office because of neurological symptoms that began six years previously. An avid gardener living in rural Delaware, she recalled feeling tired and unmotivated during that summer six years ago. She recalled no tick bite or rash. In addition to ongoing severe fatigue, a few months later she began having vision problems and strange electrical sensations involving her back, legs, and feet. Next, her knees and leg muscles began to ache, and she began to have night sweats. This was followed by balance and walking problems shortly afterwards.

Susan's doctor appropriately referred her to a neurologist. She underwent extensive testing—including MRIs, a Lyme screening test, and lumbar puncture (spinal tap)—all of which were normal. The conclusion was that she had "atypical multiple sclerosis." However, the treatment Susan was prescribed caused her symptoms to become even worse. One of her friends who had been diagnosed and treated for Lyme convinced her to get a second opinion concerning Lyme disease. Our laboratory tests confirmed that Susan had both disseminated Lyme disease and the co-infection, Babesia. (I will discuss this organism below.)

We treated the Babesia first, using atovaquone and azithromycin. This was followed by treatment for Lyme disease with intravenous ceftriaxone, along with oral clarithromycin and metronidazole. (This combination is used to attack Lyme in its three different structures: spirochete form, "L" form, and "cystic" form.) After a total of several months of antibiotic treatment, combined with the natural therapies you will learn about later in this book, Susan's symptoms completely resolved.

Lyme and Psychological Disease: A variety of mental and emotional (psychiatric) conditions can also be caused or severely exacerbated by Lyme disease. It is estimated that 50 percent of Lyme patients have psychiatric manifestations. These include behavioral disorders (including impulsive acts of aggression and violence), bipolar disorder (manic depression), chronic depression, dementia, eating disorders, hallucinations, mood swings, panic attacks, paranoia, schizophrenia, and other personality disorders and even suicide. Jill was one patient who suffered serious psychological problems because of Lyme.

Before she came to me for treatment, Jill had been in and out of psychiatric hospitals, where she was treated unsuccessfully for suicidal depression. Her deteriorating mental and emotional state first began shortly after she gave birth to her child. Initially, she experienced what she thought were symptoms of the flu. But soon thereafter, she began her mental and emotional decline. She was told she had severe post-partum depression, but her doctors were unable to help her. After she was properly diagnosed with Lyme disease and was treated with intravenous and oral antibiotics, she made a remarkable recovery and received her life back.

Dr. Virginia Sherr is a psychiatrist practicing in Holland,

Pennsylvania. She has published numerous articles in medical journals on Lyme disease and is an authority on the psychological manifestations of Lyme disease. She recently reported in the *Journal of Psychiatric Practice* three cases of panic disorder that were actually psychiatric manifestations of Lyme disease. In each of the cases, the patients presented to her with body symptoms that were not typical of primary panic disorder alone. These symptoms included foggy thinking and memory loss; joint pains; light and sound sensitivity; and bizarre, shifting, and even excruciating nerve pain. She was able to recognize that some other systemic disorder was occurring in each of these patients. After the appropriate diagnoses of Lyme disease (and co-infections) were made and treatment completed, the panic symptoms of each of the patients were totally eliminated.

Lyme and Heart Disease: One of the little known facts about Lyme disease is that it can cause a number of serious cardiovascular problems that can lead to or worsen heart disease. The reason for this is that, as Lyme disease spreads through the body, weakening other body systems, it can create an ongoing strain on the heart and overall cardiovascular system. Left unchecked, Lyme disease can also cause permanent damage to the heart and even death by heart attack.

Dr. Phillip W. Paparone, an infectious diseases specialist in New Jersey, is an expert on heart problems as they relate to Lyme disease. According to Dr. Paparone, "The potentially fatal cardiac involvement of Lyme disease remains the least well-documented complication of this multi-system illness." Medical research published in 1990 indicates that between 8 and 10 percent of all Lyme disease patients have symptoms that indicate heart involvement. He believes that the percentage of heart disease patients with Lyme disease may actually be higher due to how easily Lyme disease can escape detection or be misdiagnosed. For this reason, Dr. Paparone recommends that all patients suffering from symptoms of heart disease who live in geographic regions where Lyme disease is most prevalent be screened for the *Bb* bacteria. Frederick's case dramatically illustrates what can happen when Lyme screening does not take place.

Frederick began noticing peculiar symptoms at the age of thirty-eight. His feet began swelling, he suffered from shortness of breath with minimal exertion, and at times he would awaken in the middle of the night gasping for air. His worsening symptoms motivated him to visit his family doctor. The doctor sent him for a chest X-ray and immediately recognized that Frederick was having serious heart problems.

He was referred to a cardiologist (heart specialist) who discovered that he had "congestive heart failure." This is a condition in which the heart muscle becomes weakened to the point that it cannot pump out enough blood to meet the demands of the body. The problem was that the doctor could not figure out why Frederick had this fairly sudden onset of poor heart muscle function. At that time, he underwent heart catheterization. It showed normal coronary arteries, but a very poor heart muscle function. His "ejection fraction" was 21 percent, meaning his heart was able to pump out only 21 percent of the blood that was arriving to it. A normal ejection fraction is 50–75 percent. Frederick underwent a heart biopsy and was told that he had "idiopathic cardiomyopathy." His condition was deemed to be so serious that he was placed on a heart transplant list.

Frederick had acquired some other symptoms around the same time that his heart problems began. These symptoms included knee pains, numbness in his feet, and foggy thinking. Interestingly, Frederick's next-door neighbor had just moved into the neighborhood recently, and Frederick had told him his story. The neighbor asked if he had ever been tested for Lyme disease. At that point Frederick had not.

He requested a Lyme test from his cardiologist, but was refused. His neighbor then referred him to the Lyme Disease Association's Web site. (See the resources section at the end of this book.) He was able to get the names of several doctors who are able to evaluate and treat patients with chronic Lyme disease. He decided to travel to Maryland to visit our office.

From his history, Frederick did not have any tick bites or strange rashes. However, his symptoms certainly fit a possible Lyme disease pattern. We tested him for Lyme and a host of other problems. He had a very strongly abnormal Lyme Western Blot test. He was started on intravenous ceftriaxone as well as oral azithromycin and metronidazole.

Within two weeks of treatment, he began to feel hopeful that he might be able to get his heart functioning normally again. After three months of treatment, his heart symptoms and systemic Lyme symptoms were nearly resolved. Meanwhile, he had found a new cardiologist (one who was more open-minded) and had a repeat of his ejection fraction. His new ejection fraction was now 46 percent. After Frederick completed the intravenous therapy, he was continued on oral antibiotics for several more months, after which time his repeat ejection fraction improved to 58 percent. Eventually, the antibiotics were discontinued and he was released from my care. A year later he sent a letter stating that he was doing fine and was back to normal and no longer needed a heart transplant.

Heart conditions caused by Lyme disease are collectively known as Lyme "carditis." Any of the following problems can result from Lyme carditis: atrial fibrillation, cardiac failure, cardiomegaly, cardiomyopathy, chest pain, exertional dyspnea, irregular heartbeat (arrhythmia), myocarditis, palpitations, pancarditis, pericarditis, syncope, and tachycardia. Lyme carditis can also cause serious "blockages" in the electrical impulse transmission between the atrial and ventricular sections of the heart. These heart blockages may require that a heart pacemaker be placed inside of the patient. Without such a pacemaker, the patient may experience sudden cardiac death.

If you have been diagnosed with any of the above heart conditions for reasons that neither you nor your physician can explain, ask your physician to refer you to a physician who specializes in Lyme disease so that you can be screened for it. Given how potentially serious, and even fatal, Lyme carditis can be, when it comes to screening for Lyme, it's always better to be safe than sorry.

Dr. Burrascano's Symptom Checklist for Lyme Disease

One of the foremost Lyme disease medical experts is Dr. Joseph Burrascano, now retired from clinical practice. Dr. Burrascano pioneered many of the integrative treatment approaches for Lyme disease, and I am indebted to him for doing so, especially since his treatment protocols played a significant role in my own recovery from Lyme disease. Dr. Burrascano recognized the limitations of the criteria used by the Centers for Disease Control and Prevention. He developed the symptom checklist below so that patients and physicians alike could more accurately determine whether or not testing for Lyme disease should be considered. (Please see the references section of this book for source information regarding this checklist.) Although this checklist is by no means a method of making a definitive diagnosis, I find that it can be very helpful as an indicator of Lyme disease. The more "yes" answers that are made on the checklist, the more likely it is that Lyme disease is involved in patients' symptoms.

Risk Profile (Check all that apply.)

Have you spent time in tick-infested areas?	Yes __ No __
Do you engage in frequent outdoor activities?	Yes __ No __
Do you engage in any of the following?	
Hiking?	Yes __ No __
Fishing?	Yes __ No __
Camping?	Yes __ No __
Gardening?	Yes __ No __
Hunting?	Yes __ No __
Have you noted ticks on your pets or any other animals you may have come in contact with?	Yes __ No __
Do you recall being bitten by a tick or biting insect? If yes, when?	Yes __ No __
Do you remember having the bull's eye (EM) rash?	Yes __ No __
Have you had any other type of rash?	Yes __ No __
If yes, when?	

Symptom Checklist

Have you experienced any of the following symptoms?	
Unexplained fevers, night or day sweats, chills, or flushing?	Yes ✓ No __
Unexplained weight change (loss or gain)?	Yes ✓ No __
Fatigue, tiredness, poor stamina?	Yes ✓ No __
Unexplained hair loss?	Yes ✓ No __
Swollen glands? (If yes, list affected areas of your body.)	Yes __ No ✓

Sore throat?   Yes ✓ No __

Testicular pain/pelvic pain?   Yes ✓ No __

Unexplained menstrual irregularities?   Yes __ No ✓

Unexplained breast pain/milk production?   Yes __ No ✓

Sexual dysfunction/loss of libido?   Yes ✓ No __

Upset stomach?   Yes ✓ No __

Change in bowel function (constipation, diarrhea)?   Yes ✓ No __

Chest pain/soreness in ribs?   Yes ✓ No __

Shortness of breath, coughing?   Yes ✓ No __

Heart palpitations, skipping pulse, heart block?   Yes ✓ No __

History of heart murmur or valve prolapse?   Yes __ No *Needs to be checked*

Joint pain or swelling?
(If yes, list affected areas of your body.)   Yes ✓ No __
Everywhere

Stiffness of the joints, neck, or back?   Yes ✓ No __

Muscle pain or cramps?   Yes ✓ No __

Twitching of the face or other muscles?   Yes ✓ No __

Headache?   Yes ✓ No __

Neck creaking/cracking, neck stiffness, neck pain?   Yes ✓ No __

Tingling, numbness, burning or stabbing sensations, shooting pains?   Yes ✓ No __

Facial paralysis (Bell's palsy)?   Yes __ No ✓

Eyes/vision problems: blurry vision, double vision, increased floaters, sensitivity to light?   Yes ✓ No __

Ears/hearing problems: ear pain, buzzing, ringing, sensitivity to sound?   Yes ✓ No __

Increased motion sickness, vertigo, poor balance?   Yes ✓ No __

Lightheadedness, wooziness?	Yes ✓ No __
Tremor?	Yes ✓ No __
Confusion, difficulty in thinking?	Yes ✓ No __
Difficulty concentrating/reading?	Yes ✓ No __
Forgetfulness, poor short-term memory?	Yes ✓ No __
Disorientation (getting lost, going to wrong places)?	Yes ✓ No __
Speech difficulties, vocalization problems, problems writing, word block?	Yes ✓ No __
Mood swings, irritability, depression?	Yes ✓ No __
Disturbed sleep: too much, too little, fractionated, early awakening?	Yes ✓ No __
Exaggerated symptoms or worse hangover from alcohol?	Yes __ No ✓

If you scored high on this scale, Lyme disease is a definite possibility for you. However, one of the most important questions that you and your progressive Lyme-aware practitioner must determine is how much of your problem is due to chronic persistent Lyme infection (or co-infections) versus chronic inflammation/damage caused by the Lyme. In this book, we will come back to this question frequently because a comprehensive approach to Lyme disease will often involve working with both issues.

Co-infections and Lyme Disease

Co-infections are other infectious organisms that can be transmitted to a person at the time of a tick bite. It is my observation that the severity of the symptoms that patients with Lyme disease experience is directly related to the presence of co-infections. These co-infections create additional symptoms and additional burden for the body's defenses (the immune system) to bear. When the body has to deal with multiple infections (that is, Lyme plus a co-infection), it is more likely that the body systems will be unable to handle any one of those infections adequately.

Therefore, knowing whether or not such co-infections are present is also essential in order to create a proper treatment plan. This is particularly important with regard to specific co-infections that can be transmitted by the same type of ticks that transmit the *Bb* bacteria. Often both *Bb* and one or more of these co-infections are transmitted at the same time, placing an even greater burden on the body than the *Bb* bacteria alone.

What follows is a list of the most common co-infections that can be associated with Lyme disease.

Babesiosis: As mentioned, at the time of a tick bite, there may be other infections transmitted to a person in addition to *Bb* bacteria. One of the most serious of those co-infections is called babesiosis. Babesiosis is caused by a family of harmful parasitic microorganisms known as *piroplasms*. These organisms are actually cousins of malaria and many of the symptoms are quite similar to those of malaria. Both malaria and piroplasms belong to the phylum called *Apicomplexa*.

Babesia microti is the organism most commonly encountered in the Eastern United States. On the West Coast, *Babesia duncani* (WA-1 strain) is more common. (Based on travel history, it may be necessary to test for both.) Since there are several subtypes of Babesia (reportedly twenty or more), it makes laboratory diagnosis challenging. Additionally, experienced Lyme-aware clinicians suspect that *piroplasms* other than the subtypes for which tests are available may be responsible for human disease.

The incidence of babesiosis is on the rise in the United States, with the greatest number of cases corresponding to regions of the country that also have the highest concentrations of Lyme disease. Unlike cases of its fellow tick-borne organisms, Lyme and Ehrlichia, Babesia cases are not reportable to the CDC. Therefore, tracking of incidences of new Babesia cases is not currently being done. For that reason, no one accurately knows the status of the nationwide prevalence of Babesia infection. However, there is one thing that is very clear. It is absolutely not confined to persons living in or having recently visited coastal New England, although there is an unusually high amount of Babesia in that area. We have treated several well-documented cases of babesiosis (documented with positive blood smears) from other regions of the United States.

Many of the symptoms of babesiosis are similar to those that can be caused by Lyme disease, such as the following:

* ✓ Chills

* ✓ Fatigue and often excessive sleepiness

* High fever at onset of illness (Lyme will rarely, if ever, give a high fever at onset.) *Low grade often*

* ✓ Night sweats that are often drenching and profuse

* ✓ Severe muscle pains, especially the large muscles of the legs (quads, buttocks, and so forth)

* ✓ Neurological symptoms that patients often describe as "dizzy, tipsy, and spaciness," similar to a sensation of floating or of walking off the top of a mountain onto a cloud

* ✓ Depression

* ✓ Episodes of breathlessness, "air hunger," and/or cough

* ✓ Decreased appetite and/or nausea

* ? Spleen and/or liver enlargement

* ? Laboratory abnormalities that may include low white blood count, low platelet counts, mild elevation of liver enzymes, and elevated "sed rate"

* ✓ Headaches (migraine-like, persistent, and especially involving the back of the head and upper neck areas)

* Less common symptoms are joint pain (more common with Lyme and Bartonella), anxiety/panic (more common with Bartonella), lymph gland swelling (more common with Bartonella and Lyme), non-specific "sick feeling" (also encountered with Bartonella and Lyme)

The following case study is a good illustration of Babesia infection. Kathy is a personal trainer from Washington, D.C., who began to notice that she could not complete an aerobic training workout with her clients because of headaches and severe leg muscle pain. The pain seemed to be getting worse by the week. Her internist performed a variety of tests on her and could not find the reason for the unrelenting pain.

About that time, coincidentally, she had a sinus infection and was treated by her doctor with azithromycin. She noticed that her head and legs got better within a few days, but reverted to the old symptoms a week after completion of the medicine. When she asked her doctor about that seeming coincidence, it prompted him to perform some tests that included Lyme testing. Her Lyme screening test was indeed positive.

The doctor did prescribe a month of doxycycline, which helped somewhat with some of the joint problems Kathy was having, but did nothing for her muscle pain. She requested more azithromycin (which she had taken during previous sinus infections), but he felt uncomfortable prescribing that particular medication for Lyme. For that reason, he referred Kathy to our office for further evaluation.

In reviewing Kathy's symptoms, it became clear that she was dealing with more than Lyme disease alone. She was having drenching night sweats regularly and episodes of breathlessness, even when sitting in the car driving or at home watching

TV. Kathy also described strange episodes of loss of balance, lightheadedness, and feeling "spacy"—a sensation of an altered sense of perception. She related an example of this to me. One day, while driving on the highway, she suddenly had the sensation that the car was floating. Of course, it was not actually floating, and she could see that with her eyes, but she had a "feeling" as though it was.

Our diagnostic testing revealed a very high amount of antibodies against *Babesia microti* and also a positive Babesia FISH test (both of these will be discussed in chapter 3). She was placed on atovaquone and azithromycin and within two weeks was feeling dramatically better. The total treatment time for her babesiosis was five months. (I will discuss treatment of Babesia extensively in chapter 6.)

Interestingly, I queried her about her activities in the months prior to the onset of her symptoms. She had been on a camping trip with friends on the eastern shore of Maryland. She recalled no tick bite or rash, but recalled a very severe headache and fever of 102 degrees shortly after returning home from the trip. She went to the emergency room, received a spinal tap among other tests, and was told she had an "aggressive flu virus." It took two weeks, but she finally improved. Several weeks after that she noticed the gradual onset of the symptoms mentioned above.

Kathy's case illustrates a very important principle. Often, a patient's previous response to a course of antibiotics for an unrelated condition may serve as an excellent clue to Lyme disease or to a co-infection such as Babesia. I recommend the book by fellow ILADS member, James Schaller, M.D., entitled *The Diagnosis and Treatment of Babesia.*

Bartonellosis: *Bartonellae* is a family of bacteria, the most commonly known which causes a disease called "cat scratch fever." More than 20,000 cases of infection from members of the Bartonella genus occur in the United States each year, with the vast majority of them due to bites from fleas that infest infected cats or dogs. It may also occur directly from bites and scratches from infected dogs or cats. Bartonella can likely also be transmitted by ticks that transmit Lyme disease. In fact, in a study published recently, deer ticks from New Jersey were tested for microorganisms that they were harboring. That study revealed that the tested ticks had a higher prevalence of Bartonella organisms than of Lyme organisms.

At times, it is unclear whether the organism that we see transmitted along with Lyme disease is actually a Bartonella species (for example, *B. henselae or B. quintana*) or is a "Bartonella-like organism" (BLO) that is yet to be fully identified. (The term BLO was originally used by Lyme disease pioneer, Dr. Joseph Burrascano.) While it has features similar to organisms in the Bartonella family, it also has features similar to the Mycoplasma and the Francisella (causes tularemia) families. For the sake of our discussion in this book, when we refer to

"Bartonella," we mean either identifiable Bartonella or a BLO organism that is likely in the Bartonella family but is yet to be characterized scientifically.

Common symptoms of bartonellosis include the following:

* Fatigue (often with agitation, unlike Lyme disease, which is more associated with exhaustion)

* Low grade fevers, especially morning and/or late afternoon, often associated with feelings of "coming down with the flu or a virus"

* Sweats, often in morning or late afternoon (and sometimes at night), sometimes described as "thick" or "sticky" in nature

* Headaches, especially frontal (often confused with sinus) or top of head

* Eye symptoms are common and include blurred-vision episodes, red eyes, dry eyes, depth perception problems, retinal problems, light sensitivity

* Ringing in the ears and sometimes hearing problems (decreased or even increased sensitivity—so-called hyperacusis)

* Sore throats that are recurring

* Swollen glands, especially neck and under arms

* Anxiety, panic, or worry attacks; others perceive as "very anxious"

* Agitation, irritabity, rage, impulsivity, or aggression

* Episodes of confusion and disorientation that are usually transient (and very scary); often can be seizure-like in nature

* Poor sleep (especially difficulty falling asleep); poor sleep quality

* Joint pain and stiffness (often symmetrical, as opposed to Lyme which is often unsymmetrical, and often migratory)

* Muscle pains, especially in the calves; may be twitching and cramping also

* Foot pain in the morning involving the heels or soles of the feet (sometimes diagnosed as plantar fasciitis)

* Nerve irritation symptoms that can be described as burning, vibrating, numb, shooting, and so forth

* Tremors and/or muscle twitching

* Heart palpitations and strange chest pains

* Episodes of breathlessness

* Strange rashes recurring on the body often, red stretch marks, peculiar tender lumps and nodules along the sides of the legs or arms, and spider veins

* Gut symptoms, especially acid reflux problems

* Shin bone pain and tenderness

Kevin's case illustrates Bartonella infection. Kevin is a research scientist working in western Massachusetts. He was well until three years prior to coming to our office when he began to notice classic symptoms of Lyme disease with migrating joint pains, fatigue, foggy thinking, and sleep problems. He was properly evaluated for Lyme disease and was effectively treated with doxycycline by his primary care doctor in his hometown. Two years later he developed a new set of symptoms— symptoms that were different from the Lyme symptoms that he previously had. At this time, he noticed unrelenting headaches (especially forehead), low grade temperature with sweats in the morning and often in the late afternoon, morning pain and stiffness of his hands, painful soles of the feet in the morning upon arising, swollen lymph glands in the neck, severe anxiety reactions bordering on panic attacks, tremors of his hands and head, muscle cramping, and frequent heart palpitations.

This time when he went to his doctor, the doctor drew a Lyme test and started him immediately on doxycycline. This time the doxycycline only partially helped. His Lyme test was again convincingly positive. After two months of doxycycline and only partial improvement, his doctor decided to treat him with intravenous ceftriaxone. He responded well with about 75 percent improvement in his symptoms. However, within a week of discontinuing the intravenous medicines, his symptoms returned with a vengeance. He was prescribed several different additional antibiotics by his primary care doctor, without improvement from any of them. After continued poor response to the antibiotics, he was finally referred to an infectious diseases specialist. This specialist told him that he had been adequately treated for Lyme and that he had "post-Lyme syndrome." He was then referred to a rheumatologist to help manage his muscle and joint pain and to a psychiatrist to help manage his psychological symptoms.

Kevin was not happy with the direction that his medical team was taking and began to search the Internet for answers. After finding our office through a Lyme-referral site, he made an appointment with us. After evaluating him, I was convinced that he had Bartonella (or BLO). Although his Bartonella blood tests were normal, I was still convinced clinically that he had Bartonella/BLO.

He was agreeable to a trial of levafloxacin for this diagnosis. A week later he called the office and was very excited that he was feeling dramatically better. His headache and anxiety were much improved, and his joints were starting to feel better. By the time I saw him again a month after we started the antibiotic, he stated that he was 80 percent better. After three months of total therapy with levafloxacin, his symptoms were completely resolved and he had had no further problems.

Kevin's case is a classic example of how well-intended doctors treated his Lyme aggressively, but there was very likely a co-infection that also needed attention before the patient could recover his health.

Ehrlichiosis/Anaplasmosis: These two disease conditions are caused by two different organisms in the same bacterial family. Human monocytic ehrlichiosis (HME) is caused by the organism *Ehrlichia chaffeensis* and is most commonly transmitted by the lone star tick. Human granulocytic anaplasmosis (HGA), which was formerly known as human granulocytic ehrlichiosis, is caused by the organism *Anaplasma phagocytophilum*. HGA is most commonly transmitted by the blacklegged tick (deer tick) that also transmits *Bb* and Babesia. Both of these organisms are in the same family as the bacterium (*Rickettsia rickettsii*) that causes Rocky Mountain spotted fever.

Ehrlichiosis and anaplasmosis are both on the rise in the United States and often co-existent with Lyme disease. Symptoms, though usually of a more abrupt nature, are also very similar to those of Lyme disease and usually more severe than Lyme disease alone (especially violent headache and high fever). In addition, ehrlichiosis and anaplasmosis can also impair liver function and cause an abrupt and precipitous drop in white blood cell and platelet levels, both of which play an important role in your body's immune system. They may cause a rash at the onset and very often will cause muscle symptoms (less commonly, joint symptoms.) Chronic headache is often a consequence of ongoing untreated ehrlichiosis or anaplasmosis. It is important to understand that either of these infections (especially HGA) when acute are very serious illnesses and may be life-threatening, and require prompt medical attention. Treatment needs to begin *immediately* even prior to laboratory confirmation.

Compounding the problem of ehrlichiosis and anaplasmosis is the fact that these organisms can be resistant to some antibiotics to which Lyme disease usually responds, such as amoxicillin, cephalosporins, macrolides, and fluoroquinolones. Therefore, if you are being treated for Lyme disease with antibiotics, especially in its early or localized stage, and not responding, be sure to be screened for ehrlichiosis/anaplasmosis, as well. Fortunately, the antibiotic that is most commonly used for the treatment of Lyme disease is doxycycline, and it is the drug of choice for ehrlichiosis/anaplasmosis and should cover either adequately. (Since doxycycline also covers HME and HGA, this is perhaps the most important reason for using it as the drug of first choice when treating Lyme disease.)

The following case is a good example of these infections. Russ is a landscaper working in western Maryland. At the time I saw him, he recalled a tick bite during the summer two years ago. A few days following that bite he remembered a severe headache, high fever, and muscles pains. He was evaluated in the emergency room where he received a spinal tap and an MRI, both of which were unremarkable. He was then admitted to the hospital for observation. He remembered that the doctors were very concerned that his white blood count was low, his platelet count was low, and his liver enzymes were somewhat high. The doctor's final conclusion was that he had a severe viral illness, and he was sent home for bed rest.

His fever subsided, but he was left with ongoing headaches and muscle pains and some joint pain, also. We saw him two months later and tested him for Lyme and for all the co-infections. (His livelihood of landscaping in an "endemic" state made him especially high risk for the tick-borne infections.) His test results indeed showed Lyme disease but also a very high level of antibodies against the bacterium that causes human monocytic ehrlichiosis. After two months of doxycycline, his symptoms completely resolved.

Southern Tick-Associated Rash Illness (STARI): This potential co-infection with Lyme disease was originally described in the early 1990s by Dr. Ed Masters of Cape Girardeau, Missouri. It is most often caused by the bite of the "lone star tick" (*Amblyomma americanum*). These ticks are known for their aggressive behavior in seeking out hosts for their blood meal.

STARI gets its name from the fact that the vector, the lone star tick, is most commonly found in southern states, in Texas and Oklahoma and the Southeast and spreading up the Atlantic coast as far as Virginia. However, the infected tick has also been found as far north as the state of Maine.

Usually within seven days following infection with STARI, a rash similar to the EM rash that is associated with Lyme develops. The STARI rash is reddish in appearance and, like the EM rash, usually shaped as a bull's eye that can expand to a diameter of three inches or more. The rash is often accompanied by symptoms such as fatigue, fever, headache, and joint and muscle pain. STARI will usually test negative for Lyme and, therefore, will look as if it is a case of Lyme with a negative blood test. Generally, STARI responds to treatment with a course of oral antibiotics similar to those used for Lyme disease.

Tick-Borne Relapsing Fever (TBRF): Caused by three strains of spirochete bacteria (*B. hermsii, B. parkerii, and B. turicatae*) that are different from the *Bb* strain, relapsing fever is a systemic condition that can quickly take hold in the body. Its symptoms, which typically include chills, fever, headache, and joint pain, can last for a few days to a week, then disappear, only to reappear later, with this pattern repeating until relapsing fever is properly treated. Doxycycline is an effective antibiotic treatment.

Rocky Mountain spotted fever (RMSF): Once known as "black measles" because of the darkish rash that is one of its symptoms, Rocky Mountain spotted fever typically first manifests on the hands and feet, before spreading to the torso. Additional symptoms include chills, high fever, headache, mental confusion or "brain fog," muscle aches and pains, and sensitivity to light. Untreated, RMSF has a significant mortality rate. Treatment for RMSF is with the tetracyclines, such as doxycycline. In suspected cases, treatment with antibiotics should begin *immediately* without waiting for laboratory confirmation. With treatment, symptoms should begin to subside in 24 to 72 hours.

Tularemia: Also known as "rabbit fever" and "deerfly fever," tularemia is a potentially serious infection caused by a bacterium called *Francisella tularensis*. About half of the cases are as a result of tick bites, including bites of lone star ticks and American dog ticks. Deerfly bites, eating or handling infected meat (such as rabbit or muskrat), or drinking contaminated water are other methods of transmission. Symptoms may include sudden fever, chills, headache, diarrhea, muscle and joint aches, dry cough, swollen lymph glands, eye symptoms, and progressive weakness. Treatment is best accomplished with the antibiotics streptomycin or gentamycin. Oral alternatives include doxycycline or ciprofloxacin. A vaccination is available for people whose jobs place them at high risk for infection.

The tick-borne co-infections discussed above represent the major challenges that are seen in the offices of doctors who work extensively with tick-borne diseases. There are several other potential co-infections that deserve to be mentioned. These include:

* West Nile virus (a mosquito-borne flavivirus found also to be present in ticks, but transmission to humans via ticks is uncertain at this time)

* Colorado tick fever

* Q fever (which may cause heart complications particularly in persons with heart valve abnormalities)

* Powassan encephalitis (caused by another tick-borne flavivirus)

* Tick paralysis (caused by a nerve toxin in the tick saliva, not by infection per se)

Other infections that are not necessarily tick-borne should also be considered in patients with chronic tick-borne illness. These include species of mycoplasma, brucella, chlamydia, salmonella, leptospirosis, and several viral diseases (including enteroviruses, herpes simplex viruses such as Epstein-Barr virus, and others). However, further detailed discussion on these infections and other tick-borne co-infections is beyond the scope of this book.

Summing Up

Let's review the key points of this chapter by examining the most commonly asked questions about symptoms of Lyme disease, as well as its related co-infections.

Why do symptoms of Lyme disease present such a challenge when it comes to diagnosis?

The answer to this question has multiple parts. The first reason is that there is only one sign of Lyme disease that is considered indisputable—the EM rash. However, less than 50 percent of all adults with Lyme disease ever develop a rash. And among those who do develop an EM, the rash often goes unrecognized by patients and doctors alike. In addition, a person's *symptoms* (refers to a patient's subjective experiences) may not always be specific enough to clearly indicate Lyme illness. Lyme disease can manifest in many different ways, making it easy to confuse with other illnesses. Therefore, a doctor evaluating a patient will seek to find *signs* (objective evidence) of Lyme. As mentioned, the only universally accepted sign of Lyme disease is the EM rash. But since the rash is so often not part of patients' presenting symptoms, you can see the challenge this presents to both the patients and their physicians. Without other conclusive physical signs on patient examination, the doctor will turn next to diagnostic testing to confirm the presence of *Bb*. We will discuss the complex topic of diagnostic testing in chapter 3.

What are some of the possible symptoms of Lyme disease?

At the localized stage of Lyme disease, aside from the EM rash, the other most common possible signs include headaches, mild aches and pains, low grade fever (rarely over 101 degrees F), and mild flu-like symptoms (especially occurring out of season for the flu).

Once Lyme becomes disseminated or chronic, however, the range of possible symptoms can greatly vary and they can mimic other disease conditions. Symptoms of chronic Lyme include arthritis-like joint pain and swelling (particularly migrating pain which changes location), "brain fog" which can involve poor attention and focus (similar to attention deficit disorder), poor memory (especially short term), sleep disturbance, back pain and tenderness, sensitivity to light and/or blurred vision, decreased hearing (and often ringing in the ears), night sweats (especially in the early stages), chronic fatigue state, facial paralysis (most commonly Bell's palsy but may involve other cranial nerves), fibromyalgia, gait and balance problems, headache, impaired muscle coordination, impaired reflexes, and nerve pain (especially arms/hands and legs/feet often described as burning, tingling, vibrating, shooting in nature).

A major clue that Lyme is the cause of the above symptoms is a tendency for these symptoms to progressively worsen over time and to wax and wane in a cyclical fashion. That is, generally every three to four weeks, it seems that all the symptoms get worse for a few days, after which they resume the previous pattern. Other symptoms of chronic Lyme disease include neurological problems that can mimic or exacerbate conditions such as multiple sclerosis (MS), Lou Gehrig's disease, and Parkinson's disease; psychological symptoms, including severe depression and suicidal tendencies; and heart problems, including the extremely serious problem of Lyme carditis, which can be fatal.

How common are co-infections with Lyme disease?

Co-infections can be quite common among patients with Lyme disease, especially when symptoms are chronic and severe. Based on my clinical experience treating Lyme disease, I can say that the severity of the symptoms that patients with Lyme disease experience is directly related to the presence of and number of co-infections that are also present.

What are the most common co-infections associated with Lyme disease?

The most common co-infections are those transmitted by ticks and various insects. They include babesiosis, bartonellosis, ehrlichiosis and anaplasmosis, Southern tick-associated rash illness (STARI), tularemia, Q-fever, relapsing fever, and Rocky Mountain spotted fever. Each of these conditions, as well as their most common symptoms, is described above. Other co-infections include the mycoplasmas, brucellas, chlamydias, salmonellas, leptospirosis, and various chronic viral infections, especially the herpes family of infections.

In the next chapter, I will discuss the diagnostic testing involved in evaluating a patient who may have Lyme disease. Included will be a detailed discussion of the laboratory tests available and the pitfalls often associated with testing. Tests for other conditions that might be confused with Lyme will also be discussed.

Chapter Three

Effectively Diagnosing Lyme Disease and Its Co-infections

※

One of the most crucial elements in the successful treatment of Lyme disease is an accurate diagnosis of Lyme and of its potential co-infections. The sooner the diagnosis can be made from the time of the initial infection with Lyme or its co-infections the better. As we have discussed in previous chapters, treating Lyme disease when it is still in a localized condition offers the best hope of a long-term recovery. However, accurately diagnosing this disease is not always an easy task. Symptoms of Lyme disease manifest in a wide variety of ways, making its detection more challenging. In addition, the most commonly used diagnostic screening tests for Lyme can often yield unreliable results. They often fail to indicate Lyme when it is present in the body, with up to one third of cases of the infection being missed due to a high rate of "false negative" results. For these reasons, I recommend that all patients who suspect that they have Lyme disease seek out doctors who are most knowledgeable about Lyme disease and its co-infections for accurate diagnosis and effective treatment.

Diagnosing Lyme Disease

The most challenging problem with Lyme disease is that there is no universally accepted method for making its diagnosis. The only exception is the presence of the erythema migrans (EM) rash. This rash is considered prima facie evidence of the infection, and Lyme's presence does not require further confirmation with diagnostic tests to undergo a full course of Lyme disease antibiotic therapy. Although there are a variety of diagnostic tests that are available to evaluate a possible case of Lyme disease, there is no single perfect test. Even the more accurate types of available tests can still fail to detect Lyme disease because of the manner in which the *Bb* bacteria can "hide" as its spreads throughout the body. I want to next discuss some of the key issues concerning Lyme testing.

Pitfalls of Lyme Testing

As we have previously discussed in this book, the standard Lyme screening tests have a major problem of "false negatives." That is, they have a large potential to miss cases of true Lyme disease by calling the person "negative" when the person does in fact have active Lyme. However, not all positive test readings for the disease mean that Lyme is an active problem at this time. In some cases, positive readings are only an indication that at some point in a person's past he or she was infected with the *Bb* bacteria, at which time the body developed antibodies to combat it. In other words, the antibodies may have been produced by the body during its successful past campaign to destroy and eliminate the *Bb* bacteria. However, the continued presence of these antibodies against Lyme may mistakenly be taken by a physician as a sign that the disease is still active. Also, there are times when viral illnesses (such as those of the herpes family) or other infections (such as syphilis, gingivitis, bacterial endocarditis) may trigger the body to make antibodies against Lyme, even though there is no active Lyme infection itself. Either of these scenarios, in turn, could lead to unnecessary treatment with antibiotics.

Lyme-aware physicians rely not only on diagnostic tests, but also on their own clinical judgment and experience. Fundamentally, Lyme is a "clinical" diagnosis. This means that an accurate diagnosis depends on the astute physician's wisdom as he/she puts together the whole clinical picture—symptom patterns, risk factors, exposure history, examination findings, test results, and other clinical indicators such as response (or lack of response) to treatment. One of the most useful tools for helping you to decide whether Lyme is a possibility for you is the Symptom Checklist that I shared with you in chapter 2.

Politics of Lyme Testing

There is a significant problem of inaccurate diagnostic testing for Lyme disease. This is a major contributing factor to the lack of consensus that exists about Lyme disease. There is clearly a need for a high quality diagnostic test on which health professionals can agree. This dilemma is well recognized even at the highest levels of our federal government. In late 2001 both the House and the Senate passed legislation that calls for the development of an accurate, uniform diagnostic test for Lyme disease. Congress further instructed the Centers for Disease Control and Prevention (CDC) to correct the misuse of its surveillance criteria for Lyme disease as a method of diagnosis. The legislation, known as Public Law 107-116, was signed into law by President George W. Bush on January, 10, 2002. In part, the wording that was included in Public Law 107-116 reads:

The Committee recognizes that the current state of laboratory testing for Lyme disease is very poor. The situation has led many people to be misdiagnosed and delayed proper treatment. The vaccine clinical trial has documented that more than one third (36 percent) of the people with Lyme disease did not test positive on the most sophisticated tests available. The ramifications of this deficit in terms of unnecessary pain, suffering and cost is staggering. The Committee directs CDC to work closely with the Food and Drug Administration to develop an unequivocal test for Lyme disease.

The Committee is distressed in hearing of the widespread misuse of the current Lyme disease surveillance case definition. While the CDC does state that "this surveillance case definition was developed for national reporting of Lyme disease: it is NOT appropriate for clinical diagnosis," the definition is reportedly misused as a standard of care for health care reimbursement, product (test) development, medical licensing hearings, and other legal cases. The CDC is encouraged to aggressively pursue and correct the misuse of this definition. This includes issuing an alert to the public and physicians, as well as actively issuing letters to places misusing this definition.

The Committee recommends that the CDC strongly support the re-examination and broadening of the Lyme disease surveillance case definition by the Council of State and Territorial Epidemiologists. Voluntary and patient groups should have input into this process. Currently there is just one definition ("confirmed case") of seven possible categories. By developing other categories while leaving the current category intact, the true number of cases being diagnosed and treated will be more accurately counted, lending to improved public health planning for finding solutions to the infection.

The CDC is encouraged to include a broad range of scientific viewpoints in the process of planning and executing their efforts. This means including community-based clinicians with extensive experience in treating these patients, voluntary agen-cies who have advocacy in their mission, and patient advocates in planning committees, meetings, and outreach efforts.

Interestingly, despite the recommendations of Public Law 107-116, as of this writing, six years after its passage, there is not an improved standard diagnostic screening test for Lyme disease. There has been little, if any, progress made. The testing issue to which Congress is referring is called the "two-tiered" diagnostic system for Lyme disease. This two-tiered system is still in place, and CDC continues to use it for its "surveillance case definition" of Lyme. Let me explain to you how the CDC two-tiered testing process works.

The two-tiered approach begins by screening a person with the ELISA/IFA test. If the screening test is positive, the test is "confirmed" with the standard Western Blot. While this approach may work well for CDC's "epidemiological" purpose, it is totally inappropriate for clinical diagnostic purposes because it misses too many cases of persons with Lyme disease. I will explain the inadequacies of this testing approach later in this chapter.

Types of Diagnostic Tests

There are two categories of diagnostic tests most commonly used by most physicians to screen for Lyme disease: (1) those that test for the presence in the blood of antibodies directed against the *Bb* bacteria and (2) those that seek to directly detect *Bb* in the blood, urine, or other body tissue. Of these two categories, antibody testing is used more frequently because it is widely available and relatively inexpensive.

What are antibody tests? To understand how antibody tests work, you need to first understand what antibodies are. Simply put, whenever your body is exposed to an infectious agent, such as a bacteria or virus, the body's immune system goes to work immediately. One of the first things that happens is that your immune system sends out cells (called macrophages) to capture and process the harmful agent (in the case of Lyme disease, the *Bb* bacteria).

The immune cells that are involved in this capturing of the microorganism then signal other cells in the immune system to do certain defensive things in order to destroy the attacking germs. One of the most important things that the other immune cells (called lymphocytes) do is to produce antibodies. Antibodies are a specialized class of proteins. They are like very specific bullets from a gun. Their job is to attack and eliminate infectious agents before they can cause harm.

The first antibody produced by the body's immune system when harmful microorganisms invade is known as immunoglobulin M (IgM). In most cases, IgM appears within the first four to six weeks following the body's exposure to the infectious agent. While IgM is doing the initial job against the invading organism, the immune cells of the body are creating an even more specific, "tailor-made" antibody against the organism called immunoglobulin G (IgG).

At the time of emergence of IgG, the levels of IgM begin to fall. The levels of IgG antibody can and often do remain elevated indefinitely following the harmful microorganism's attack on the body. However, in the case of chronic unresolved Lyme, it is common to find ongoing elevation of IgM antibodies often along with IgG antibodies. (This occurs because of active, chronic, and ongoing "antigen presentation" by the macrophages to the lymphocytes, thereby inducing the body to make IgM constantly. In other words, IgM will often be made until the chronic infection is either effectively treated or is under control by the immune system.)

Antibody tests are indirect tests. That is to say, they do not screen for the actual infectious agents themselves. Instead they look for the presence of these specific IgM and IgG antibodies targeted against the infectious agent in the blood. The rationale behind such tests is this: When antibody levels are high, it is a reliable sign that the infectious agent is, or has been, present in the body.

What are the types of antibody tests? The three most common antibody tests for Lyme disease are the ELISA test, the IFA test, and the Western Blot test. It is important to understand the background regarding these tests. In 1995, the CDC began recommending a "two-tiered" antibody testing approach for reporting active cases of Lyme disease, as well as for reporting cases of previous infection. It is important that you understand the logic of a two-tiered (or two-step) testing approach.

In the first tier a *sensitive* test is used that is able to correctly diagnose nearly all (95 percent or greater) of the actual cases of the disease, even if it over-diagnoses some cases. By over-diagnose, I mean some people without the disease are falsely identified as positive. In the second tier, a more *specific* test is used for everyone who tested positive on the first test. This second tier test sorts out the cases that tested falsely positive (and who don't really have the disease) from those who really do have the disease.

This two-tiered approach required that a positive *sensitive* screening antibody test (ELISA or IFA) be followed by a confirming *specific* antibody test (Western Blot). "Sensitive" screening tests mean that such tests "rarely miss a true positive case of disease," while "specific tests" "never falsely call a non-case a case of disease," meaning that specific tests can sort out true positive cases from false positive cases.

Can you help me understand what these two-tiered tests mean? This is such a key point to understand, let me illustrate it with an example. Let's say that there is a new virus that has been detected in our population. For the sake of illustration, let's call it "Virus X." We want to do a test that will detect Virus X in the population. When we administer this new test, there are only four different results possible of our test:

- Test is Positive in persons that HAVE Virus X (True Positive).

- Test is Negative in persons that HAVE Virus X (False Negative).

- Test is Positive in persons that DO NOT HAVE Virus X (False Positive).

- Test is Negative in persons that DO NOT HAVE Virus X (True Negative).

Let's further define the situation. We have developed a set of two tests that we think will reliably tell us who has Virus X and who does not have Virus X. (It will separate the "haves" from the "have nots," so to speak.)

- Test #1—Screening Test (This is given to everybody in the target population who is at risk for getting the virus.)

- Test #2—Confirmatory Test (This is given only to those who were positive with Test #1 to sort out which really have it from those that don't have it.)

Here is how it is done. Test #1 is given to everyone in the population. We call that our "screening test" because we hope it will separate out most of the people who have Virus X from those who do not. Test #1 is not a perfect test—it will "underdiagnose" some people who actually have Virus X (remember, we call those people False Negative). It will also "over-diagnose" some people who don't have the virus (and we call those people False Positive).

Therefore, because of Test #1's inaccuracies, we have to administer a second, more accurate test, Test #2. This is our "confirmatory test." Its purpose is to confirm that everybody that Test #1 said has Virus X really has it. By doing this test we weed out all the people who may have been falsely diagnosed with Virus X by Test #1. In medical testing, Test #2 is always used to sort out the positives diagnosed by Test #1 in order to determine which are True Positives and which are False Positives. If you are positive with Test #1 and negative in #2, you are considered negative. If you are positive in Test #1 and #2 both, then you are considered positive and have the disease.

Now we understand the purpose of each test—one is to screen and the other to sort out the positives that came from the screening test. Remember, neither test is perfect, but Test #2 is clearly the most accurate. The most critical piece of the puzzle that we must now put into place is to define exactly the accuracy of the tests. This issue of accuracy is the key to whether our two tests are useful clinically, or not useful. What I will now explain will help you to understand why CDC's two-tiered approach is quite adequate for public health surveillance purposes in the population that CDC targets, but totally misses the mark with the clinical population that we physicians see in our offices.

In terms of accuracy, let's say that the Test #1 is 65 percent sensitive and 50 percent specific. Sensitivity means how often a test will accurately detect those who truly have Virus X. In our case, if 100 people who have the disease are tested, 65 percent *sensitivity* translates into 65 of those 100 diseased people being correctly called "true positive." On the other hand, 35 people have been missed by the test and now fall into the category of "false negatives." Further in our case, let's say that there are 1,000 people who do not have the virus that are being screened with Test #1. In this case, 50 percent *specificity* means that the test will call 500 of that 1,000 people correctly as "true negatives." On the other hand, it will call the other 500 of that 1,000 who don't have the disease incorrectly as positive, which we label as "false positive." The main purpose of Test #2 in this situation is to try to sort out who of all those 565 positive tests from Test #1 (65 true positives, 500 false positives) are really infected with Virus X and which are not. Therefore, Test #2 has to be a very specific test in order to accomplish that separation process.

Let's apply this now to Lyme disease. The accuracy of the CDC two-tiered system totally depends on how much Lyme exists (also called the "prevalence") in the population being tested. Without going into the mathematical specifics, let me explain how this works:

- If the population being tested for Lyme is *low* risk, or low probability, or low prevalence (they all mean essentially the same), the accuracy of the CDC criteria is quite good—in the 90 percent or more range.

- If those same tests are given to a population at *high* risk, high probability, high prevalence for Lyme, the accuracy drops dramatically—to 70 percent or less. In other words, the *more* likely that the population being tested actually has Lyme, the *less* accurate the test is because the screening test (Test #1, also known as ELISA/IFA) has poor sensitivity.

It is the people of this second "high risk" category that often are mislabeled as not having Lyme disease when they, in fact, do have the infection. Who are the individuals in the high risk group in regards to Lyme? In clinical practice, this means persons who have a high probability of having active Lyme infection. The following is a partial list of risk factors that may place a person in the high prevalence or high probability group. I believe people in this category are not good candidates for two-tier screening. This group includes people who:

- have symptoms and/or diagnoses that are consistent with the possibility of Lyme disease

- live and work in endemic areas

- work in a profession, occupation, or recreation that places them at high risk (such as landscapers, home construction workers, golfers, hunters, and hikers)

* have had previous tick bites (or bites of insects that may possibly transmit Lyme)

* have an infected family member and/or infected pets

* have a history of previous Lyme disease or a tick-borne co-infection

To test this group would require that a very sensitive (and specific) test be used. We will see below that the Western Blot qualifies as the most accurate (of currently available test methods) for a population in which there is a high probability or high risk of Lyme disease.

Why does the CDC use the two-tier approach? The CDC's intention for recommending this two-tiered approach was, appropriately, for the purpose of public health surveillance and disease prevention. The two-tier approach works well for their surveillance and "disease trends" usage. The tracking of infection trends is a vital public health function, and we need to be grateful to the CDC for performing this valuable function. The CDC needs to know that, if they designated a case of Lyme disease as a "true positive" case, that it is a definitive case and is not disputable. Unfortunately, the CDC's recommendations have become the standard form of testing for Lyme disease. It is used by most physicians and health researchers, as well as most insurance companies. Yet the CDC has always maintained that Lyme disease is a clinical diagnosis.

The tests employed in the CDC's two-tiered recommendations do not meet the standards of clinical diagnosis when it comes to Lyme disease because they have a high degree of inaccuracy when applied to a population in which the probability of the disease is high. Using the CDC criteria to define a clinical case of Lyme will result in a very high number of false negatives. My own case of misdiagnosed Lyme is an excellent example of how that can happen.

What are the screening tests used in the two-tiered approach? The most commonly used screening or first test in the CDC two-tiered approach is the ELISA test. The ELISA (enzyme-linked immunosorbent assay) test relies on enzymes to detect antibodies to the *Bb* bacteria. However, the ELISA test has a sensitivity of 65 percent (like Test #1 above) and, therefore, is inaccurate 35 percent of the time when it comes to detecting Lyme disease. This means that the ELISA test fails to detect Lyme disease in 35 out of every 100 people who are infected by it. (This is in contrast to the sensitivity of the screening test for HIV that has a sensitivity in the 95 percent or higher range.)

The other commonly used screening or first test utilized in the two-tiered approach is the IFA. The IFA (indirect fluorescent antibody) test has about the same inaccuracy rate as the ELISA test when it comes to Lyme disease. The IFA test was the original test used by physicians to diagnose Lyme. It uses a fluorescent dye that is placed on a slide containing a blood sample mixed with a dead specimen of the *Bb* bacteria. It is read by a trained technician (as opposed to a machine like the ELISA), thus possible human subjectivity increases the likelihood of error.

There are a variety of reasons why both the ELISA and IFA tests fail to detect Lyme disease 35 percent of the time. According to Karen Vanderhoof-Forschner, cofounder of the Lyme Disease Foundation, the reasons include:

* Samples that are tested too soon after infection, before the immune system is fully able to produce enough antibodies to defend against the *Bb* bacteria. (In cases of Lyme disease in which the EM rash appears, it often requires four to six weeks after the rash's appearance before sufficient amounts of antibodies are produced at a detectable level.)

* Laboratory error

* The strain of *Bb* bacteria involved is not something that the testing lab is capable of detecting because it differs from the reference strain that the lab is using. It is even possible that reference strains being used by some labs may not even originate in the United States, making it very likely that many strains native to this country could be missed by that lab's test.

* The antibodies that are produced by the immune system bind to the *Bb* bacteria, creating what is known as a "complexed antibody." When this occurs, there is not enough free-floating antibodies left in the bloodstream to be detected.

* The immune system is not producing enough antibodies due to impaired immune function. (The relationship between the immune system and Lyme disease is discussed in detail in chapters 4 and 5.)

* Early antibiotic use caused the production of antibodies to be halted or reduced to below detection.

* The *Bb* bacteria have altered their surface characteristics, thus escaping detection by the immune system, which therefore does not produce antibodies. (This process of the *Bb* bacteria altering their makeup is known as *pleomorphism*. Although pleomorphism is a common characteristic of many infectious microorganisms, it is often overlooked by physicians and not taken into consideration by most conventional diagnostic tests.)

* The *Bb* bacteria have cloaked themselves within immune cells, making it difficult for the immune system to detect them.

* The person affected with Lyme disease is genetically predisposed to cause antibody blood tests to produce false negative results.

To be clinically effective, antibody screening tests such as the ELISA and IFA tests should have a sensitivity rate of at least 90 to 95 percent (meaning that they only miss 5 to 10 percent or less of all cases of Lyme). Clinicians and the CDC alike desire sensitive tests for all diseases being evaluated. As screening tests for Lyme, neither the conventional ELISA nor

IFA works to accomplish that objective. A sensitivity rate of 65 percent would not be acceptable for screening for HIV viruses (that cause AIDS), and therefore, it is not appropriate for Lyme patients to settle for an inferior test for clinical use.

Is there a better test than the ELISA and IFA? Because of its higher accuracy, the Western Blot test is usually used as a confirmatory test in follow-up to the ELISA and IFA tests. However, it actually would be the superior screening test. Although the Western Blot test is more sensitive and specific than the ELISA and IFA tests, there is one major problem when it comes to detecting Lyme disease. The problem is that the commercially available Western Blot test omits the two very important antibodies for Lyme, which are known as "band 31" and "band 34." By omitting these two bands, the commercial labs decrease the sensitivity of the Western Blot.

Most Lyme-aware doctors use laboratories that report all bands, including bands 31 and 34. Studies have shown that the most Lyme-specific Western Blot "bands" are: 18, 23–25, 31, 34, 39, and 83–93. Any one of these, along with band 41 (which appears early and is specific for all borrelia including Lyme), strongly suggests Lyme exposure. In my Lyme disease treatment experience, I prefer seeing at least a positive band 41 (along with at least one specific band) for me to consider the Western Blot positive. If other specific bands are positive, but not the band 41, it makes me strongly consider this may be a "false positive" Western Blot (caused perhaps by viruses). When a person is found to have a "true positive" Western Blot it confirms exposure to Lyme, but Lyme active infection is a clinical determination to be made by a Lyme-aware doctor based on symptoms and other criteria.

A logical question at this point would be: If the sensitive Western Blot with bands 31 and 34 is better, why don't CDC and the commercial labs use it? This problem is best explained on the Web site (www.ilads.org) of the International Lyme and Associated Diseases Society (ILADS), which states:

> For "epidemiological purposes" the CDC eliminated from the Western Blot analysis the reading of bands 31 and 34. These bands are so specific to Borrelia burgdorferi [the Bb bacteria] that they were chosen for vaccine development. Since a vaccine for Lyme disease is currently unavailable, however, a positive 31 or 34 band is highly indicative of Borrelia burgdorferi exposure. Yet these bands are not reported in commercial Lyme tests.

In conclusion, the CDC two-tiered approach is inappropriate for general diagnostic clinical use. The following key points should be considered:

* The screening tests (conventional ELISA/IFA) are inadequate with a sensitivity of only 65 percent, meaning that 35 percent of cases will be missed. This is unacceptable for a high prevalence population with a high probability of being infected with Lyme.

* The standard, conventional confirmation test (Western Blot without bands 31 and 34) is incomplete. Since the Lymerix vaccine is no longer a factor, omitting band 31 does not make logical sense. The reporting form to the CDC filled out by the reporting doctor asks if the patient has received the vaccine. If the doctor answers "yes" then, and only then, should the CDC be justified in dismissing the band 31. If the answer is "no" then the band 31 would be extremely useful in correctly diagnosing Lyme disease. Likewise, the band 34 was omitted because it does not occur early in the course of Lyme disease. But because of that, however, it would logically serve as a useful marker for later or chronic Lyme cases rather than being totally discarded.

* If a person is tested for Lyme using the two-tiered approach, and the test confirms Lyme, then the person should be treated for Lyme. However, if a symptomatic person tests negative, and that person is in a high risk group, further Lyme evaluation needs to be aggressively pursued such as a sensitive Western Blot test that includes the 31 and 34 bands.

Are there more accurate methods for detection of Lyme? More definitive laboratory methods for direct testing for Lyme exist. Among those methods currently available is the growing of the *Bb* bacterium in "culture." This test is absolute proof of Lyme disease. In studies where cultures have been done, it is interesting and significant that 20 to 30 percent of persons with a positive culture have negative antibody tests, meaning that it is even more accurate than antibody tests.

Culturing Lyme means creating favorable laboratory growth conditions for *Bb* in what is called a "culture medium." This involves taking a sample of a patient's blood and placing that sample into a nourishing growth substance where Lyme can grow. There are many inherent difficulties with culturing as a test for Lyme, however, including the fact that *Bb* is not consistently present in patients' blood. Further, it must be grown on special culture media that are not readily available to commercial clinical laboratories and, therefore, is not practical to consider in the setting of the clinical office.

Another definitive method for diagnosing Lyme would be the demonstration of Lyme in the biopsy of body tissue. Biopsy involves taking a blood and tissue specimen from a patient for microscopic examination. However, because there is not always a detectable number of *Bb* spirochetes present in the biopsy specimen, they are very easy to miss. Additionally, there are very few pathologists (doctors who examine biopsy specimens) who are able to perform accurate Lyme analysis on biopsy specimens.

As an alternative to culturing *Bb* and biopsying body tissue, the next best laboratory option is to test for pieces of the *Bb* bacteria's DNA. The test used for this procedure is known as a PCR (polymerase chain reaction). It is frequently used by researchers and physicians in the field of infectious disease to track and identify various infectious agents, including HIV and hepatitis. This test is well respected for its ability to provide definitive evidence of infection. However, the PCR test is expensive and often not covered by a patient's insurance. In addition, it too can result in a false negative reading for Lyme because it relies on finding the DNA of the organism it is testing for in the blood (and sometimes urine). The *Bb* bacterium, however, is not primarily a blood-borne organism and is more commonly found in tissue that contains collagen, such as the joints, tendons, fascia, and other connective tissues. For this reason, the PCR test may not be able to detect *Bb* even when it is definitely present.

Are there other tests that can be done to detect the presence of Lyme? Two other diagnostic tests that can be used to evaluate suspected Lyme disease are Brain SPECT scans and lumbar puncture (also known as spinal tap). A SPECT (single photon emission computer topography) scan is a diagnostic test that reveals the distribution of a radioactive tracer in a targeted area (that is, it shows how blood flows to tissues and organs, including the brain). In this test, physicians can determine how well organs and tissues are functioning. (This is in contrast to X-rays, CT scans, and MRIs, which reveal the condition of an organ or tissue's structure.)

Some Lyme authorities believe that many patients suffering from chronic Lyme disease, particularly those who evidence cognitive impairment (e.g., "brain fog") and chronic headaches, have abnormalities in their blood flow as revealed by Brain SPECT scans. SPECT scans cannot provide a definitive diagnosis of Lyme disease, but they can provide objective evidence that a person's symptoms are real and not just psychogenic. (However, Brain SPECT scans can be abnormal in purely psychiatric states such as depression.) Additionally, as Dr. Burrascano states in his 2005 monograph, *Diagnostic Hints and Treatment Guidelines for Lyme and Other Tick Borne Illnesses*, if the SPECT scan is found to be abnormal, it can help to quantify the abnormalities. Furthermore, repeat scans after a course of treatment can be used to assess treatment efficacy.

Most of the time, SPECT scans reveal only nonspecific findings for most patients with Lyme disease who have neurological symptoms. For this reason, many Lyme-aware physicians limit the use of SPECT scans to those patients who present with profound neurological deficits or to those patients where differentiation from psychiatric disorders is important. Should patients with Lyme choose to have a SPECT scan performed, I recommend that they choose a testing facility that has experience with Lyme disease. In addition, patients should be aware that changes in SPECT scans often lag well behind the clinical improvements of their condition, often by many months.

A spinal tap, also known as a lumbar puncture, is a procedure that involves inserting a sterile needle into the lower spine (the lumbar region) to collect cerebrospinal fluid that is then analyzed for various abnormalities, including Lyme disease. Spinal taps can be useful in helping Lyme physicians in three situations: (1) achieve a clearer diagnostic picture of Lyme patients with significant neurological symptoms (that is, offer further confirmation that Lyme is indeed the culprit behind the neurological symptoms and not a different medical reason for the symptoms), (2) help assessment of patients who test negative in their blood for Lyme disease yet still are exhibiting neurological symptoms associated with Lyme disease, and (3) help determine why treatments fail for Lyme patients with neurological symptoms. It is important to keep in mind that the sensitivity of the lumbar puncture for detecting Lyme disease is not very good—10 to 20 percent or less.

When used for Lyme patients, the primary goal of a spinal tap is to rule out other potential causes of neurological problems, such as multiple sclerosis or even infections other than Lyme and its co-infections. Of course, it is also useful to determine if the *Bb* bacteria or any co-infections (particularly Bartonella) are present in the cerebrospinal fluid. (When *Bb* is present in spinal fluid, it can be a sign of Lyme meningitis.) Despite the low yield in terms of Lyme sensitivity, it is probably wise to consider a diagnostic spinal tap for cases of Lyme where moderate to severe neurological symptoms exist. For most cases of Lyme disease with milder neurological symptoms, however, spinal taps are generally not necessary, especially when antibody confirmation of Lyme has already been accomplished.

How does a Lyme-aware doctor decide that I have Lyme disease? Because of all the diagnostic issues discussed above, the diagnosis of Lyme disease is often difficult. The task of the Lyme-aware physician is to gather as much evidence as possible from multiple sources in order to make a diagnosis of Lyme disease. This information-gathering work includes:

* A thorough medical history (which may include a review of the Burrascano symptom checklist from chapter 2) and performance of a comprehensive physical examination

* Assessment of a person's probability of having Lyme (that is, the prevalence status of the person based on risk factors and so forth)

* Lab testing that provides the most sensitive and specific results for Lyme. In our practice we use a "sensitive Western Blot test," with bands 31 and 34 also reported, as our screening test. The reasons for using this test were discussed earlier in this chapter.

* The addition of the PCR, SPECT scans, lumbar puncture, biopsy, neuropsychological testing, and so forth, when appropriate

* It is crucial that medical disorders other than Lyme be considered, and those alternative possibilities be evaluated also. Remember, Lyme symptoms are often not specific. For example, everyone with chronic fatigue and fibromyalgia does not have Lyme.

* Assessment of possible co-infections

* Other tests that help assess vital body functions (These will be discussed later in this chapter.)

In summary, the diagnosis of Lyme disease is similar to the work of a detective. Lyme-aware doctors must rely on their clinical experience, in addition to using the most accurate tests. Remember, even the best of laboratory testing will result in 20 to 30 percent of Lyme patients being missed.

Diagnosing the Co-infections

As discussed in chapter 2, many Lyme patients are also infected with co-infections. These microorganisms may be transmitted to a person at the same time that Lyme is transmitted, or they may enter the body at a different time than does Lyme. A high percentage of so-called "Post-Lyme Disease Syndrome" individuals that present to the offices of Lyme-aware doctors have undiagnosed co-infections. As with Lyme disease, the diagnosis of these organisms can be very challenging. Many times the diagnosis of a co-infection is made by an experienced physician based purely on clinical grounds. This frequently happens when laboratory testing does not confirm the diagnosis. Dr. Kenneth Liegner, co-author of *Coping with Lyme Disease*, clearly states the problem encountered by physicians who are attempting to sort out the confusing clinical picture of Lyme and the other tick-borne diseases (TBDs):

With tests for several tick-borne illnesses not always reliable, and with overlapping non-specific symptoms, the treating doctor is often confronted with a dilemma. The problem faced by the doctor, responsible for improving the health of an often very seriously ill or debilitated patient, is that he or she must often resort to empiric treatment based on educated guesses, inferential reasoning, and observation of response (or lack of response) to trials of therapy. In other words, often the doctor must rely on "playing the percentages" in terms of what most likely is going on with the patient. While this approach may seem "unscientific," this analytic approach is often necessary given the unsatisfactory diagnostic testing tools available today.

I agree with Dr. Liegner that often in order to help severely ill patients with Lyme and other TBDs, doctors must rely on their clinical experience and judgment, rather than testing alone, in order to help patients recover their health.

The following diagnostic tests are recommended when screening Lyme patients for the possible tick-borne co-infections. Let me reemphasize that it is very important for these infections to be considered because they are such important co-factors in a patient's symptoms. I will discuss the diagnostic approach to the major co-infections.

Babesia: This is the parasitic organism that causes babesiosis. Babesia is rarely detected using one diagnostic test alone. To effectively screen for Babesia, Lyme-aware physicians generally screen for 2 strains—*Babesia microti* and WA-1 (*Babesia duncani*)—by testing for antibodies (by IFA or ELISA testing) made by the body against those organisms.

Another very useful test for Babesia is known as the FISH (fluorescent in situ hybridization) test. The FISH test is performed on thin blood smears (tests used to detect germs in white blood cells) and is able to detect the RNA (genetic material) of Babesia. If this test is positive, it is very strong evidence of the presence of active Babesia. The advantage of the FISH test is that it will detect other subspecies of Babesia in addition to *B. microti and B. duncani.* (A direct thick and thin blood smear using a staining technique called "Giemsa" can also be done by one's local or commercial labs to look for Babesia organisms in red blood cells; however, it is an insensitive test except during acute Babesia, particularly when fever is present.)

A final potentially useful test is the Babesia PCR (polymerase chain reaction). Unfortunately, in my experience it is also not a sensitive test and is the least useful of the three tests mentioned.

All three of these tests—Babesia IFA, FISH, PCR—are available through IgeneX, a laboratory specializing in Lyme disease and other tick-borne organisms. Medical Diagnostics Laboratory (MDL) has two of the tests—Babesia ELISA and PCR. Both labs are excellent and I utilize both regularly. (See the resources section for more information.) However, as mentioned, Babesia can frequently escape detection by diagnostic tests. Therefore, many times babesiois must be a clinical diagnosis made by physicians who are experienced in its detection and treatment.

Bartonella: This bacterium is perhaps the most challenging of all the co-infections to identify. Common strains of Bartonella, such as *B. quintana and B. henselae*, can usually be detected using antibody tests that are available at most medical laboratories. The PCR test can also be used to screen for Bartonella. See the resources section to learn of labs that perform Bartonella PCR testing.

Antibody tests may fail to detect Bartonella even when it is present by PCR testing. Many times the diagnosis of Bartonella (or BLO as we discussed in chapter 2) is a clinical diagnosis, in that it is based on a patient's symptoms, the doctor's examination, and the elimination of other possible diagnoses.

There is one test that may be useful in screening patients suspected of being infected with Bartonella. This test may also be particularly useful in the follow-up of patients with Bartonella/BLO. This blood test is called "vascular endothelial growth factor" (VEGF). This test measures a substance that is produced by the Bartonella microbe in order to facilitate its entry into the body tissues it likes to inhabit. Elevated levels of VEGF often (but not exclusively) mean that a patient is infected with Bartonella. By monitoring VEGF levels during the course of treatment, physicians can monitor the progress of treatment (antibiotics). When VEGF levels return to normal, it generally means that the antibiotics have been successful and can be discontinued. The VEGF test is available from standard commercial laboratories.

Ehrlichia and Anaplasma: These organisms are in the family of bacteria known as *Rickettsia*. Remember, as I discussed in chapter 2, the diagnosis and treatment of these microorganisms should be prompt and based on clinical grounds. Treatment should not be based on test results alone, which results may be negative early in the course of the infections. As far as lab reliability, standard commercial lab tests generally do a good job of detecting antibodies (IgM and IgG) for both human monocytic ehrlichiosis (HME) and human granulocytic anaplasmosis (HGA), formerly known as human granulocytic ehrlichiosis. In some cases, however, blood smears or the PCR test may be considered, as well.

Rocky Mountain Spotted Fever (RMSF): This infection is caused by another organism in the family of bacteria known as *Rickettsia*. In general, it is believed that RMSF only rarely, if ever, becomes a chronic infection. Therefore, unless there is a clinical history that strongly suggests RMSF, most Lyme-aware doctors do not screen for RMSF. However, if it were going to be tested, standard commercial laboratories do an adequate job in detecting RMSF. Remember, as with HME and HGA, treatment must begin with suspicion of the infection and not upon confirmation with antibody testing.

Mycoplasma: Most people have been exposed to a small "atypical" bacterium called Mycoplasma. Interestingly, many of the symptoms of chronic Mycoplasma are similar to Lyme symptoms. From the standpoint of testing, serology for Mycoplasma has only limited usefulness; however, PCR is useful to detect active cases of Mycoplasma.

Acute and Chronic Virus Infections: Often patients who are chronically ill and who test negative for Lyme and other co-infections are suffering from chronic viral infection. There are well-documented times when viral infections have been known to cause "false positive" Lyme antibody tests. For this reason, I recommend that chronic viruses be considered as possible offenders when one is undergoing evaluation for tick-borne illnesses. There are several common culprits that may require testing, including the following:

* West Nile virus

* Cytomegalovirus (CMV)

* Epstein-Barr virus (EBV)

* Herpes zoster virus (HZV)

* Herpes simplex 1 (HSV-1)

* Herpes simplex 2 (HSV-2)

* Human herpes virus 6 (HHV6)

* Parvovirus B19

* Colorado tick fever

* Powassan encephalitis

* Eastern equine encephalitis (EEE) and Western equine encephalitis (WEE)—these should be suspected in cases where meningitis is suspected.

* HIV

* Hepatitis viruses—B and C

Other Recommended Tests
(In Addition to Tick-Borne Infection Testing)

As I mentioned earlier in this chapter, it is important to be tested for a variety of medical conditions in addition to tests for the infectious organisms. Additionally, it is important that a thorough dental examination be accomplished on patients suspected of having chronic Lyme or other tick-borne illnesses. In this section I will discuss some of the key tests that need to be completed as part of a thorough evaluation for Lyme disease and the co-infections. I will divide these tests into two parts: (1) essential tests that are highly recommended and (2) very useful tests that are optional but potentially helpful.

(1) Essential Tests (highly recommended):

* Complete blood count (CBC). This test examines the blood cells—red cells, white cells, and others. All the tick-borne organisms can affect the CBC. For example, Ehrlichia commonly causes a low white blood count. This test needs to be followed regularly if a patient is on antibiotics, because medications can affect the CBC (and may need to be changed if the CBC is significantly altered by a medication).

* Comprehensive metabolic chemistry profile. This test examines key chemical components of the blood, including minerals, proteins, liver function, kidney function, and others. Several of the tick-borne organisms may have an adverse effect on vital organs, and these effects may be detected on this test. The classic example is Ehrlichia and Anaplasma, which commonly cause an elevation of the liver enzymes. As with the CBC, this test needs to be followed regularly (at least monthly) while the patient is on any antibiotics for any length of time.

* Electrocardiogram. The standard EKG needs to be done at some point in the evaluation of Lyme, even if heart symptoms are not present. If you are on certain antibiotics (like the macrolide and ketolide groups that include Ketek, Biaxin, and Zithromax), an EKG is very important.

* Urinalysis. The basic urine test is important to obtain as a baseline.

* Syphilis test. This test should be done in the evaluation of any infectious disorder, because syphilis (a cousin of Lyme) can look like so many different medical disorders.

* C-Reactive protein (CRP). Inflammation is an important problem with tick-borne infections. This test is a useful determination of inflammation in the body. This test can be followed during the course of therapy.

* Sedimentation rate (sed rate). This test, like the CRP, may be very useful to follow if the value is elevated at the onset of treatment. It also measures inflammation in the body.

* Anti-nuclear antibody (ANA). This test screens for certain autoimmune disorders such as systemic lupus erythematosis ("lupus"). Often autoimmune disorders can be triggered by Lyme or the co-infections.

* Rheumatoid factor (RA factor). This test screens for other types of autoimmune disorders such as rheumatoid arthritis.

* Vitamin B12 level. Low levels of B12 can be a very serious problem in Lyme patients. Supplementation with B12 can be very useful in Lyme. (This is discussed in chapter 6.)

* Vitamin D (25-hydroxy vitamin D or 25-OH vitamin D). There is growing evidence that vitamin D plays a major role in the autoimmune disorders. Many of my Lyme patients have abnormally low levels of this criti-

cal substance. Therefore, measurement of 25-hydroxy vitamin D level can be very useful. The use of sunlight and vitamin D supplementation can be very helpful in Lyme disease. Some advocates recommend testing of blood levels of 1,25-dihydroxy vitamin D in addition, but I do not recommend this because the reliability of 1,25-dihydroxy vitamin D is highly questionable. (Vitamin D and the immune system are discussed in chapters 4 and 6.)

* Magnesium level. The usual serum magnesium level is of little value because the vast majority of magnesium is inside of cells. Better tests would be red blood cell magnesium or ionized magnesium and these are the ones you should request. (These tests are also discussed in chapter 6.)

(2) Useful but Not Essential Tests:

* VEGF. This test was discussed earlier in this chapter in relation to Bartonella testing.

* CD 57. This test is being used by an increasing number of Lyme-aware doctors. It is a measurement of a certain type of white blood cell called a natural killer cell. It may prove to be useful in evaluating a person on antibiotics to help a doctor know when the patient has completed Lyme antibiotic therapy. (This test is discussed in chapter 4 in greater detail.)

* TSH, free T4, and free T3. Hormonal abnormalities are common in the setting of the tick-borne infections. Thyroid abnormalities are among the most common hormonal problems encountered.

* Adrenal function tests. Another of the hormonal organs that often require evaluation are the adrenal glands. When the function of the adrenal glands is totally deficient, it is a medical condition called adrenal insufficiency or Addison's disease. Addison's is a very serious medical disorder that may be fatal if untreated. However, short of Addison's disease, many Lyme patients experience overstress and fatigue of their adrenal glands due to chronic illness, lack of sleep, and stress. There are several ways to evaluate adrenal function. Perhaps the best and most commonly used test is 24-hour urine testing. However, because of expense and convenience, I use a different screening method called salivary hormone testing. Studies have shown that salivary levels correlate with free hormone blood levels. (See references section, articles by Vining and by Lac.) Therefore, if I suspect adrenal problems, I order the saliva test called an adrenal stress profile by either Genova Labs or Metametrix. (See the resources section for lab details.) In lieu of that test, an "8 A.M. morning cortisol" and a DHEA-sulfate level can be done as a screen. (In chapter 7, I will discuss adrenal and other hormonal issues in much greater detail.)

* Insulin (fasting). A fasting insulin test looks at the function of the pancreas and also how well the body is handling sugar in the blood. (More details will be discussed in a later chapter.)

* Other hormones. Depending on the clinical situation, it is often very useful to look at levels of progesterone, pregnenolone, estrogens, testosterone, and melatonin.

* Angiotensin converting enzyme. This test is useful for detecting and for monitoring a disorder called sarcoidosis. If sarcoidosis is found to be present, it is advisable not to supplement vitamin D even if blood levels are low.

* Cardiolipin antibodies (IgM and IgG). This test is useful if a history of abnormal blood clotting is present or if the platelet count is low. It is abnormal in autoimmune disorders.

* Toxic mineral analysis. Certain heavy metals, such as mercury, arsenic, cadmium, and lead, may have a major impact on the course of Lyme infection. Levels can be tested by blood or urine. (More information will be presented about this later in this book.)

* Sleep study. This test may be very valuable to evaluate the role of a sleep disorder in symptoms of Lyme. Some patients with chronic fatigue and fibromyalgia actually have a treatable sleep disorder like sleep apnea.

* Celiac profile. Screening for an intestinal condition called celiac disease is very useful. It should be done frequently, especially when abdominal symptoms are a prominent part of the Lyme picture.

* Food allergy testing. In certain patients it is useful to do laboratory testing for food allergies. ELISA testing may be a useful technique.

* HLA genetic testing. Certain genetic types (HLA DR2, DR4, and B27) may have a more severe clinical course during Lyme infection. Some experts believe that genetic patterns (HLA, DRB, and DQB) are associated with reduced ability to rid the body of Lyme toxins and may help predict who might benefit from medicine to help the body detoxify itself from Lyme toxins.

* Urine porphyrins. This test is useful to diagnose a group of conditions (genetic and acquired) called "porphyrias," which are caused by the accumulation of precursor substances for the manufacture of heme. Heme is essential for the function of many proteins in the body related to oxygen transport, toxin removal, and energy production. Porphyria symptoms may include neurological, psychiatric, skin, gastrointestinal, and other body organ dysfunction symptoms. Toxic minerals such as mercury may play an important role in this disorder. Metametrix performs an excellent test for the evaluation of the porphyrias.

* Inflammatory markers. Although mainly used for research and investigational purposes, the balance of Th1 and Th2 can be tested, and this evaluation may at times be clinically useful. Other useful immune system tests may include C3a, C4a, MMP9, TNF-alpha, IL2, IL6, and IL10. Testing for important "T cell regulators" will have an increasingly important place in our evaluation for these tick-borne disorders, especially when chronic inflammation becomes a major issue. (This is discussed further in chapter 4.)

Summing Up

Let's review the key points of this chapter by answering some of the most common questions people have about diagnosing Lyme disease.

Why do you recommend that patients work with doctors who are Lyme-aware (LAMP) or Lyme-literate when it comes to diagnosing Lyme disease?

The reason for this recommendation is simple—not all physicians are versed in recognizing the wide variety of symptoms and presentations of Lyme disease. Additionally, many physicians continue to use the CDC two-tiered diagnostic approach that is often unreliable for screening for Lyme in people for whom the infection has a high likelihood.

This recommendation does not mean that physicians who are not Lyme-aware physicians are not excellent and highly responsible medical practitioners. It simply means they do not specialize in Lyme disease and related illnesses. Because of this, working with a Lyme-aware doctor makes good sense. This is similar to a person's need to seek out a specialist in another medical field in order to diagnose and treat other diseases. Another important point about Lyme-aware doctors is that some of them have had Lyme disease themselves. Therefore, they are familiar with the special needs and considerations Lyme patients may have.

If ELISA or IFA tests are so inaccurate for detecting Lyme disease, why are they still so commonly used?

As I discussed above, the original purpose behind the CDC's recommendation for these tests was for public health surveillance, not for diagnostic purposes. In fact, the CDC has always maintained that Lyme is a clinical diagnosis. Unfortunately, soon after the CDC recommended its two-tiered surveillance approach, its recommendations became the standard form of testing for Lyme disease. It was inappropriately adopted by some physicians and health researchers, as well as most insurance companies, as the sole basis for making a diagnosis of Lyme disease.

What about routine lab testing and testing for co-infections?

In addition to tick-borne infection testing, patients need to have a variety of other testing performed. This testing is necessary in order to rule out other conditions that might be causing the symptoms. Co-infections are quite common among patients with Lyme disease. For this reason, I recommend that virtually all Lyme patients suffering from chronic symptoms be tested for co-infections also.

I hope this chapter helps you realize why a clinical diagnosis remains the best approach for determining whether or not a patient has Lyme disease in view of the challenges presented by all the various factors discussed above. Also, given the high degree of inaccuracy of the most commonly used diagnostic tests for Lyme and the other TBDs, I hope you understand why working with a Lyme-aware physician is so essential. Now that you understand the key elements that are involved in diagnosing Lyme disease, it's time to turn our attention to how to most effectively treat it. The answers to this question are covered in depth in parts 2 and 3, beginning with the next chapter, which takes a more comprehensive look at the importance of your body's immune system in terms of Lyme and your overall health.

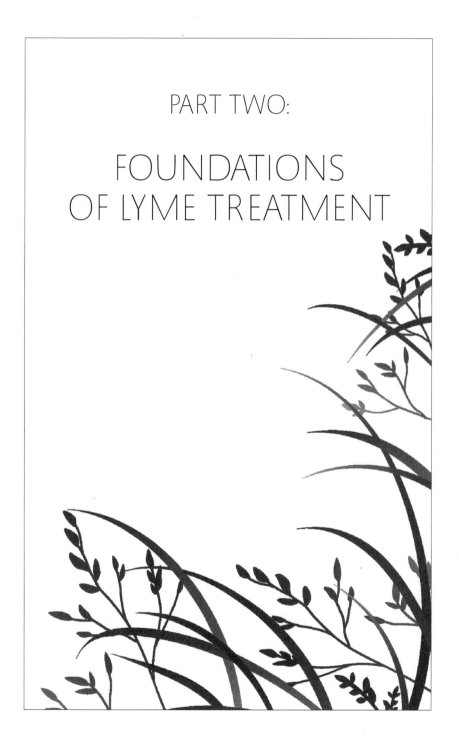

PART TWO:

FOUNDATIONS OF LYME TREATMENT

.

Chapter Four

Lyme Disease and Your Immune System

＊

Beginning with this chapter, I want to present an exciting, practical approach to your healing and recovery from the ravages of Lyme disease and other tick-borne illnesses. There is much that you can do to help yourself get well again. My goal is to help reintroduce hope into your life and to provide you with self-help tools that will allow you to be a full participant in your health recovery.

Upon completion of this book, I want you to feel confident that you are the captain of your health care team. And, as captain, you are empowered to choose your pathway and your team members who will assist you on your journey back to health and wholeness of body, mind, and spirit.

In chapter 1, I told you that "Knowledge is power." Now I would like to add this thought: "The power that comes from knowledge only works when you wisely apply that knowledge to solve problems." In this chapter and throughout the remainder of this book, I will focus on the specific how-to information you can use to recover your health if you are willing to diligently apply this knowledge to your situation. This knowledge begins with an understanding of how your body works to keep you healthy and of the important role your immune system plays in that process.

A Balance of Opposites

Your body is constantly seeking to maintain a delicate balance between opposites. This regulation of opposites is known as *homeostasis*, a term first coined in 1932 by William Cannon, M.D., Ph.D., in his book *The Wisdom of the Body*. Homeostasis is essential for good health and involves the regulation and delicate balancing of many bodily systems and functions, including body temperature, the endocrine (hormone) system, the body's acid-alkaline balance (pH), and the levels of various chemicals in the bloodstream. Prolonged imbalances in any of these areas creates stress that causes the immune system to become compromised.

The body's inherent wisdom allows it to know when it needs to "fight" and when it needs to "retreat." Your body knows when it needs to be active or restful. To better understand this "dance of cooperating opposites," consider the tides of the ocean. Low tide is when the water has receded from the beach, and high tide is when it has risen to cover a larger part of the beach. Let me say at this point that the metaphor breaks down a bit because in most parts of the world there are two low tides and two high tides per day, and the times of day of tides will vary. But for the sake of the analogy, I want to take "literary license" and assume that there is only one morning low tide and only one evening high tide, and these tides occur at the same time every day.

During a daytime low period, the tide is down and everything is alive and active. The beach is teeming with birds and people. Sandcastles are being built. Vendors are selling trinkets. Surfers try to catch the perfect wave. Athletes engage in games of soccer and volleyball. By the end of the day, the sand is torn up and totally disordered from the daytime activities. Then comes the nighttime high period, and the high tide arrives. Everything becomes quiet and is at rest. Birds are not hunting. The sandcastles are washed away as the sand is smoothed out. By morning the quieting repair work of the high tide is completed, the low tide returns, and the beach becomes alive again. This ebb and flow of activity and restful repair is also what occurs in our bodies throughout the course of the day. The following table illustrates a few of these opposites to which I am referring:

Daytime Low Tide	Nighttime High Tide
Sunshine	Moonlight
Summer	Winter
Fire	Water
Work (humans and many animals)	Rest (humans and many animals)
Stimulation	Relaxation
Fight, Flight	Sleep, Safety
Yang	Yin
Sympathetic Nervous System	Parasympathetic Nervous System
Immune Activation	Immune Suppression
Oxidation	Reduction (anti-oxidation)
Thyroid	Adrenals
Estrogen	Progesterone

The key thing to remember here is that your body has been designed by our Creator to maintain a delicate balance and regulation of these opposing forces. When the regulatory mechanisms of the body are working well, we have health. When they are in a state of "dysregulation," the result is disease. Therefore, one of your primary self-care goals in treating and recovering from Lyme disease is doing all you can to re-establish your normal God-given capacity to self-regulate. Achieving this goal begins with your immune system which, when attacked, can be likened to the following analogy.

The Castle Under Seige

There once was a king who lived in a large castle seated in a lush valley. Surrounded by rival kingdoms, the king realized his vulnerability to attack and so provided the best security that money could buy. He had a deep moat which encircled the property, stocked with crocodiles. The windows were fortified with iron bars. Nothing was spared in securing his fortress.

One night, however, an enemy quietly laid a long plank across the moat and its army got onto the property. Moving stealthily, the invading army then managed to get inside the castle undetected. The night watchman, however, while routinely patrolling, came across one of the invaders. The protocol was very clear—when you come across the enemy you must send out several signals.

The first signal was to wake up the artillery team, the second was to let the firefighters know that there was probably going to be lots of fire (so get the water ready), and the third was to give certain of the fighters detailed information about the enemy, so that they could prepare very specific strategies for their attack. As these signals were sent, other night watchmen joined the first one and began to engage the enemy with powerful weapons of their own. Others magically cloned themselves in an attempt to outnumber the enemy.

Very soon, the night watchmen were joined by a team of knights who had amazing swords that could instantly kill the enemy with one blow. As this first team of knights did their job, another team of knights covered each of the remaining enemy soldiers with a substance that clearly identified their where-abouts. As a result of this tagging procedure, a team of archers could send flaming arrows into the enemy soldiers identified by these markings. And, because the firefighters had been called, when a fire accidentally got out of hand, the fire could be con-tained with water before it destroyed any of the castle.

By morning the chief of knights could see that the enemy was contained enough to allow his troops some rest and nour-ishment for a short period of time. Regularly scheduled breaks allowed his soldiers to regroup, rearm, and recoup their strength. In a very short time, the battle was over and the enemy was suc-cessfully repelled, with minimal damage to the castle.

This oversimplified illustration shows how the body repels invaders. There is always vigorous attack, followed by controlled rest, during which time cleanup and repair and fire control are accomplished. With this descriptive tale in mind, let's turn our attention to the immune system itself.

Immune System Basics

When dangerous foreign materials or infections attempt to invade your body, many excellent built-in external and inter-nal defenses go to work to defend you against them. The most important and effective of the external defenses is actually the largest organ of the body—the skin. If this skin barrier defense has been breached by a tick bite, it then becomes the job of the internal defense mechanisms to step forward and prevent damage and infection from occurring in your body. This internal defense system is called the immune system.

Your immune system is a very finely balanced combination of white blood cells, proteins, hormones, messenger molecules, and many other components that are designed to rapidly spring into action to do three things: (1) recognize a threat, (2) aggressively respond to that threat, and (3) back off for cleanup and repair when the threat is contained. The immune system can be divided into two branches—the *innate* system and the *adaptive* system. It is important that you understand the difference between these two branches.

The Innate System

This is the first line of immune system defense for your body. The innate system is a primitive, yet very vital, aspect of the immune system. Its role is to be constantly on guard for trouble in the form of infections, tumors, and any other foreign invader that the innate system considers "not self." The job of the innate system is to be the first-responder to the scene of trouble. That response is nonspecific in that it attempts to eliminate anything it considers to be foreign to the body. When this system encounters trouble, it normally has a great capacity to deal with the trouble immediately and powerfully by using a number of different mechanisms. It may do this through white blood cells that can kill an invader, the production of proteins that are able to neutralize it, and by many other methods.

However, because the problem may be potentially over-whelming (and life-threatening), the innate system immediately begins to send out signals and messages that attract other helpers into the vicinity to help with the crisis. The result of the innate system's encounter with the presence of a foreign infectious agent or other abnormality (like a cancer cell) is to begin a process that is called "inflammation." The job of inflammation is to contain and destroy the invading enemy.

As I mentioned, your body is constantly seeking balance. In keeping with the example of the tides, the innate system realizes that balance is necessary. Too much inflammation can be destructive. Therefore, while inflammation is ongoing, the innate system sends out messages to other parts of the body to prevent excess destruction from the ongoing inflammatory process. By bringing in such anti-inflammation assistance, the destructive process will not be allowed to get out of control and thereby cause unnecessary damage to body tissues (and possibly death).

The Adaptive System

The signals that are sent out by the innate system bring in a vast array of helpers that enhance the ability of the immune system to become much more specific in its fight against the enemy. This new, and even more powerful, specific approach that is added onto the innate system is called the adaptive system. It is a tailor-made program for the problem at hand.

With the addition of this new participant (adaptive system) in the attack, the immune system can deal so specifically with the enemy invasion that it will normally be able to resolve the attack quickly, effectively, and with minimal long-term damage. Additionally, the adaptive immune system will have a memory of the invasion so that if a repeat attack occurs, it can spring into action even more quickly and decisively like experienced "knights" (using our castle analogy). However, when infectious-invading microorganisms (such as the *Bb* bacteria) can resist the defensive measures of the immune system, immunity becomes impaired, setting the stage for disease to occur. This is why improving your body's immune response is so essential to effectively dealing with Lyme disease and other tick-borne illnesses.

Now let's take a closer look at how your immune system works by introducing you to the key immune agents involved in your body's immune response to Lyme and related diseases.

Key Players of the Innate System (Nonspecific Immunity)

The Macrophage. The macrophage is a type of white blood cell whose function is similar to that of a member of a scouting party. The macrophage's job is to roam or "scout" around the body looking for trouble, such as foreign invaders like Lyme spirochetes. Some macrophages are stationed in specific organs (such as Kuppfer cells in the liver). Others, called "monocytes" in your white blood cell blood test, roam around freely in the blood, from which they can go into body tissue when needed. If the macrophage encounters an invader while making its rounds, its duty is to sound the alarm, send out distress messages, and begin the battle while help is on the way.

The Natural Killer Cell. The natural killer cell, also known as the "NK" cell, is a critical member of the innate system team because it is able to independently seek out infected cells and, in many cases, cause instant destruction of foreign invaders. That is to say, the NK cells do not require recognition of a specific foreign antigen in order to attack and kill the enemy. The NK cells are said to be "cytotoxic," meaning that they kill cells. In fact, they can instantly kill any cell containing a foreign invader or a tumor cell.

The NK cells fall into the category of white blood cells called "lymphocytes" on your white blood cell lab test. Lyme probably cannot be adequately controlled by the body unless the NK cells are performing their function adequately. Many Lyme-aware physicians believe that the blood level of a specific NK cell called the CD57 cell is an excellent predictor of when a person can come off of antibiotics. When the CD57 is high, then the NK cells (and the rest of the immune system) can handle Lyme without further need for antibiotics. When the CD57 is low, then the immune system is not strong enough to handle Lyme without the help of antibiotics. We will have much more to say about the NK cell later in this chapter.

The Cytokines. Cytokines are chemicals that are secreted by various cells of the immune system. Both innate and adaptive cells can produce these substances. One of the first things that macrophages do is to secrete several types of cytokines to attract help from other members of the immune system. Therefore, cytokines act as messenger molecules (like telegrams) that help direct various components of the immune system. They also serve other functions, including helping white blood cells to grow and mature, all aimed at mounting the necessary attack to repel the enemy.

When it comes to Lyme disease, there are two vital opposite functions of cytokines: pro-inflammatory cytokines and anti-inflammatory cytokines. By definition, the pro-inflammatory cytokines increase inflammation in the area of infection in order to help the immune cells get rid of the infectious organism. The anti-inflammatory cytokines reduce the inflammation in order to reduce collateral damage to self. From start to finish of an infection, the body is constantly secreting both of these types of cytokines in a very delicate balance in order to eradicate the invader with minimal harm to the body.

Going back to our tidal example, when the pro-inflammatory cytokines are dominant, the body is at daytime low tide (which is "seek and destroy" time). When the anti-inflammatory cytokines are dominant, the body is at nighttime high tide (which is "repair and replenish" time). Some of the major components of this cytokine group include:

Pro-inflammatory cytokines	Anti-inflammatory cytokines
Interleukin one (IL-1)	Interleukin ten (IL-10)
Interleukin two (IL-2)	Interleukin four (IL-4)
Interleukin twelve (IL-12)	
Gamma interferon (IFN-g)	
Tumor necrosis factor (TNF)	

Adaptive System Key Players (Specific Immunity)

T Lymphocytes. Shortly after the battle begins, under the direction of the macrophages (and their cytokines), certain other white blood cells in the lymphocyte family are stimulated to form specific T lymphocytes. The process is somewhat complex.

As I stated, the job of the innate system's scout, the macrophage, is to gather information. Armed with that information, the macrophage wants to facilitate the active involvement of the more powerful adaptive system. The way the process occurs is that the macrophage first ingests and then digests some of the foreign invaders. It then is able to convey (or present) the specific information about that enemy to a T lymphocyte cell. The T lymphocyte that this information is presented to can then mature (or differentiate) in one of two directions, becoming either "helper" T cells (also called CD4 cells) or "suppressor" and "cytotoxic" T cells (also called CD8 cells).

In the discussion of Lyme disease, we are primarily interested in the helper T cells, also known as the CD4 cells. The helper T cells (CD4) can further divide into one of the following three kinds of CD4 cells:

* Th1 cells (which stands for "T helper one" cells), which secrete the pro-inflammatory cytokines mentioned above and are very effective at killing invading germs (even those inside of cells), but may cause potentially damaging excessive inflammation

* Th2 cells (which stands for "T helper two" cells), which secrete the anti-inflammatory cytokines mentioned above and also direct the cells that produce antibodies to begin their antibody production

* Treg cells (which stands for "T regulator" cells), which "regulate" the balance between Th1 pro-inflammation and Th2 anti-inflammation

All three CD4 components are critical to the successful control of Lyme disease. At the onset of Lyme infection, the Th1 response is vital to controlling Lyme. But the Th2 response is important to "cool off" the Th1 and to produce antibodies for help to control Lyme. Finally, the Treg response is absolutely necessary to keep the system balanced. That is to say, the Th1 system tends to suppress the Th2 system and vice versa—a process similar to a see-saw. The Treg system keeps things in balance.

Here are some examples of how problems can occur when the T cell system does not work properly.

Example one: When Lyme invades the body, it wants to avoid the Th1 response, because that is the most deadly immune system attack on it. Therefore, Lyme actually induces the body to make IL-10 (an anti-inflammatory cytokine) for the purpose of suppressing the Th1 response. If the body's Th1 system is not strong enough to overcome the premature Th2 (IL-10) suppressive action, then Lyme can penetrate deeper into the body tissues. Therefore, a Lyme-weakened Th1 (from excess IL-10) response will allow Lyme to successfully invade the body.

Example two: As previously stated, Lyme causes excess IL-10 production. But there are situations in which the body may already be in a state of overproduction of IL-10. This pre-existing excess IL-10 condition is called "Th2 dominance." Th2 dominance is a setup for a poor outcome from Lyme. Conditions such as chronic fatigue syndrome, chronic viral infections (like Epstein-Barr virus), mercury overload, parasitic infections, and chronic allergies all lead to the Th2 dominant state. In that state, the Th1 is suppressed not only by Lyme but also by the other situations that we just mentioned. Once again, the Th1 is limited in what it can do and Lyme is able to establish itself in the body.

Example three: In either of the above examples, if Lyme has successfully invaded, the Th1 system continues to try to attack

Lyme but unsuccessfully. In this circumstance, there are four possible reasons. The first reason for this lack of success could be due to Th1 weakness/exhaustion (for example, if nutritional deficiencies are present). The second is that it could be due to ongoing suppression of Th1 by Th2. The third possibility is that a person has ongoing co-infections such as Babesia or Bartonella. Finally, it could be due to Treg's lack of regulation of the process. I believe that the unfortunate result is that the weakened and inadequate Th1 system loses its ability to distinguish infected tissue from "self tissue." This leads to what we call "autoimmunity" and chronic inflammation (which I will discuss in the next chapter). This is very frequently the picture of a typical Lyme patient when coming into a Lyme-aware doctor's office—a long history of inadequately treated, active, or persistent Lyme with accompanying autoimmune manifestations.

The Antibodies. Most of the time when we think about Lyme and the immune system, we have the tendency to think about antibodies. This is because the blood tests that are done to detect Lyme most often involve measuring levels of antibodies directed against Lyme. The antibodies measured by Lyme testing involve two classes of antibodies—(1) the IgM antibody, which is large in size (limiting its tissue accessibility), potent in enhancing the immune response, and produced in the first two to three weeks of Lyme infection and (2) the IgG antibody, which is smaller (and more accessible to tissue), more specific to the infecting antigen, and comes later when the body is nearer recovery.

By definition, antibodies (also called immunoglobulins) are proteins produced by cells in the body called "B cells." The goal of an antibody is to seek out and then attach itself to an invader like the Lyme spirochete. After antibody attachment, the other immune components then spot the tagged invader and come in to finish the job by destroying the germ. Most of the antibodies are produced in the adaptive immune system under the direction of the Th2 system and are very specific for a particular germ's body parts (called "antigens").

As an interesting sidebar, in addition to the Th2-directed antibody production in the adaptive system, there are also "natural IgM antibodies" produced by the innate system. The cells that produce these nonspecific antibodies are innate system cells called "B-1 cells." It may be that these nonspecific antibodies are very important in the initial control of Lyme, even while the spirochete is still inside the tick. Some Lyme experts believe that high levels of these natural IgM antibodies may be the reason some people do not contract clinical Lyme when exposed to it by a tick bite. When the innate system is working well, with macrophages, NK cells, and the B-1 cells all able to do their job effectively, the body has an excellent chance of winning the war it faces, from infections to cancer. When both the innate and the adaptive systems are functioning efficiently, the body has an advantage over any potentially lethal foreign invader.

Additional Key Players

In addition to the immune system itself, healthy immune function is supported by other components in the body. Two particularly key players in this regard are the adrenal glands and chemical messengers known as endorphins.

The Adrenal Glands. The adrenal glands play a key role in the balance of the immune system because of their production of cortisol. Cortisol is a hormone that helps to "cool down" the immune system after it has accomplished its tasks in defending against harmful, invading microorganisms. This cool-down occurs in the following way.

One of the cytokines secreted by macrophages is known as IL-1B. Among its many functions, IL-1B sends messages to the brain's hypothalamus, instructing it to release corticotropin-releasing hormone (CRH). CRH then stimulates the pituitary gland to produce adrenocorticotropic hormone (ACTH). ACTH, in turn, instructs the adrenal glands to secrete cortisol to help regulate the inflammatory response that the macrophages are involved in. If we did not have this mechanism in place, we could die of overwhelming inflammation when we contracted an infection.

However, there are two potential problems with regard to cortisol production. The first problem is that, due to stress, the adrenal glands go into overdrive, overproducing cortisol. This condition is called "adrenal stress." This scenario can result in excessive immune system suppression due to too much cortisol being produced. This resulting suppression can help Lyme bacteria to escape detection by the immune system, thereby helping the bacteria to survive.

The second problem occurs due to chronic stress, which can cause the adrenal glands to become overworked and exhausted. This condition is called "adrenal fatigue." This scenario can result in inadequate cortisol production which, in turn, can lead to damage to healthy tissues due to uncontrolled inflammation. In this case, it may require taking *physiologic* doses of cortisol by mouth to help the adrenals until they can recover.

For both of these reasons, it is important that adrenal function be assessed in most patients with chronic Lyme disease. When adrenal function is impaired, adrenal support may be necessary. This support can be achieved using certain herbal remedies, as well as other natural supplements. The key items that are clinically useful include vitamin C, vitamin B5 (pantothenic acid), magnesium, eleutherococcus (Siberian ginseng), schisandra seed, rhodiola, green tea, grape seed and skin, licorice, and others. Again, when documented by laboratory testing, it may also be necessary to use temporary low dose oral natural cortisol (using adrenal replacement doses, *not* immunosuppressive doses) until the exhausted adrenal glands can recover enough to do their own job. Another key component of adrenal support is adequate uninterrupted sleep. (I recommend ideally seven to nine hours per night with at least five of those hours uninterrupted.) I will discuss adrenal and other endocrine gland issues in more detail in chapter 7 and the major problem of sleep deficiency in chapter 8.

The Endorphins. As with the adrenal glands, endorphins also play an important role in maintaining healthy immune function and are critical to the control of Lyme disease. Endorphins are natural opiate-like substances produced by the body to help control pain. They are produced in the body during nighttime, with peak production occurring between 2 and 4 A.M. During waking hours, they are used by the body in various bodily systems including the nervous system, endocrine system, and immune system.

In addition to their pain-relief properties, endorphins also have very powerful immune system effects. For instance, the natural killer (NK) cells have endorphin receptors on their surfaces. When endorphins are present, the NK cells increase in number and in function by as much as 300 percent. Exercise is known to enhance NK function. The NK immune enhancement that derives from exercise is totally mediated by the effect exercise has on increasing endorphins. In fact, studies have shown that the administration of an endorphin receptor antagonist (which blocks the effects of endorphins on the NK cell) to a person exercising totally eliminates any immune system NK enhancement induced by exercise. In addition to exercise, endorphins may be increased also by massage and touch therapy, acupuncture, laughter, core body temperature elevation, and dark chocolate (without sugar please).

It is my belief that many patients with chronic Lyme disease are "endorphin-dysregulated" (that is, the production of endorphins has become chaotic and unregulated). For this reason, Lyme patients are, therefore, more susceptible to Lyme-related autoimmune disorders. Because this is so, restoring healthy endorphin production is essential when treating Lyme disease. In chapter 7, I will discuss a novel treatment for endorphin-dysregulation that has dramatically helped many of my Lyme patients.

Strategies for Immune System Enhancement and Regulation

As previously mentioned, when the body is under attack, it goes into defensive mode by mobilizing various immune agents against the enemy. The body truly believes that the best defense is a good offense. During the time of "taking the fight to the enemy," three things are happening: the *pro-inflammatory* system is turned on maximally, the *pro-oxidant* system is also turned on maximally (peroxides and other oxidants that are highly toxic to invading germs), and *pro-coagulant* systems are turned on (allowing the body to manage the blood vessels in the area of the attack). And, as I said, there are regulatory mechanisms in place that prevent over-inflammation, over-oxidation, and over-coagulation.

When we are healthy and following a lifestyle that supports health, then the battle is usually short-lived and the body wins the war. However, the combination of chronic infection (as with Lyme and co-infections), chronic stress, and unhealthy lifestyle presents a major dilemma to the body. In such a setting, homeostasis is next to impossible without help and without important lifestyle changes.

This help may come in the form of antibiotics to lower the numbers of invaders. It should also include lifestyle changes, including dietary nutritional changes, as well as psychological, emotional, and spiritual changes that may need to be considered. (For more on this subject, see chapter 9.) Depending on the severity of the health challenges caused by Lyme disease, the lifestyle changes may sometimes need to be drastic.

The targeted use of nutritional and herbal supplements, in particular, is often extremely helpful in assisting the body in its effort to get the "upper hand" on Lyme disease. I will discuss these nutrients in more detail in chapter 6. Additionally, because the field of nutritionally oriented medicine changes rapidly, I also refer you to my Web site (www.lymedoctor.com) for up-to-date details about therapies that I am currently recommending in my practice.

Let's examine Lyme disease and the immune system from

three standpoints: (1) lyme prevention, (2) early stage lyme disease, and (3) late stage lyme disease.

Lyme Prevention
(To help avoid active Lyme)

In the prevention of Lyme disease, it is critical that the innate immune system be strong and fully functional. The key innate system components that require support are the *macrophages*, *NK cells*, and the *cytokines* (*IL-2 and IFN-g*). When the macrophages and NK cells are active and healthy, and when the body is making adequate amounts of the cytokines IL-2 and IFN-g, the body has an excellent chance of handling Lyme effectively. Let's discuss natural approaches that help support the essential innate immune system.

(1) Macrophages

Macrophages are the true workhorses of the innate immune system. They seek out the enemies of the body, signal other immune components to join in the process of attack, and even begin the process of destroying the enemy invaders by the use of a substance inside of them called nitric oxide. IL-12, IL-10, IFN-g, and TNF-a all assist the macrophages in their quest to jump-start the immune defense process. The following natural substances have been useful in the support of macrophages:

* Beta 1,3 glucan 10–250 mg per day (depending on brand)

* Aloe vera (The active ingredient is acemannan.)

Beta glucan is a natural product that comes from several dietary sources. My favorite supplement source is from the cell wall of certain types of yeast (Saccharomyces cerevisiae). However, there are many good products on the market, some of which are from other sources, such as oats. It is the "insoluble" form that has been shown to work most effectively for our immune systems.

When taken into our body, beta glucan is primarily ingested by the macrophages of our immune system. It will help to do two things once inside the macrophage. It will help it do its germ-killing job more effectively, and it will adjust the activity of the immune system so as not to cause excessive inflammation. In its germ-killing role, the macrophage needs to be able to produce several chemicals, including nitric oxide and several of the cytokine messengers that we discussed earlier in this chapter. Beta glucan helps the macrophage produce everything it needs to do this job. Additionally, beta glucan helps to reduce the chances of excessive inflammation, of autoimmunity, and of free radical damage to body tissues.

Acemannan is an active ingredient from the aloe vera plant. It has been shown to be useful for the activation of macrophages. It stimulates nitric oxide and TNF-a in macrophages, which improve their killing power. It can be taken in the form of high quality aloe vera liquid or, preferably (and more palatably), as a standardized oral product in capsule form.

(2) Natural Killer Cells (NK cells)

NK cells are perhaps the most lethal weapon in our innate system's arsenal against Lyme disease and related co-infections. NK cells are able to identify foreigners that are "not-self" and instantly destroy them on contact in defense of "self." The foreign invaders could be infectious in nature or malignant tumors. The NK cells in our bodies are absolutely critical to our survival upon exposure to any of these invaders. Because of this fact, we should be doing all that we can to support these immune system "warriors." As I mentioned above, many Lyme-aware doctors believe that the NK cell is the major key to a successful outcome with Lyme treatment. Because of this fact, we often measure the levels of one of those NK cells called the CD57 on a regular basis when we are treating chronic Lyme disease.

There have been many studies that have shed light on NK cells. As a result, we know much about both the helpful and the unhelpful factors related to these cells. Factors that have been found to be unhelpful (and actually harmful) to NK cells include exposure to environmental chemicals, such as pesticides and herbicides. Even general anesthesia may temporarily lower NK function, which explains why many people catch colds soon after a surgical procedure. Chronic viruses frequently cause problems with NK cells (such as Epstein-Barr virus and HIV virus). Chronic fatigue syndrome and various autoimmune disorders have also been associated with NK cell abnormalities.

The normal aging process and chronic stress also appear to have an adverse effect on NK cells. Excessive strenuous exercise of greater than one hour may have a temporary negative effect on NK cells. Nutritional deficiencies have clearly been shown to cause poor NK numbers and function, especially deficiencies of vitamin C, B12, B6, beta carotene, and zinc.

Finally, anything that depletes the cells' reserves of an important antioxidant called glutathione (GSH) may have an adverse effect on the killing power of the NK cell. The most notorious culprits for glutathione depletion are alcohol consumption and misuse of acetaminophen (the active ingredient in Tylenol). Acetaminophen should be used in low doses only and never on an empty stomach or with alcohol.

Another problem for the immune system is cigarette smoking. Smoking depletes the body of vitamin C. When cigarettes and alcohol are used together, the result is depletion in the body of both vitamin C and glutathione. This combination results in a severe compromise of two of the body's most critical antioxidants. This will often severely impair the NK cell function, which greatly reduces the immune system's ability to fight invaders.

Thankfully, there are many helpful factors for the NK cells

also. As you can imagine many of these positive factors are the opposite of the negative ones. The first, and arguably the most important, is exercise. Mild to moderate exercise is a critical positive factor for the NK cells. In my clinical experience, I have seen many patients in whom regular exercise played as important a role as did their antibiotics in the successful treatment of their disease. Earlier in this chapter, I discussed the fact that the immune enhancement that is derived from exercise comes from endorphins. As a brief review, in addition to exercise, other factors that favor endorphin-related NK cell improvement include laughter, acupuncture, massage (for example, Swedish massage weekly), and dark, organic sugar-free chocolate.

One's nutritional status is another key NK issue. The quality of the diet and the use of superior vitamin and mineral supplements are both important features to be considered. Proper nutrition and supplementation must include an excellent source of beta carotene. It turns out that beta carotene is one of the true champions of NK cell function. A study performed in 1996 among elderly men showed that beta carotene restored their NK function to normal levels. Other related supplements that may play a very useful role for NK cells include the major antioxidants, vitamins C and E. I mentioned the important role of glutathione above. Selenium, B-complex vitamins, N-acetyl cysteine (NAC), alpha lipoic acid, and glutamine all support the crucial manufacture of glutathione.

Finally, spicy foods play a wonderful supporting role for our NK cells. One of the best is the substance called curcumin. This is found in the spice curry, and I recommend that this spice be included in the diet regularly if possible. If you prefer, it may also be taken as a supplement. Curcumin not only enhances NK cells, but also supports macrophages without causing unwanted excess inflammation. In fact, curcumin works in the body as an anti-inflammatory nutrient. Garlic is another food that should be used very liberally in order to support the NK cells of the body. As with curcumin, garlic may be taken as a supplement also.

There are four natural products/activities that are of particular usefulness for supporting NK cells and therefore for the prevention of Lyme and the co-infections:

* Beta carotene (along with other vitamins and minerals)—10,000 IU per day

* Exercise

* Lifestyle—avoidance of cigarettes, alcohol, and acetaminophen when used improperly

* Foods—garlic and curry

Beta carotene is well known as an antioxidant nutrient. It is also a precursor of vitamin A in the body. Its effect on the NK cell appears to be, however, independent of its vitamin A activity. In my practice, my preference is to recommend beta carotene as part of an excellent multiple vitamin and mineral supplement. Incidentally, beta carotene always works best when combined with other antioxidants. Therefore, I would advise against taking beta carotene alone as a supplement without other antioxidants accompanying it. (In the next chapter, on Lyme nutrition, we will deal with nutritional sources of beta carotene, such as carrots and other orange and yellow foods.)

Exercise is another important key to a strong immune system. The patients that I have cared for who have had the best outcomes with Lyme disease are those who had a pre-existing regular exercise program. Leslie's case is a typical illustration of this point.

Leslie is a 42-year-old woman who ran competitively for many years. One year before seeing me, she had a tick bite and rash that was not typical of Lyme. She received two weeks of doxycycline and was told she was cured. This was not the case, however, and soon she became progressively worse with fatigue, brain fog, sleep problems, and joint pains.

After appropriate examination and testing, I made the diagnosis of Lyme and Bartonella. I informed Leslie that the normal treatment would usually last from three to six months. We started a comprehensive program including levafloxacin and doxycycline. She came back one month later, and to my utter surprise, she was completely well. At that time we discontinued the medications and a month later repeated the CD57. The CD57 count had increased significantly and she remained totally symptom-free. My last visit with her six months later demonstrated that she was still doing quite well. I am convinced that her healthy lifestyle, particularly the exercise component, placed her in a position to recover completely in a relatively short period of time with our treatment.

Therefore, my strong advice is that you get on a regular exercise program and stay on it. As with Leslie, those people who adopt a good activity program invariably do better than those who are not on a good program. It has been said that the best exercise program is that program which a person is willing to do. There are so many good exercise video resources and quality exercise equipment available today. However, the most common three forms of exercise today still remain: swimming, cycling, and running (or brisk walking). In chapter 6, I will discuss in much more detail the question of exercise programs for patients with Lyme disease.

Lifestyle is the final critical piece of the puzzle for proper NK function. Most of this is common sense, and I am sure you have heard it many times before. However, please understand that it is imperative that you make the lifestyle changes that I mentioned above concerning smoking and alcohol usage. You will have a much more difficult time avoiding Lyme and a much more difficult course of treatment if you do not live a healthy lifestyle. In chapter 5, I will deal extensively with nutrition and dietary lifestyle issues, including recommendations concerning how to make necessary changes. In chapter 9, I will deal with stress, psychological, and spiritual lifestyle issues.

In addition to the recommendations I have made about avoidance of certain chemicals, I wish to add that proper sleep is essential for proper immune functioning. Many good things happen related to the immune system while we sleep, and, therefore, we should never shortchange our sleep schedule. In chapter 8, I will discuss sleep extensively, including natural and pharmacologic ways to deal with the poor sleep quality that is so common in patients with chronic Lyme disease.

(3) Cytokines

There are two cytokines that appear to be key to the prevention of Lyme disease: IL-2 and IFN-g. The herb astragalus, which is widely used in traditional Chinese medicine (TCM), does an excellent job in helping the body produce both of these key substances and also acts as a powerful immune system tonic. I agree with Stephen Harrod Buhner, author of *Healing Lyme*, that the daily use of astragalus for individuals living in a Lyme-endemic area makes good sense. Therefore, I recommend its use during the high risk seasons.

* Astragalus (during the highest risk seasons) 1,000 mg per day

Lyme Prevention in Summary

To help prevent Lyme disease, the preceding recommendations should be followed by anyone living in an area of the country where Lyme disease is endemic. Here is a review of the key elements.

* Healthy lifestyle, including avoidance of alcohol, tobacco, overuse of acetaminophen (especially on empty stomach or with alcohol), and adequate sleep

* Use of a daily excellent multiple vitamin/mineral, along with a healthy diet, rich in spicy foods like curry and garlic (discussed in the next chapter)

* Regular exercise (see chapter 6.)

* Daily use of either beta glucan 10–250 mg a day (or aloe vera) during high risk seasons or high risk behaviors, like gardening, hiking, and hunting

* Daily use of astragalus, 1000 mg a day during high risk seasons or high risk behaviors

Early Stage Lyme Disease
(The first few weeks after
contracting Lyme)

If you are unable to avoid contracting Lyme, your innate immune system will require help from the adaptive immune system. In early stage lyme, you will need to continue the things we discussed above, and you will also need to employ additional therapies to help your body cope with Lyme. Those additional therapies primarily involve supporting the T lymphocytes and the adrenal glands. The goal of these therapeutic approaches is twofold.

* Augmenting the innate immune system's ongoing battle by bringing in the "cavalry"

* Supplying the necessary ingredients so that the proper tidal ebb and flow pattern can be maintained. This regulatory pattern of the body will effectively eliminate invading microorganisms, while minimizing collateral body tissue damage.

(1) T Lymphocytes

You will recall from our discussion earlier in this chapter that the body constantly seeks to maintain a balance that we call homeostasis. It does this by going into an *attack mode* followed by a *cooling off mode* when exposed to harmful microorganisms. In its wisdom, the body does this in a cyclical fashion similar to the tides of the ocean. In terms of the adaptive immune system regarding Lyme, the same principles apply. When the T lymphocytes of the CD4 variety are in an attack mode, we call that a "Th1 response." When in a cooling off mode, we call that a "Th2 response."

Astragalus supports the Th1 response and should be continued during early or acute Lyme. The following additional therapies for two months support the Th1 *attack mode*:

* Cat's claw (*Uncaria tomentosa*) liquid: work up to 10 drops twice a day or capsules: 500 mg, 2 capsules 3 times per day. Cycle on 12 days and off 2 days.

* Resveratrol (Japanese knotweed): 500 mg, three times per day

* Andrographis: 500–1,000 mg two to three times a day, use with caution (For full discussion of Andrographis, see chapter 6.)

* Alpha lipoic acid (enhances production of glutathione): 200–300 mg per day (**Caution:** if you have diabetes, please be aware that alpha lipoic acid may affect blood sugars by lowering them, and therefore, let your physician know you are taking it. If desired, you may substitute N-acetyl cysteine at a dose of 300–500 mg twice a day.)

Most often I will use a combination of two to three of the four supplements on the above list when a patient presents to my office with early Lyme. While the antibiotic regimen will usually be effective alone in the early stages, it seems prudent to enhance the immune system's capacity to control the infection. If I suspect Bartonella (or BLO) in addition to Lyme, one of my choices will definitely be resveratrol in the form of Japanese knotweed. If glutathione levels are likely to be low (for example, if a person drinks alcohol regularly), often alpha lipoic acid will be added as one of the choices.

If CD57 levels are low, then cat's claw is recommended. Cat's claw (*Uncaria tomentosa*) is a very special herb that originates from the rain forests of the Amazon River region of South America. It is a weed-like vine that has projections that look like the claws of a cat and, therefore, was named "uña de gato" (claw of the cat) by the natives of the Amazon rain forest. I have found this herb, taken properly, to be very useful in the treatment of Lyme disease. It works by several mechanisms: (1) helps control excessive inflammation by controlling a substance called "nuclear factor kappa beta" (NF-kB), (2) strengthens and increases the number of lymphocytes and NK cells (including the CD57 cells), and (3) seems to have direct anti-Lyme effects. In chapter 6, I will discuss at length the way to properly use cat's claw because taken incorrectly it can cause problems for you.

The following therapies support the Th2 cooling off mode:

* Vitamin A: 5,000 IU per day

* Vitamin D: 400–2000 IU per day (based on measurement of 25-hydroxy vitamin D levels)

It is also very important to avoid key nutritional deficiencies. Make sure that you get adequate supplementation support of vitamins A, B complex (including niacin or niacinamide), and, very importantly, vitamin D. Concerning vitamin D, it is interesting that the vast majority of my patients experience improvement of Lyme symptoms with sunlight exposure. This implies that vitamin D (which is manufactured in the skin upon sunlight exposure) may be playing a healing role in some way. My theory is that vitamin D works in support of one of the major T lymphocyte regulator cells, called the CD25 regulatory cell. Research suggests that this cell utilizes vitamin D to help cool off Th1 if necessary. Therefore, proper vitamin D support is necessary for immune regulation.

It has been suggested, by some advocates of restriction of vitamin D in Lyme disease, that vitamin D is overly suppressive of the immune system and, therefore, should be avoided so that the immune system can do its job against Lyme. The apparent evidence, according to the proponents, is that patients who have low vitamin D levels have exaggerated temporary Lyme die-off symptoms (called a "herx" response) to even low doses of antibiotics. This supposedly implies that vitamin D (which structurally is related to "steroid" hormones) is suppressing the immune system and preventing it from doing its job properly.

The reality is that the exaggerated antibiotic "herx" seen with vitamin D deficiency is more likely a result of a dysregulated immune system, where a damaging pro-inflammatory state exists because of vitamin D deficiency. (The exception to what I just stated is an uncommon condition called sarcoidosis, where abnormally high levels of CD25 cells exist, resulting in immune suppression rather than regulation). As I will discuss in chapter 5, a chronic pro-inflammatory state often leads to a host of dangerous adverse health effects secondary to chronic inflammation.

(2) Adrenal Glands

Often during the early phase of Lyme disease, the adrenal glands will be under great pressure from several sources. The first source is the immune system itself, particularly the cytokines

IL-1 and IL-6. Further pressure comes from the pituitary gland to make hormones to deal with the infection. Finally, the stress of being sick and feeling constantly ill adds another pressure to the overburdened adrenal glands. As I stated above, in chapter 7, I will discuss adrenal support in much more detail.

At this point in early stage Lyme disease, my approach is to use nutritional and herbal supplements to help the adrenals to cope with their overuse due to stress. Natural products that contain eleuthrococcus and rhodiola are most useful. Licorice is another valuable herbal product. There are many good products available on the market. It is also important at this point to ensure that you are receiving adequate basic nutrition support for the adrenal glands in the form of vitamin C (500–2,000 mg per day); vitamin B5 as pantothenic acid or, better yet, pantethine (300–900 mg per day); and magnesium (400–1,000 mg per day). Proper exercise, rest, and sleep are also important factors for adrenal support.

Late Stage Lyme Disease (Six months or more after contracting Lyme)

Late stage or chronic Lyme disease is much more complicated to deal with because the immune system, at this point, is invariably dysfunctional and unable to adequately perform its job. The goal of therapy at this point, in addition to antibiotics to lower Lyme load in the body, is to accomplish the three "R's."

* Reduce inflammation that is causing misery and tissue destruction

* Restore the immune system to its strong yet regulated state of homeostasis, hopefully with reduction in auto-immune phenomena

* Repair the nervous system, the energy systems, and the musculoskeletal system

This is a tall order, yet much can be done using several helpful modalities. Except for the use of antibiotics, these methods fall outside of the realm of conventional allopathic medicine, but vast experience using them says that they are very safe and very effective. Chapters 6, 7, and 8 contain a full discussion of the treatment modalities (including dosage ranges) that are used for chronic or late Lyme disease. Briefly, the following are the most useful additional immune-impacting techniques that we have to offer:

* High dose essential fatty acids—both pure fish oil as a source of EPA and DHA and borage oil (or primrose oil) as a source of GLA. This combination is very helpful in reducing chronic inflammation.

* Glutathione (GSH) as intravenous (IV) or transdermal—in addition to oral support with N-acetyl cysteine and lipoic acid—It is common to need several weeks of intravenous GSH in order to restore cellular stores of this vital antioxidant to assist with NK cell function.

Recently an effective oral preparation of glutathione called "acetylglutathione" has been found to be useful at a dose of 100 mg two to three times per day.

* High dose methylcobalamin—vitamin B12 in its most healing form for the neurological system. Sometimes intramuscular injections for a period of several weeks, followed by sublingual or intranasal B12, can produce very strong results in terms of energy and neurological healing.

* Alpha glycans—The source of this substance that I have used clinically is a rice product imported from Thailand that seems to have healing properties for the immune system and the nervous system. Some of the results of this whole foods vegan product have been impressive. Briefly, alpha glycans are very small complexes of two substances: carbohydrates (called polysaccharides) and proteins (called peptides). These "polysaccharide peptides" can penetrate into cells resulting in excellent detoxification of cells, repair of genetic material in cells, and improvement in energy function of cells.

* Endorphin support—one of the most exciting new therapies that I have recently introduced into my practice. The product that is used is a prescription for a very low dose of a very safe and non-toxic drug compound called naltrexone. This inexpensive product is taken at night before falling asleep and works by causing a temporary blockage of the body's endorphin receptors. The body

responds by making more endorphins. The resulting endorphin production helps re-establish the endorphin cycle and raises body endorphin production by as much as threefold. This improved endorphin production has a profound effect on the immune system, essentially helping to both strengthen and regulate it. This is one of the most promising new therapies for Lyme patients. I will discuss the protocol that we use for this therapy in chapter 7. Please keep in mind that this therapy must be prescribed by and supervised by a licensed physician. To read more about this useful, novel therapy go to www. lowdosenaltrexone.org.

Summing Up

Let's review the key points of this chapter by answering the most commonly asked questions about Lyme disease and the immune system.

Why is the immune system so critical for Lyme disease and other tick-borne illnesses?

Along with your skin, the immune system is your body's first and most important line of defense when it comes to protecting you against harmful microorganisms, including *Bb* and other tick-borne bacteria. Therefore, healthy immune function is absolutely essential in helping your body resist and recover from Lyme and related conditions.

How does the immune system work to protect against Lyme and related diseases?

The actions of the immune system when exposed to invading microorganisms are many and consist of three general goals: 1) recognizing the threat the invaders pose, 2) aggressively responding to that threat, and 3) returning to normal function once the threat has been contained so that your body can then begin the processes of clean-up and repair.

The actions initiated by the immune system when the body is under attack are orchestrated by two subcategories of immune function, the *innate* system and the *adaptive* system. The innate system is the first line of defense for the body. Its primary initial goal is to constantly be on guard against trouble in the form of infectious agents, tumors, and other foreign invaders. When such harmful invaders are detected by the innate system, it springs into action, employing a variety of mechanisms, including inflammation, to attack the invaders while simultaneously signaling the body to send other immune agents to the scene of the crisis.

While the innate system is doing its job, the adaptive system also comes into play, creating specific immune responses that are tailor-made for combating the problem at hand. Additionally, the adaptive system creates a "memory" of the invaders so that, should they return, it will be able to recognize them and spring into action quickly and decisively.

Since the immune system is designed to respond so quickly and effectively to harmful microorganisms, why do so many Lyme patients suffer from poor immune function?

Like all other systems of your body, the immune system can only optimally function when the body is in a state known as homeostasis, which is responsible for maintaining a delicate balance of opposites. Put another way, homeostasis is necessary for regulating all the body's systems. In the case of the immune system, homeostasis is what instructs the immune response to attack and to rest so that the body's clean-up and repair mechanisms can function.

Homeostasis can become chronically upset due to Lyme disease. When this happens, the ability of the body to regulate the immune system and other body systems becomes impaired. This, in turn, results in impaired immune function, making it more difficult for the body to resist and recover from harmful invaders such as the *Bb* bacteria.

Additionally, many other factors can result in diminished immune function. These include poor diet, nutritional deficiencies, stress, lack of exercise, and unhealthy sleep patterns. Disturbances in the adrenal gland function and in the body's ability to manufacture endorphins may also adversely affect immune function.

What can be done to improve immune function, both to prevent Lyme disease and to help the body recover from it?

In addition to working with a Lyme-aware physician, there are a number of effective self-care measures that you can take to help achieve and maintain healthy immune function. The use of natural therapies, such as herbal and nutritional immune-supporting supplements, can be very helpful. For a more detailed discussion of herbal alternatives, I refer you to the excellent book by Stephen Buhner, *Healing Lyme*. Various alternative therapies can also be helpful, such as acupuncture and massage, both of which can improve your body's ability to increase endorphin production. Laughter is also an excellent producer of endorphins, as is dark, organic chocolate with no added sugar.

Adopting a healthier lifestyle is the most important change that you may need to make when it comes to immune function and your overall health. In particular, I recommend that you avoid smoking and exposure to secondhand smoke. Alcohol should also be avoided, as should the overuse or improper use of drugs that contain acetaminophen, both of which deplete the body of glutathione, an important antioxidant that is vital for the proper function of the immune system's natural killer (NK) cells. Additionally, stress management, regular exercise, healthy eating (which we will discuss in chapter 5), and proper sleep are all vitally important to achieving a healthy immune system.

What role do antibiotics play in aiding immune function?

Antibiotics are essential in treating Lyme and related diseases because of their ability to kill off the harmful invaders that cause these conditions. In that regard, antibiotics can be an important ally to the immune system as it does its job. However, antibiotics alone are often not enough to adequately treat Lyme disease, especially once it has moved beyond its earliest stage to spread deeper throughout the body. This is why many Lyme-aware physicians advocate a comprehensive and integrative treatment approach for Lyme that treats the "whole person" (body, mind, and spirit). Moreover, effective though they may be, antibiotics should never be considered as a substitute for healthy immune function. Nor should any of the other treatments recommended in this book be thought of as a replacement for a healthy immune system. The goal of treatment should always be first and foremost to restore immune function to its optimal level. Once this is achieved, in most cases the need for antibiotics and other therapies will eventually come to an end.

Now that you understand how vitally important your immune system is, it's time to turn our discussion to a related important factor that influences how well or poorly your body is able to respond to Lyme. I am referring to the problem of chronic inflammation. In the next chapter, you will discover the reasons that bringing chronic inflammation under control is so important. Additionally, I will introduce you to the Lyme Inflammation Diet, a powerful tool for helping you achieve this important goal of controlling chronic inflammation.

Chapter Five

The Lyme Inflammation Diet®

❋

In this chapter, I'll be discussing the most vital self-care step that all patients with chronic Lyme disease can take in reclaiming their health. This step is the healthy eating approach that I call the Lyme Inflammation Diet (or LID for short). In recent years, more research attention has been paid to the role that chronic low-grade inflammation plays in causing a number of serious health disorders. It is also a primary causative factor in a number of our most deadly diseases including cancer, heart disease, and the "autoimmune disorders" like lupus, rheumatoid arthritis, and multiple sclerosis.

Based on a large volume of scientific studies, one thing is now very clear—when inflammation becomes unchecked in the body, illness becomes inevitable. However, many people do not realize the important role that inflammation plays in Lyme disease. This lack of awareness about inflammation in relationship to Lyme is unfortunate. Simply put, *the degree to which chronic low-grade inflammation exists in the body is directly related to the severity of symptoms that Lyme patients experience.* This explains why the severity of symptoms for people with disseminated Lyme disease can vary so greatly, with some people nearly incapacitated by Lyme and others only mildly affected by it.

Understanding Inflammation

Inflammation is the body's natural healing reaction in its response to various occurrences including injury, exposure to infectious microorganisms (bacteria—including the *Bb* bacteria and the co-infections associated with Lyme disease—viruses, and fungi), and exposure to allergy-causing substances known as allergens. Inflammation that occurs as a result of these occurrences is a good thing because the body's inflammatory response helps to properly repair injured bones, joints, organs, and tissues. At the same time, it also helps to mount a defense against invading microorganisms and allergens. In a state of overall good health, the inflammatory response is only temporary. Once the body has the circumstances that trigger inflammation under control, the inflammatory response subsides.

Such incidents of normal, healthy inflammation are known as *acute inflammatory responses*. One common example of an acute inflammatory response is the process that occurs when you accidentally cut yourself. Your body's immune system immediately directs various healing agents to the site of the cut in order to seal it off and protect it from possible infection. Should potentially harmful microorganisms be present at the wound site, immune cells go to work to attack and eliminate them. Simultaneously, other immune cells work to rid the site of cellular debris and waste by-products caused by the cut.

During this process, the area of the body surrounding the cut will usually redden and swell to some extent. You may experience sensations of heat and pain. Depending on the severity of the cut, a temporary loss or impairment of function in the affected area may also occur. But once the healing process is underway, a healthy immune system recognizes that its job is done and puts an end to the inflammatory response. (I discussed the mechanisms for regulation of the immune system in the previous chapter.) At this point, symptoms such as swelling, heat, and pain begin to subside, and full function of the affected area begins to return.

Most cases of acute inflammation are short-lived, usually lasting only for a few days or less. But when the inflammatory response continues beyond the originally intended purpose, the stage is set for potential health problems. If left unchecked, serious, and in some cases even life-threatening, health issues can develop. Such ongoing inflammation is known as *chronic inflammation*.

Unlike acute inflammation, which is usually an immediate and short-term response, chronic inflammation is generally of a more low-grade nature and is ongoing or recurring. Because it is low-grade in nature, the symptoms of chronic inflammation aren't always noticeable. When they are, they most commonly occur as pain and swelling that are continuous or which flare up intermittently.

In some cases, there are no obvious symptoms of chronic inflammation. Yet, though patients may believe themselves to still be healthy, inside their bodies internal damage caused by an ongoing inflammatory response can be taking place. This, in turn, can cause a cascade of internal events that can lead to serious degenerative disease. Often, however, it can be years before such degeneration becomes noticeable. For example, a common result of chronic inflammation is silent damage to the arteries and other blood vessels, which can lead to sudden heart attack without any warning signs.

Causes of Chronic Inflammation

Chronic inflammation can either be caused as a result of an unresolved acute inflammatory response, or it can develop on its own. In either case, the immune system perceives that the body is under continuous attack. In most cases, this perception is accurate. Obviously, this is an accurate perception in the case with untreated Lyme disease. Yet in other cases, the perception

of attack by the immune system is faulty (or perhaps we just
don't know the cause), with the result being that the immune
system literally starts to attack parts of the body, such as joints,
organs, and other tissues. This inappropriate activity on the part
of the immune system is known as "autoimmune dysfunction."
Autoimmune dysfunction is an increasingly common cause of
chronic inflammation among many people today.

In addition to Lyme, other causes of chronic inflammation
include the following:

* **Allergies and sensitivities:** Often the terms allergy and
sensitivity are used interchangeably, but actually they
are quite different. As I mentioned above, allergens are a
common trigger for the inflammation response that we
call allergy. Technically, allergy occurs as a result of an
immediate reaction to the allergen caused by a specific
kind of antibody called IgE. (An example of a food
allergy is peanut allergy, which causes a severe, immediate, often life-threatening reaction.) In the case of sensitivities, the immune system response is delayed, rather
than immediate, and is caused by a different immune
mechanism than IgE. An example of food "sensitivity"
is celiac disease where a non-allergic immune reaction
occurs to gluten resulting in chronic inflammation if a
patient continues to consume gluten-containing foods.
Most triggers of chronic inflammation fall into the realm
sensitivities rather than allergens. In the case of chronic
inflammation, exposure to the sensitizing substance is
persistent, preventing the immune system from shut-

ting down the normal inflammation process. There are two classes of sensitizing substances that can trigger an immune response: (1) environmental substances, such as chemicals and environmental pollutants and toxins and (2) foods and food products.

* **Environmental toxins and pollutants:** In addition to triggering sensitivity immune reactions, toxic environmental chemicals can cause a variety of other health problems, including cancer. When such toxins and pollutants become lodged in the body, the immune system struggles to eliminate them. The end result is chronic inflammation. Also, as we discussed previously, these toxins can cause a reduction in the critical natural killer (NK) cells of the body. There are times when the NK counts (such as the CD57 count) will not rise until after we have done a body cleansing of toxins and heavy metals. We will deal with the question of toxic chemical and heavy metal elimination (called "detoxification") in chapter 8 of this book.

* **Cigarette smoking:** Previously we discussed the role of smoking and its effect of reducing immune function. In addition, this unhealthy lifestyle choice is another significant cause of chronic inflammation. For those two reasons alone, it would be beneficial for you to quit if you smoke. Another important reason to quit is that the *Bb* organisms do not like oxygen. When you smoke, you deprive the body of one of its most useful tools to fight Lyme—oxygen. In my clinical experience, Lyme patients who stop smoking have a much better outcome

than Lyme patients who do not stop smoking. Therefore, if you smoke, seek help in quitting.

* **Free radical damage:** Free radicals are normally occurring unstable atoms and atom groups in the body. When the body becomes overloaded with free radicals it leads to a condition called "oxidative stress." Oxidative stress is a major contributor to chronic inflammation. The tidal analogy we used in chapter 4 applies here also. Normally, the body has a process that uses oxygen called *oxidation* (low tide). However, excessive oxidation is always balanced by the opposite reaction called *reduction* or *antioxidation* (high tide). In other words, free radicals are created as part of normal oxidation processes, but these potentially damaging particles are always balanced by the presence of antioxidants. When unchecked free radicals circulate throughout the body; they cause damage to the cells resulting in chronic inflammation. An unbalanced diet that is deficient in foods containing antioxidants (fruits and vegetables) and high in foods that contribute to excessive oxidation (processed and fried foods) is a major contributor to chronic inflammation.

* **Obesity:** Fat cells may release chemical substances known as cytokines that can cause inflammation. For most people who are obese or overweight, chronic inflammation is often a problem. Many obese people also suffer from two other significant contributors to chronic inflammation—namely, insulin resistance and leptin resistance, which will be discussed later in this chapter. Interestingly, approximately 80 percent of Lyme

patients in the United States who suffer from chronic Lyme symptoms are also overweight or obese.

* **Advanced glycation end products (AGEs):** AGEs are unstable and toxic compounds that can be very harmful to the body. These substances form when excessive simple sugars (most commonly glucose and fructose) bind abnormally to proteins. The resulting end product is called an "advanced glycation end product." These AGE substances are seen by the body as "foreign," and the body then mounts an immune attack against them, resulting in inflammation. For that reason, chronic exposure to these AGEs can be a major contributor to chronic inflammation. AGEs have been associated with a number of diseases that have been linked to chronic inflammation, such as Alzheimer's disease, arthritis, atherosclerosis (hardening of the arteries), diabetes, high blood pressure, and certain types of vision problems, such as cataracts and macular degeneration. There are two sources of AGEs. The first source is "exogenous," meaning they are already formed and present in food we eat. We take in these exogenous sources of AGEs when we eat poor-quality carbohydrates (such as cakes and donuts) and fried or high-temperature-cooked foods (such as barbecued meats). The second source is "endogenous," meaning they are created internally in the body after we ingest certain foods. The internal source of AGEs is, most commonly, the excessive use of sugar (such as sucrose and glucose) and fructose (such as high fructose corn syrup). These sugars bind to proteins like enzymes, causing them to function poorly. In summary, whether the source is

external or internal, AGEs stimulate chronic inflammation. Ultimately the key source of all pro-inflammatory AGEs is a bad diet. A poor diet of unhealthy carbohydrates, sugar, and overcooked foods clearly leads to excessive AGEs. This diet also leads to a related condition called "insulin resistance" which I will discuss next.

* **Insulin resistance:** Insulin resistance is an increasingly common problem in our society, primarily due to unhealthy eating habits. Insulin is a hormone produced by the pancreas in order to help the body's cells utilize glucose, a type of sugar that is the chief source of fuel in the body. The primary source of this essential fuel, glucose, is from carbohydrates in our diet. (Incidentally, the body requires a *proper* amount of glucose and is so critically dependent on glucose that it can even manufacture glucose from protein in an emergency situation.) Without insulin, glucose would not be able to pass from the bloodstream through the cellular walls and into the cells themselves. Insulin resistance occurs when the amount of insulin normally produced by the pancreas becomes insufficient for unlocking the receptor sites on the cell walls that allow glucose to pass into the cells. When the cells resist or do not respond to insulin, levels of glucose in the blood become elevated. This causes the pancreas to produce even more insulin in an effort to balance glucose levels in the blood. When this balance becomes disrupted, it can result in high blood sugar (hyperglycemia) or type 2 diabetes. In addition, insulin resistance can significantly contribute to or exacerbate

chronic inflammation. At the same time, chronic inflammation can also cause insulin resistance, resulting in a vicious cycle of unhealthy consequences.

* **Leptin resistance:** Leptin resistance results when leptins are no longer able to properly perform their job in the body. What are leptins? Leptins belong to a special class of hormones known as adipokines that are produced by your body's fat cells. Leptins help the brain know how much body fat you have and act to reduce appetite and increase metabolism so that your body does not become overweight. In women, leptins also help to regulate fertility and the functioning of the ovaries.

Scientists have discovered that most people who are overweight or obese have elevated leptin levels. In such cases, the leptins are unable to regulate appetite and metabolism the way they should. The problem isn't that the leptins are malfunctioning, but that the fat cells aren't properly responding to the messages the leptins are sending them. Therefore, the body produces even more leptins. This, in turn, can help contribute to chronic inflammation. At the same time, just as with insulin resistance, chronic inflammation can also cause leptin resistance, setting up another vicious cycle of unhealthy conditions in the body.

* **Standard American diet:** This is our biggest hurdle to overcome. It's only too appropriate that the acronym for the standard American diet is SAD. Such a diet, which consists of processed fast foods and other nutrient-deficient food products, is the number one lifestyle

choice responsible for our nation's health care crisis. This resulting crisis now costs more than $1.9 trillion in health care-related costs. The standard American diet is also a primary source of the following: free radicals, food allergens, oxidized fats (such as fried foods), excessive omega-6 fatty acids (and deficient omega-3s), empty calories, sugar, AGEs, and many, many other unhealthy ingredients. All these potentially harmful products can either cause or prolong chronic inflammation. Let's look at an example. Omega-6 fatty acids (such as grain oils like corn oil), while essential to good health, are usually consumed to excess by most people. Too much omega-6 fatty acid in the diet results in the production of arachidonic acid and other compounds that can cause, intensify, and prolong inflammation. Fortunately, by taking responsibility for your diet and following the guidelines of the Lyme Inflammation Diet that I share with you below, there is much you can do on your own to significantly reduce and eventually eliminate chronic inflammation. Taking this step is absolutely essential for helping your body more effectively cope with and reverse Lyme disease, the co-infections, and the resulting chronic inflammation.

* **Fatigue and lack of sleep:** Fatigue that is persistent or chronic creates stress and low energy levels, which in turn can contribute to chronic inflammation. Failing to get at least seven or more hours of sleep on a regular basis also creates stress and, therefore, chronic inflammation. Sleep disruption may alter the endorphin cycle.

"Nighttime high tide" is the time period when endorphins are *produced*—from around 2:00 A.M. to 4:00 A.M.
"Daytime low tide," the remainder of the 24 hours, is
the time period when the endorphins are *utilized* by
the body for immune support and other vital functions.
Proper adrenal function is also dependent on obtaining
proper sleep.

* **Lack of regular exercise:** Exercise, in addition to its many
  other health benefits, helps to reduce stress. Conversely,
  lack of exercise can contribute to stress buildup, thereby
  leading to chronic inflammation. Additionally, exercise
  strengthens and regulates the immune system by increasing the body's normal production of endorphins.

* **Infectious microorganisms:** Bacteria (including the
  Bb bacteria and the various potential co-infections of
  Lyme disease), mold, fungi, parasites, and viruses all
  cause the body to initiate an inflammation response
  that can become chronic if the immune system is not
  able to eliminate such microorganisms. There are also
  times when organisms actually disrupt the body's normal inflammation control mechanisms for their own
  protection from the immune system. A good example of
  this dilemma is the Lyme bacterium, which induces the
  manufacture of IL-10 in order to suppress the immune
  system's Th1 response (as we discussed in chapter 4).
  Therefore, whenever we are dealing with chronic infections like Lyme, we must be careful not only to treat a
  person with appropriate antibiotics, but also to address
  the chronic inflammation problems that have been trig-

gered by Lyme. This chapter addresses the crucial role that nutrition plays in this ongoing battle to restore normalcy to the body dealing with chronic Lyme infection and inflammation.

The Effects of Chronic Inflammation

To better understand why chronic inflammation is so hazardous to your health, let's take a look at what happens inside your body when inflammation becomes chronic. At the beginning of the inflammation response, your immune system releases specific hormones (histamines) and proteins (kinins) that act in unison with each other to cause blood vessels to dilate. This causes increased blood flow and tissue swelling in the area of the body that the immune system is attempting to heal.

Very soon after histamines and kinins are released, a flood of other chemicals (cytokines, eosinophils, prostaglandins, leukotrines, and interleukins) are also unleashed by the immune system and sent to the area of the body in need of healing. The arrival of these chemicals to the targeted body site causes a further progression of the inflammation process, resulting in further tissue swelling, redness, and possibly sensations of heat and pain.

In time, the body makes proteins called antibodies. The role of the antibody (which is directed specifically at the invader, which we call an "antigen") is to seek out the foreigners in the body and attach to them. When the antibody and the antigen come together, they form what are called "circulating immune complexes" (CICs). There are two possible types of CICs.

The first type occurs when the amount of antibody (beneficial protein) in the blood directed against the antigen (enemy invader) is sufficient to *exceed* and overwhelm the invader. When this happens, this type of CIC causes a chemical reaction to occur that allows the other white blood cells to eat (or "phagocytize") the foreigners. This is a good reaction and the CICs are "cleared" from circulation, and minimal inflammation occurs.

The second reaction is a problematic one. In this scenario, there is *insufficient* antibody to overwhelm the invaders and the result is that the CICs have more antigen than antibody. When this happens, the CICs become deposited in tissue instead of being cleared by the white blood cells. The result of this deposition in tissue is inflammation.

Poor diet, when combined with an invader like Lyme, increases the risk of CICs developing to the point where the body cannot eliminate them. For this reason, the Lyme Inflammation Diet is such an important part of a comprehensive treatment program for Lyme disease, because it is effective in reducing chronic inflammation. Because it is such a health-promoting nutrition program for everyone, the Lyme Inflammation Diet can significantly improve the health status of those suffering from the many other degenerative diseases. Some of the health conditions currently shown by scientific research to be directly linked to chronic inflammation are listed below:

* Alzheimer's disease

* blood sugar problems (especially hyperglycemia, which may result in diabetes mellitus)

* cancer

* candidiasis (systemic yeast overgrowth)

* cystic fibrosis

* fibromyalgia

* food addictions and possibly eating disorders

* gout

* headaches (including migraines)

* heart disease

* inflammatory bowel disease
  (ulcerative colitis, Crohn's disease)

* kidney disease

* liver disease

* lupus (systemic lupus erythematosus or SLE)

* multiple sclerosis

* obesity

* Parkinson's disease

* respiratory conditions
  (such as asthma, chronic bronchitis, emphysema)

* rheumatoid arthritis and perhaps osteoarthritis

Chronic Inflammation and Lyme Disease

The links between chronic inflammation and the above conditions are well-studied. While less is known about the role that chronic inflammation plays in Lyme disease, many of us who work with Lyme have seen many indications that it plays a major role. In the case of many of my patients, I am convinced that there is an ongoing combination of both active *Bb* infection and uncontrolled chronic inflammation. As I mentioned, Lyme disease and chronic inflammation together produce a very unhealthy double-edged sword. On the one hand, untreated disseminated *Bb* bacteria (or the co-infections) cause chronic inflammation as the body attempts to battle these invading microorganisms. On the other, as a direct result of ongoing chronic inflammation, the body's immune system becomes poorly regulated and ineffective in its response to the infestation of Lyme and other co-infections. This ineffectiveness in turn enables these infections to gain stronger footholds in the body, thereby causing increasingly severe health symptoms.

An apt analogy that illustrates the vicious cycle of Lyme disease and chronic inflammation is that of adding fuel to a fire. Obviously, doing so only makes matters worse. To put out the fire, you need to stop adding fuel and start using water. Continuing this analogy, this is precisely what you will accomplish as you begin to follow the principles of the Lyme Inflammation Diet. Following these dietary recommendations faithfully will over time produce powerful anti-inflammatory effects. The result will be a reduction in the burden on your body's immune system, as well as on other organ systems, so that it can more effectively begin to target and eliminate *Bb* bacteria and its co-infections.

Assessing Your Risk for Chronic Inflammation

A simple and inexpensive blood test can help your physician determine whether or not you suffer from chronic inflammation. It also helps you know the extent of inflammation. It is known as the CRP blood test. CRP stands for *C-reactive protein*, a type of protein that is present in small amounts in the blood of all people. As chronic inflammation sets in, levels of CRP in the bloodstream become elevated. This is because the liver produces more C-reactive protein in response to chronic inflammation (especially IL-6 and TNF-alpha). You can ask your doctor about the CRP test, which is widely available across the country.

In addition to the CRP test, the following questionnaire focuses on factors that can improve or make worse inflammation. It is an effective self-assessment tool you can use to quickly determine whether or not you are at risk for chronic inflammation. The good news is that every bad thing is reversible and every good thing is capable of being added to your program. This test is very easy. Simply write down the numbers that indicate "positive" or "negative" for each item. Then add the positives together. Then add the negatives together. The final score is the sum of positives and negatives, and this total will tell you where you rate.

Positive (Anti-Inflammatory) Daily Dietary and Lifestyle Factors

Award yourself the indicated positive (+) number for each of the following items that are part of your *average* daily or weekly dietary and lifestyle routine. If the item does not apply to you, leave that particular score blank.

Fruit Consumption:
(5 points for each serving of fresh, frozen, or dried organic fruit you consume each day; 3 points for each serving of unsweetened fruit juice) _____

Vegetable Consumption:
(5 points per each serving of raw or steamed vegetables) _____

Daily Vitamin/Mineral/Antioxidant Supplementation:
(5 points) _____

Consumption of Oily Fish (e.g., Salmon) or Omega-3/Fish Oil Supplements:
(7 points for consumption four or more times/week; 4 points for consumption 1–3 times/week) _____

Organic or Range-Fed Meat Consumption:
(5 points) _____

Regular Use of Olive Oil and/or Other Healthy Oils for Cooking:
(5 points) _____

Regular Exercise:
(3 points for each 10 minutes of exercise performed per day) _____

Consumption of Pure, Filtered Water:
(1 point for each eight-ounce glass of water; 8 points total for eight glasses or more) _____

Laughter:
(2 points per good, hearty laugh each day, up to 6 points total) _____

Positive Attitude/Gratefulness/Giving Spirit:
(7 points)   ____

Daily Prayer or Meditation:
(7 points)   ____

Daily Exposure to Sunlight for 10 or More Minutes:
(5 points)   ____

Daily Exposure to Fresh Air/Deep Breathing Exercises:
(4 points)   ____

Healthy Relationships and Social Networks:
(5 points including church groups, therapy, and so forth)   ____

Daily Giving and Receiving Hugs:
(2 points per hug; 6 points maximum total)   ____

Total Positive Score:
(add all the above scores)   _____

Negative (Pro-Inflammatory) Daily Dietary and Lifestyle Factors

Give yourself the indicated negative (-) number (e.g., -5) for each of the following items that are part of your regular dietary and lifestyle routine. If the item does not apply to you, leave that particular score blank.

Smoking:
(-10 points per pack smoked)   ____

Overweight:
(-7 points up to 50 pounds overweight;
-10 points for over 50 pounds)   ____

Consumption of Wheat, Dairy, or other Sensitivity-Causing Foods:
(- 5 points per food consumed daily—e.g., eating bread daily = -5) ____

Use of Trans-Fatty Acids (margarine, hydrogenated
and partially-hydrogenated oils):
(-5 points for each time used per day) ____

Exposure to External AGEs (fried foods, doughnuts, pastries, etc):
(-5 points for each exposure per day) ____

Consumption of Sugar or Artificial Sweeteners
(aspartame, splenda, and so forth):
(-3 points for each time used per day) ____

Excess Omega-6 Fatty Acid (Arachidonic Acid) Consumption:
(Food sources of omega-6 fatty acids include corn, peanut,
safflower, and sesame oils: −3 points for each time consumed per day) ____

Use of Cooking Oils Other Than Olive and Other Healthy Oils:
(-5 points) ____

Alcohol:
(-7 points for each alcoholic beverage consumed per day) ____

Negative/Pessimistic Attitude-Victim Mentality:
(-7 points) ____

Tendency Towards Unforgiveness:
(-7 points) ____

Averaging Less Than Seven Hours of Sleep:
(-7 points) ____

Poor Water Intake:
(Less than six eight-ounce glasses per day; -7 points) ____

Chronic Exposure to Mold in Home or at Work:
(-5 points) ____

Less Than Ten Minutes of Daily Sun Exposure:
(- 4 points) ____

Total Negative Score: ____
(add all the negative scores)

Combine both of your positive and negative scores
to tally your NET SCORE: _____

Rating

50 or above = Excellent
(Very low risk of chronic inflammation)

25 to 49 = Very Good

0 to 24 = Fair

-1 to -24 = Poor

-25 to -49 = Very Bad

-50 or below = Emergency
(Extremely high risk of chronic inflammation)

Adopting the Lyme Inflammation Diet

In the Foreword of this book, written by Dr. James A. Duke, he equated your body to a lovely garden. Just as a garden requires an adequate supply of sunlight, water, and regular care, so too does your body need a daily supply of life-supporting foods in order to flourish. This is the goal of the Lyme Inflammation Diet. By following it, you can help to reverse chronic inflammation and boost your immune system's ability to fight *Bb* bacteria and other infectious microorganisms. In addition, this nutrition program will help you to significantly reduce or eliminate both insulin resistance and leptin resistance. The dietary recommendations that I outline below will help you to create a foundation of wellness by supplying your body with a rich supply of nutrients—the fiber, vitamins, minerals, antioxidants, essential fats, and other vital substances that it needs in order to function optimally and to flourish as a well-cared-for garden.

The Lyme Inflammation Diet consists of four phases:

* Induction Phase

* Early Reentry Phase

* Late Reentry Phase

* Maintenance Phase

Each of these phases should be followed according to the guidelines below. If you stick to these guidelines, I can assure you that, over time, you will begin to notice improvement in your Lyme symptoms. You will also notice improvement in your overall health. Here is an example of how powerful the Lyme Inflammation Diet can be in providing health benefits.

Ed is a patient who came to our office after suffering from severe Lyme arthritic symptoms for several years. He was a very hard working man who awakened at 4:00 every morning, left the house at 4:30 A.M., and arrived at the workplace by 5:00 A.M., daily. On the way to work, his habit was to stop at the corner fast-food store in order to get his coffee, donut or pastry, and sometimes fried "tater tots." At lunch, he would usually have a diet cola (extra large), along with two hotdogs on white buns smothered with pickles, mayonnaise, ketchup, and mustard. Usually, he would have an order of french fries in addition. For dinner, his wife would prepare potatoes and steak, along with one vegetable and several dinner rolls. Always for dessert he would have ice cream. While watching TV in the evening he would usually have two or three beers and nachos with a cheese dip or with guacamole.

As he described his diet to me, I was shocked by several things: the complete lack of fruit, the nearly complete lack of fiber, the relative lack of vegetables, the excess of sugar and fried foods, and, finally, the use of coffee, colas, and beer instead of water. I told him that if he wanted to get well, he would have to make some major changes in his dietary program. I told him that if he would be willing to follow the Lyme Inflammation Diet, I would promise that he would feel significantly improved by the time he came back to my office in one month for his follow-up visit. (At that follow-up we would be starting antibiotics.)

His wife, sitting beside him, began to smile. She said that he could never take this radical approach to his diet. However, she misjudged Ed, who is the kind of man who loves a challenge. He said he would do it, and he did it. A month later he returned, saying that his joints were 75 percent better, his energy was 50 percent better, and his thinking processes were also 50 percent better. His wife nodded in confirmation and then remarked that he wasn't as grouchy as usual either. Remember, this all happened *before* we started Ed on antibiotics. It happened because the Lyme Inflammation Diet not only greatly reduced his inflammation, but it also supplied necessary antioxidants and vital nutrients that his body had been craving for years.

Ed's positive experience after adopting the Lyme Inflammation Diet is quite common among my other patients with Lyme disease. Now let's explore each of the four phases of the diet in more detail.

Phase One—The Induction Phase (one week)

Phase One of the Lyme Inflammation Diet is to be followed for one week. Its goal is to quickly help your body to shut down the mechanisms of chronic inflammation and begin detoxifying the body. This is accomplished by a primarily vegetarian diet that consists of eating safe foods that are low in what I call "universal negative inflammation triggers" (UNITs). Examples of UNIT foods would be trans-fatty acids, AGEs, and refined sugar.

Eating during Phase One may be tough for you. Consuming these Phase One fiber-rich foods exclusively will help to quickly and effectively begin to control inflammation. During this time, you should also avoid eating all foods that you know you are allergic or sensitive to even if they are on this list. (If you are uncertain about whether you have food allergies or sensitivities, consider being tested. For lab tests that are most accurate for screening for food allergies and sensitivities, see the resources section.)

What follows are the top seventy foods and beverages that I recommend that you consume during Phase One. For best results, choose foods of highest quality such as those that are organically raised. If possible, fish should be caught in the wild rather than farm-raised. Farm-raised fish usually contain dyes and are laced with antibiotics and other potentially harmful agents.

Beverages: Your best choice of beverage during Phase One is pure, filtered water. Avoid drinking tap water unless you allow it to sit for 30 or more minutes (allowing the chlorine amount to lessen). Also be wary of bottled water that comes in plastic containers, as the chemicals in plastics can leach into the water. If you must drink bottled water, use water that comes in glass containers or hard plastic, which are less susceptible to chemical leaching. If you can afford it, a reverse osmosis water system in your home is an excellent investment.

Other healthy beverages you can drink during Phase One are unsweetened acai, blackberry, blueberry, cherry, cranberry, pomegranate, and raspberry juices. The ideal method is to juice these items yourself. However, this may not be practical for most people. Therefore, use only the highest quality brands that have the fewest added substances. It is important that you become an avid label reader. Be especially careful concerning commercial name brands, as these can often contain sugars and other sweeteners, as well as other artificial ingredients. Consume the following beverages during this phase:

* Pure water

* Seven healthy unsweetened fruit juices: acai, blackberry, blueberry, cherry, cranberry, pomegranate, and raspberry

Fruits: I recommend eight fruits during Phase One. Avocado is a fruit that is a rich source of vitamins B6 and E, as well as healthy essential fatty acids. It is also rich in glutathione, making it a particularly good choice for you. Other recommended fruits during this one-week period are blackberries, blueberries, cherries, coconut, cranberries, pomegranates, and raspberries. Try to eat two to three servings of these fruits each day during Phase One:

* Avocado
* Blackberries
* Blueberries
* Cherries
* Coconut (or coconut milk)
* Cranberries
* Pomegranate
* Raspberries

Nuts and Seeds: For Phase One, the three best food choices in this category are almonds, walnuts, pine nuts, as well as freshly ground flaxseed, all of which are rich sources of anti-inflammatory oils and other nutrients.

* Almonds (or unsweetened almond milk)
* Flaxseed (keep refrigerated and grind fresh daily)
* Pine nuts
* Walnuts

Vegetables: Non-starchy vegetables are your best choices for this category. The best vegetables to eat during Phase One are arugula, artichoke, asparagus, beets, bok choy, broccoli, Brussels sprouts, cabbage, carrots, cauliflower, celery, chard, collard greens, cucumber, kale, leeks, mustard greens, onions, Romaine lettuce, scallions, shiitake mushrooms, spinach, sprouts, string beans, and watercress. Try to eat at least five to eight servings of these vegetables each day, either raw or lightly steamed.

* Arugula
* Artichoke
* Asparagus
* Beets
* Bok choy
* Broccoli
* Brussels sprouts
* Cabbage
* Carrots
* Chard
* Celery
* Collard greens
* Cucumber
* Kale
* Leeks
* Mushrooms (shiitake would be best choice)

* Mustard greens

* Onions

* Romaine lettuce

* Scallions

* Spinach

* Sprouts

* String beans

* Watercress

Grains: The only grain foods that I recommend during Phase One are organic brown rice and wild rice.

* Brown rice (organic)

* Wild rice

Herbs and Spices: The following herbs and spices can all be used according to your taste preference during Phase One—sea salt, basil, cardamom, chives, cilantro, cinnamon, cloves, curry, ginger, garlic, parsley, oregano, rosemary, and stevia. (Stevia is a healthy alternative to sugar and other sweeteners and is found in most health food stores.)

* Sea salt

* Basil

* Cardamom

* Chives

* Cilantro

* Cinnamon

* Cloves

* Curry

* Ginger

* Garlic

* Parsley

* Oregano

* Rosemary

* Stevia

Protein Sources: Other than egg whites, the fish food group is your primary source of protein during Phase One. Many fish are also a rich source of omega-3 oils and other essential fatty acids that act as powerful anti-inflammatory nutrients. The best types of fish during Phase One are flounder, mackerel, salmon, sardines, sole, and tilapia. Except for sardines, which are usually purchased canned, select fish that are wild-caught rather than farm-raised. Farm-raised fish are often full of antibiotics and coloring dyes. Also *do not* fry eggs or fish, as fried foods significantly contribute to inflammation in the body.

* Eggs (organic, free-range highly recommended; egg whites are high in quality protein; the yolk in phosphatidylcholine, lutein, and zeaxanthin)

* Flounder

* Mackerel

* Salmon

* Sardines

* Sole

* Tilapia

Other: Extra virgin olive oil and sesame oil can be used to prepare foods and as a dressing. Apple cider vinegar is also recommended as a healthy alternative to other types of vinegar. Clarified butter (ghee) is allowed in Phase One. Vanilla extract and a small amount of raw honey are also permissible during Phase One.

* Apple cider vinegar

* Extra virgin olive oil (mixed with small amount of sesame oil is acceptable)

* Ghee (clarified butter)

* Honey, 2 teaspoons per day (unheated raw honey)

* Vanilla extract

A Sample Daily Menu for Phase One

To help you create meal plans during Phase One, here is a sample of breakfast, lunch, and dinner menus that you can consider. For menu items listed, you'll find a full list of recipes in the appendix. Remember to drink lots of water between meals on this first phase.

Breakfast

* Fruit juice "smoothie"—8 ounces combo of frozen raspberry, blueberry, cherry, pomegranate juice, and coconut milk blended with 1 teaspoon of honey

* Vegetable omelet with egg whites, onions, scallions, and mushrooms, lightly cooked with olive oil

* 10-12 almonds and/or walnuts

Lunch

* Salad with arugula, carrots, cucumbers, leaf spinach, sprouts, broccoli, walnuts, pine nuts—with apple cider vinegar/olive oil/garlic vinaigrette dressing

* 4-ounce salmon fillet

* Asparagus spears

Dinner

* Brown rice

* Mixed vegetable stir fry medley—onions, cabbage, cauliflower, broccoli, and carrots using olive oil

* Baked flounder

* Dessert—fruit "compote" of blueberries, cherries, raspberries

Phase Two—The Early Reentry Phase (three weeks)

Phase Two of the Lyme Inflammation Diet is to be followed for the next three weeks, once Phase One is concluded. During this phase, your goal is to slowly reintroduce healthy foods that have a low risk of triggering inflammation. You will do this by *gradually* adding each food group's new foods to your diet. (For example, try adding the group's new food every other day like this: Day One, add back the new fruits, Day Three, add back the new nuts, and so on.)

It is vitally important that you do not rush the reintroduction of the foods listed below. If you experience any symptoms of inflammation after the foods are reintroduced, this is a sign that you should continue to avoid them for the time being. Otherwise, the following healthy foods can be reintroduced during Phase Two. Be aware that the foods that carry the highest risk of triggering inflammation are nuts and certain fruits, such as mangos. If you continue to do well, try adding *one* of the following food groups every other day to the foods already permitted in Phase One:

Beverages: Choose from green tea or vegetable juice (with the exception of tomato juice). For best results, use organic juice, preferably freshly squeezed if possible, and carbonated water, such as Perrier.

* Green tea

* Vegetable juice without tomato

* Carbonated water such as Perrier

Fruits: Fruits that are permissible during Phase Two include apricot, cantaloupe, date, fig, pear, pineapple, prune, and watermelon. Mango is also permitted so long as symptoms of inflammation do not recur.

* Apricot

* Cantaloupe

* Date

* Fig

* Mango

* Pear

* Pineapple

* Prune

* Watermelon

Nuts and Seeds: Nuts and seeds are very healthy foods. Brazil nuts, cashews, pecans, pumpkin seeds, sesame seeds, and sunflower seeds can be reintroduced during Phase Two. For best results, eat them roasted or germinated.

* Brazil nuts

* Cashews

* Pecans

* Pumpkin seeds

* Sesame seeds

* Sunflower seeds

Vegetables: Veggies that you can add to your diet during Phase Two include pumpkin, squash, sweet potato, and tapioca.

* Pumpkin

* Squash

* Sweet potato

* Tapioca (cassava)

Grains: At this stage of the Lyme Inflammation Diet, you can add oatmeal (preferably organic and slow-cooked).

* Oatmeal

Beans and Legumes: This food category, which is not included in Phase One of the Lyme Inflammation Diet, is an important vegetarian source of protein, which your body needs to maintain and rebuild bone and soft tissues and to properly regulate other important body functions. Permissible beans during Phase Two include black beans, kidney beans, navy beans, and pinto beans. Soy beans should *not* be eaten during Phase Two. Other permissible legumes include chickpeas (garbanzo beans), lentils, and peas.

* Black beans

* Chickpeas

* Kidney beans

* Lentils

* Navy beans

* Peas

* Pinto beans

Meat: During Phase Two you can now add organic lamb to your diet, while continuing to also eat the permissible fish listed for Phase One above.

* Lamb

Other: Other foods and beverages that you can include in Phase Two are black pepper, coconut kefir, and *non*-partially hydrogenated margarines. Xylitol and sorbitol may be used as sweeteners. Pure maple syrup and agave nectar can also be used in small amounts during this time.

* Black pepper

* Coconut kefir

* Maple syrup and agave nectar (in small amounts)

* Margarines *without* transfats
  (such as Earth Balance, Smart Balance, and Benechol)

* Xylitol and sorbitol

A Sample Daily Menu for Phase Two

To help you create meal plans during Phase Two, here is a sample of breakfast, lunch, and dinner menus that you can consider.

Breakfast

* Fruit medley—cantaloupe, watermelon, blueberry, pine-apple combo

* Oatmeal with maple syrup

* Two eggs with yolk scrambled lightly with olive oil

* Perrier

Lunch

* Large salad with cauliflower, romaine lettuce, chickpeas, kidney beans, pine nuts, carrots, and broccoli with raspberry vinaigrette dressing

* 4-ounce tilapia filet with spicy cilantro sauce

* Wild rice with almonds and cranberries

* Green tea with honey, ginger, and cloves

Dinner

* Roast leg of lamb

* Brown rice

* String beans with slivered almonds

* Lentil soup

* Dessert—chilled mango slices with shredded coconut

Phase Three—The Late Reentry Phase (four weeks)

Phase Three of the Lyme Inflammation Diet lasts for the next four weeks. Before beginning it, make sure that the foods you reintroduced in Phase Two have not triggered new bouts of inflammatory symptoms. If symptoms do recur, wait until they subside before moving on to Phase Three.

During Phase Three, your goal will be to reintroduce additional foods that are normally healthy, but which can trigger inflammation in some people. All these foods have a greater risk of doing so than the foods listed in Phase Two, so you must proceed cautiously, once again reintroducing Phase Three foods no sooner than every other day. Should health problems occur as a result of eating these additional foods, quickly stop and go back to Phase Two until you feel better.

The food and beverages that pose the highest risk of triggering inflammation during Phase Three are listed below in *italics*. As you did during Phase Two, proceed slowly. For instance, try adding only one food group of those listed below every other day.

Beverages: Organic apple juice can be reintroduced during Phase Three, as can unsweetened *citrus juices* and *coffee*.

* Apple juice

* *Citrus juices*

* *Coffee (organic)*

Fruits: Fruits that you can add back to your diet during Phase Three include apple, banana, *grapefruit*, *lemon*, *lime*, nectarine, *orange*, peach, and *strawberry*.

* Apple

* Banana

* *Grapefruit*

* *Lemon*

* *Lime*

* Nectarine

* *Orange*

* Peach

* *Strawberry*

Nuts: Peanuts can be reintroduced at this time, but only if you do not have a history of peanut allergy. If you do have an allergy, avoid peanuts.

* *Peanuts*

Soybeans: At this point, you can include soybeans in your diet, but avoid soymilk, textured soy protein meat substitutes, and soy powders, as these products are generally less desirable. Instead, use fermented soy foods, such as miso, natto, and tempeh. Tofu is permissible, as well, but fermented soy foods are better choices.

* Miso
* Natto
* Tempeh
* Tofu

Grains: As a food class, grains carry a greater than normal risk of inflammation compared to most other food groups, particularly those with the highest gluten content (*wheat, barley, rye*). Therefore, proceed with caution as you reintroduce grains to your diet. Acceptable grain choices during Phase Three are *barley*, buckwheat, *corn*, oat groats, millet, quinoa, oats, *rye*, and *wheat (including durum, semolina, spelt, kamut, einkorn, and faro)*. Whole grain pasta made from these items is acceptable if you do not react adversely to them.

* *Barley*

* Buckwheat

* *Corn*

* Sprouted grain breads (such as Ezekiel)

* Groats

* Millet

* Quinoa

* Oats

* *Rye*

* *Wheat very cautiously (including durum, semolina, spelt, kamut, einkorn, and faro)*

Nightshade Foods: Avoid this category of foods altogether if you know you are sensitive to the following foods or if you suffer from arthritis symptoms that you know are aggravated by these foods. Otherwise, proceed with caution as you reintroduce *chilies, eggplant, peppers* (both red and green), *white potatoes,* and *tomatoes,* as well as the spices *cayenne, chili powder,* and *paprika.*

* *Cayenne*

* *Chilies and chili powder*

* *Eggplant*

* *Paprika*

* *Peppers (red and green, hot or mild)*

* *Potato (white)*

* *Tomato*

Dairy Products: This is another food category that has a higher-than-normal risk for inflammation, as well as for food allergies and sensitivities. If you are allergic or sensitive to dairy products, avoid them. Otherwise, proceed with caution as you reintroduce them. The healthiest dairy products to use are organic butter, organic milk and cheeses (preferably raw source), goat's milk and cheeses (feta), and unsweetened, organic yogurt. As an alternative to dairy products, consider using coconut milk and oil.

* Butter (organic)

* *Cheeses* (raw cow or goat milk sources highly preferable)

* *Milk and cream*

* *Yogurt* (plain, unsweetened, organic)

Meat: At this time, you can now start to eat organic, free-range beef, bison, chicken, turkey, and venison.

* Bison

* Beef (free-range)

* Chicken

* Turkey

* Venison

A Sample Daily Menu for Phase Three

To help you create meal plans during Phase Three, here is a sample of breakfast, lunch, and dinner menus that you can consider.

Breakfast

* Sliced apples and walnuts

* Hash brown potatoes with onions and turmeric

* Organic turkey bacon slices cooked in olive oil

* Perrier with lime

Lunch

* Miso soup

* Tofu salad on Ezekiel bread with romaine lettuce, sprouts, and avocado

* Green tea with lemon

* Pear

Dinner

* Sweet potato soufflé with apples and pineapple

* Baked chicken with onions and peppers

* Steamed broccoli with raw cheddar cheese sauce

* Small tossed salad with arugula, carrots, tomatoes, cucumbers, and celery

* Dessert—peach cobbler (honey- and nectar-sweetened)

Phase Four—The Maintenance Phase
(Six months or indefinite)

Phase Four of the Lyme Inflammation Diet begins eight weeks after you began Phase One. Should you still be experiencing symptoms of chronic inflammation, remain on the earlier phases of the diet until your symptoms subside before beginning Phase Four. Once you do begin it, strictly abide by the guidelines below for at least *six months* to ensure that you obtain the most benefit from it. My recommendation is that you continue to avoid the poor quality "universal negative inflammation trigger" foods like fried foods and refined sugar permanently if at all possible.

By the time that you begin Phase Four, you will have eliminated all foods that trigger inflammation from your diet. You should be able to determine which healthy foods you can enjoy without triggering inflammation and which foods you should avoid. After you complete six months of following Phase Four, you can begin to occasionally add back into your diet some of the foods to which you were previously sensitive (*not* allergic foods which should only be added after clearance from your physician). However, these foods should not be consumed more than once a week. Obviously, if any food causes problems, you should eliminate it altogether. As a good rule of thumb, remember: If in doubt, leave it out.

Although Phase Four provides you with more options when it comes to your food choices, compared to Phases One through Three, your goal here should be to continue to consume only foods and beverages that are healthy. This phase includes all the foods and beverages you safely consumed during the first three phases of the Lyme Inflammation Diet, plus new selections from the food and beverage categories below. Again, avoid at all times staples of the standard American diet, such as sodas, processed foods, sugar and sugar products, refined carbohydrates, and unhealthy fats and oils.

During Phase Four, all foods and beverages from the following categories are permissible so long as you do not experience symptoms of inflammation after consuming them.

Beverages: Filtered water, mineral water, unsweetened fruit juices (acai, apple, blackberry, blueberry, cherry, cranberry, purple grape, pomegranate, raspberry), vegetable juices (ideally freshly squeezed), green tea, and herbal teas. Coffee is also permitted, but if you drink coffee, try to limit yourself to two cups per day.

Fruits: Apples, apricots, avocado, bananas, blackberries, blueberries, cantaloupe, cherries, cranberries, coconut, dates, figs, grapes (purple), grapefruit, kiwi, lemons, limes, mangoes, oranges, papayas, pears, prunes, raspberries, strawberries, watermelon. Aim for three to five servings of fruit each day.

Dairy Products: Limit your intake of dairy foods to organic butter, organic milk and cheeses, goat's milk and cheese (feta), and organic, unsweetened kefir and yogurt.

Eggs: Ideally, you should only eat eggs from organically raised, free-range chickens. Eggs eaten in moderation are an excellent source of proteins and other important nutrients for most people.

Beans and Legumes: All beans and legumes listed in Phases One through Three above are permissible during Phase Four.

Grains: Barley, brown rice, buckwheat, couscous, kamut, millet, oats, quinoa, rye, whole wheat flour, and wild rice. Remember, gluten sensitivity can be a significant cause of food intolerance leading to chronic inflammation, and in some cases, many need to be permanently eliminated from your diet.

Meats and Fish: Organic, free-range beef, bison, chicken, lamb, turkey, and venison, wild-caught flounder, mackerel, salmon, sardines, sole, and tilapia.

Nuts and Seeds: Almonds, Brazil nuts, cashews, flaxseed (freshly ground), hemp seed (freshly ground), pecans, pumpkin seeds, sesame seeds, sunflower seeds, and walnuts.

Vegetables: Artichokes, arugula, asparagus, beets, bok choy, broccoli, Brussels sprouts, cabbage, cauliflower, carrots, celery, chard, chives, collard greens, cucumber, garlic, green beans, green and red peppers, kale, leeks, mustard greens, onions, peas, red potatoes, pumpkin, radishes, romaine and other dark green lettuce, scallions, seaweed, shiitake mushrooms, sprouts, squash, string beans, sweet potatoes, tomatoes, turnips, watercress, and yams. Aim for at least five to seven servings of vegetables each day. Remember, nightshade-food sensitivity is a major cause of food intolerance leading to chronic inflammation.

Spices: Black pepper, cayenne, cinnamon, curry, garlic, ginger, mints, oregano, parsley, rosemary, sage, salt (Celtic or sea salt; avoid commercial table salt), and turmeric.

Sweeteners: Raw organic honey, stevia, sorbitol, maple syrup, and xylitol are all acceptable.

Other: This is the good news—you can use dark chocolate that is 70 percent or greater cocoa content as long as it is not sweetened with sugar.

A Sample Daily Menu for Phase Four

To help you create meal plans during Phase Four, here is a sample of breakfast, lunch, and dinner menus that you can consider. All the recipes listed in the resources section may be used in Phase Four.

Breakfast

- French toast (Ezekiel bread) with maple syrup and blueberries
- Yogurt with vanilla and stevia
- Hot chocolate

Lunch

- Potato salad

- 4-ounce salmon patty

- Small tossed salad with romaine lettuce, broccoli, carrots, cranberries, pine nuts, and pecans with olive oil and apple cider vinegar dressing

- Green tea with ginger and lime

Dinner

- Spinach salad with sliced tomatoes, onions, cucumbers

- Venison stew with potatoes

- Ezekiel bread (or sprouted grain rolls) with organic butter

- Dessert—sliced pineapple with shredded coconut

Additional General Dietary Guidelines (all Phases)

The following guidelines should be followed after you complete all four phases of the Lyme Inflammation Diet so that you can maintain the health benefits you've achieved.

- Avoid sodas and all commercial beverages, including carbonated beverages that include sugar or artificial sweeteners, sports drinks with added sugar, commercial fruit and vegetable juices, and any beverage that contains salt, sweeteners, and/or other chemical additives and preservatives.

* Eat fruits fresh, not canned, and limit your intake of fruits that are high in natural sugar content, such as bananas, grapes, and raisins.

* Avoid the use of all refined carbohydrates, including white pasta and rice and white flour and flour products.

* Avoid sugary desserts, especially cakes, donuts, pastries, and other cooked high-sugar products that are high in exogenous AGEs.

* Avoid honey-glazed meats, barbecued meats, and processed commercial meat products, such as bacon, bologna, hot dogs, salami, and sausage, as well as all fast-food fish, meats, and poultry (fish, hamburgers, chicken). Pork and shellfish should also be avoided, as should farm-raised fish and non-organic beef, chicken, lamb, and turkey.

* Avoid all trans-fatty acids and hydrogenated and partially hydrogenated oils, as well as lard, margarine, and shortenings. Commercially packaged foods and fried foods should also be eliminated from your diet, as should vegetable oils such as corn, cottonseed, and safflower.

* Sources of good fats include coconut and extra virgin olive oil, organic butter (especially from pasture-fed cows), organic raw milk cheese and other cheeses from pasture-fed cows, avocado, nuts and seeds, and sesame oil.

* For cooking purposes, use olive oil (or olive combined with sesame oil) and, for high temperature cooking, coconut oil.

* Avoid the use of table salt (Celtic and sea salt are both permissible), as well as all food additives, especially aspartame, monosodium glutamate (MSG), nitrates, and sulfites.

* Be sure to have a healthy breakfast. Breakfast is considered by many health experts to be the most important meal of the day. Therefore, do not skip breakfast.

* Avoid alcohol completely during Lyme treatment and for at least three to six months after you go off of antibiotics. While I prefer that you abstain permanently, if you are going to drink alcohol, please limit yourself to one to two glasses of wine (or one to two beers) per day after the three-to six-month abstinence period has been completed.

Dealing with Sugar Cravings

One of the most common dietary issues that Lyme patients deal with is sugar cravings. It is critical that you discontinue use of sugar if you want to recover from chronic inflammation. This may be difficult, because sugar is addictive. However, there are ways to deal with these cravings successfully.

The first step is to be aware that when you stop consuming sugar you probably will feel poorly for about three days for the following three reasons: (1) the yeast in your body (such as Candida) will be dying off and you may have symptoms from yeast toxins in your body, (2) withdrawal from any addictive substance (including caffeine) causes about three days of minor symptoms, and (3) it may take a few days for insulin and other hormone levels to adjust to the change in sugar status.

The next step is to eat multiple small meals per day, making sure that you include a source of protein and quality fat at each meal. Many patients find that snacking with a few almonds is very helpful for this purpose, as almonds contain healthy protein and fat.

Finally, adding certain nutritional supplements can be very useful. Be sure to add a good quality multiple vitamin and mineral that contains B-complex and chromium. (In chapter 6, I will discuss the nutritional supplements that I recommend to my patients.) Three other supplements are also very useful: glutamine (500–1,000 mg three to four times a day), alpha lipoic acid (100–300 mg per day), and 5-hydroxytryptophan (5-HTP 50–100 mg one to two times a day).

As a general principle, about one month after elimination of sugar, you will notice some very interesting changes. You will observe that the cravings have greatly lessened and that sugar will seem extremely sweet. Also, you will feel very poorly when you attempt to eat it (especially if you try to eat it on an empty stomach). If you can avoid sugar, you should notice three benefits in about a month: your energy will increase, your gastrointestinal system will work better, and you will begin to lose undesired weight.

Going Forward

I encourage all my patients, not just those with Lyme disease, to stick as closely as possible to the healthy eating guidelines that make up Phase Four of the Lyme Inflammation Diet once they have completed the first three phases. My hope is that you will do the same. As you make your daily food choices, here are some other important tips to keep in mind.

Generally, the foods you eat each day should consist of a wide array of fresh vegetables, high-quality protein foods, whole grains, and quality fats. The foods you eat should also be consumed as close to their natural state as possible. As I've already emphasized, this means eliminating all fast foods and processed/refined foods from your diet.

As you become more conscious of the relationship between healthy eating and good health, I also encourage you to begin to get in touch with how the foods you eat make you feel. There is a big difference between the physical and emotional satisfaction derived from high-quality, nutrient-dense foods and the addictive "quick fix" feelings that come from eating unhealthy foods. By tuning into how you feel as you eat, you will start to develop an unerring instinct that lets you know what foods are most appropriate for you, as well as when you should eat them. The more you "listen" to the instinctual messages of your feelings, the more you will find yourself effortlessly gravitating towards the food selections that are best for you.

Eat from the Rainbow

The more variety there is in your diet, the more likely you are to meet your basic nutritional needs. An easy way to ensure that you achieve this variety is by including foods of every color in your daily diet. Just as the rainbow of vibrant colors is what makes a healthy garden so appealing to the eye, so too does a rainbow array of foods make for healthy eating.

In addition to the many nutritional benefits these foods provide (vitamins, minerals, enzymes, antioxidants, and other important nutrients), most of them also promote alkalinity in the body, instead of the acidic effect that is so common in the standard American diet. The health benefits of a primarily alkalizing diet are many and continue to be discovered.

One of the primary benefits has to do with the state of your body's bloodstream. In the 1930s, German researcher Dr. Otto Warburg proved that infectious microorganisms cannot long exist in an oxygen-rich environment, such as the bloodstream. Dr. Warburg also showed that cancer cannot thrive in an oxygen-rich environment. Dr. Warburg's discoveries twice won him the Nobel Prize in Medicine. Today, we know that alkalizing foods increase the amount of oxygen in the bloodstream, while acidifying foods decrease the amount of oxygen in the bloodstream, making it much easier for harmful microorganisms, including the *Bb* bacteria and related Lyme co-infections, to take hold. (For more information on the benefits of alkalizing foods, I recommend *The Acid-Alkaline Food Guide* by Dr. Susan Brown and Larry Trivieri, Jr.)

Here is a list of some of the most common healthy "rainbow" foods:

* White—coconut flesh (fresh, dried), coconut milk, and coconut oil (for cooking); organic, plain yogurt and kefir (containing active cultures and no sugar); and properly cooked eggs (soft not hard)

* Green—broccoli, celery, chard, chlorella, cucumber, dark greens, Granny Smith apples, green tea, kelp and other seaweed foods, lime, olive oil, and romaine lettuce

* Yellow—curry, dandelion, egg yolk, lemon, pineapple, yellow squash

* Orange—apricots, cantaloupe, carrots (eat sparingly due to their high concentration of natural sugars), mango, pumpkin, sweet potato, and yams

* Red—apples, cherries, raspberries, red peppers, strawberries, tomatoes, and watermelon

* Purple—plums, pomegranates, prunes, and purple grapes and raisins (eat sparingly due to high natural sugar content)

* Blue—bilberries, blackberries, and blueberries

* Brown—beans, brown rice and other whole grains (barley, Ezekiel bread, oatmeal, quinoa, sprouted grains, and so forth), fermented soy products (miso, natto, tempeh), garlic, ginger, onions, nuts and seeds, range-fed meats and poultry, and wild-caught fish low in mercury

Fruit Intake While Using Antibiotics—A Special Note

As a general rule, during antibiotic treatment, you should limit your intake of most fruits because of their naturally high sugar content. One of the unfortunate side effects of antibiotics is that they have a tendency to kill off both unhealthy and healthy bacteria. One role of healthy bacteria is to prevent uncontrolled growth of potentially harmful organisms, such as *yeast*. As a consequence of the "friendly fire" killing the healthy bacteria (such as acidophilus and bifidus), the yeast in the body may grow out of control.

Yeast are normal inhabitants in the body, but do not cause problems because of the policing presence of healthy bacteria. Yeast tend to grow more easily when sugar is present in the diet. Sugar from any form, including healthy fruit, will feed yeast.

Therefore, when implementing the LID program while on antibiotics, you should observe the following principles when doing the various phases of this program:

* Eat the Phase One fruits only two to three times a week while on antibiotics.

* Use the Phase Two fruits only one to two times a week while on antibiotics.

* In Phase Three, when lemon, lime, and grapefruit are available to you, these particular low-sugar fruits may be used daily if desired.

* In *all* phases, take a good "friendly bacteria" replacement formula (also known as a probiotic) on a regular basis as long as you are on an antibiotic.

Summing Up

Follow the above dietary recommendations to reduce the levels of inflammation, and you will be well on your way to improved health. You will experience increased energy levels and an overall feeling of well-being. This will make a tremendous difference in your journey to overcome Lyme disease and other potential co-infections. Now let's review the key points of this chapter by answering the most common questions about chronic inflammation and its relationship to Lyme disease and other co-infections.

What is inflammation?

Inflammation is a normal bodily process that is triggered by your body's immune system in response to injury, infectious microorganisms (bacteria, fungi, viruses), exposure to allergy and sensitivity-causing substances, and temporary stress. In healthy people, the inflammation process is short-lived, ending when the problem that triggered it is successfully dealt with by the body. When inflammation becomes chronic, however, a wide range of health problems can eventually arise.

What causes inflammation to become chronic?

The primary causes of chronic inflammation are allergies and sensitivities, advanced glycation end products (AGEs), environmental toxins and pollutants, persistent fatigue and lack of sleep, free radical damage, infectious microorganisms, insulin and leptin resistance, lack of exercise, obesity, and smoking, each of which is explained in more detail earlier in this chapter. But perhaps the biggest and most serious cause of chronic inflammation is poor diet.

Why does chronic inflammation have significance when it comes to Lyme disease and other co-infections?

Lyme disease and chronic inflammation act as a very unhealthy double-edged sword. On the one hand, the *Bb* bacteria that causes Lyme disease, as well as other co-infections, help to trigger chronic inflammation once they become disseminated in the body. On the other hand, chronic inflammation that already exists prior to infection by the *Bb* bacteria and other co-infections impairs the ability of the body's immune system to respond effectively to these bacteria. Because of the way chronic inflammation diminishes immune function and efficiency, *Bb* and other co-infections are able to gain stronger footholds in the body, causing increasingly severe health symptoms.

How can I determine if I am at risk for chronic inflammation?

Ask your physician to screen your blood for levels of C-reactive protein (CRP). Elevated levels of CRP are a strong indication that chronic inflammation exists. The more elevated the CRP levels in the bloodstream, the greater the degree of chronic inflammation that exists.

You can also assess your risk for chronic inflammation on your own, using the self-assessment questionnaire that I've supplied above.

What can I do to bring chronic inflammation under control?

The single most important thing that you and anyone else can do to prevent and reverse chronic inflammation is to make a commitment to eating a healthy diet, consuming foods and beverages that do not trigger the inflammation response in the body. Following the principles of the Lyme Inflammation Diet is effective in reducing chronic inflammation. I consider it to be the most essential self-care step you can take to ensure your health and the health of your loved ones. By doing so, you will also dramatically assist your body in its recovery from Lyme disease, while setting the stage for long-term good overall health.

Because of how tenaciously the *Bb* bacteria and other co-infections can take hold in the human body, many patients need to enhance the benefits of the Lyme Inflammation Diet with other medical and self-care strategies. In the next chapter, I will share with you the importance of a specific integrative treatment approach to Lyme that includes antibiotics, nutritional supplements, and alternative-medicine approaches. I will provide my recommendations for the specific effective therapies for Lyme and each of the main co-infections that we utilize in our clinical office setting.

Chapter Six

Core Treatment Strategies for Lyme Disease and Other Tick-Borne Diseases

❋

In this chapter, I want to build on the treatment measures I discussed in chapters 4 and 5 for improving immune function and reducing chronic inflammation. I will share with you the core principles of effective therapy for Lyme disease (LD) and the other tick-borne diseases (TBDs). In addition to the Lyme Inflammation Diet, the other two components of Lyme treatment include the proper use of antibiotics and the use of alternative and complementary therapies such as herbal and nutritional supplements.

The treatments discussed in this chapter can be considered as the *basic* essentials of my approach to Lyme disease and other tick-borne diseases. Depending on each patient's *specific* problems and/or needs, additional therapies may also be necessary. I will be discussing those therapies with you in the remaining chapters of this book.

Beginning Treatment—Making the Diagnosis

There are two important elements that you need to consider at the beginning of treatment. They are helping your doctor to acquire an excellent patient history, along with a detailed physical examination, and obtaining accurate diagnostic laboratory testing.

The Importance of a Medical History and Physical Examination: To make an accurate diagnosis of an illness, a doctor is trained to follow certain systematic steps. The first, and by far the most important, step in that diagnostic process is the doctor's obtaining a good patient "history." A good history is a patient's complete story of his or her illness told from onset to its current status. The skilled doctor will listen carefully to the patient as the story is being told and will then ask leading questions that prompt the patient to reveal important additional details of the story.

When the patient's entire story is completed, the doctor will then perform a careful physical examination as the next step. When both steps are complete, the doctor can then match that patient's historical and physical information with the information in the doctor's knowledge database to come up with a list of diagnostic possibilities. If the pattern of the patient's story and exam matches a recognizable pattern in the doctor's knowledge database, then the doctor is likely to head down the proper pathway of "making the correct diagnosis."

It would be ideal if all patients with suspected Lyme or other tick-borne diseases would be evaluated by an experienced Lyme-aware doctor (also known as Lyme-literate M.D. or DO). However, that possibility may not always be attainable. For that reason, it is important that you help your doctor understand your story in a way that will allow the doctor to more easily recognize the possibility of a tick-borne disease.

My recommendation to you is to use the Burrascano LD Symptom checklist and the symptom lists for the other TBDs that I provided for you in chapter 2 of this book. It is helpful when seeing a doctor to have thoroughly thought through those symptoms discussed in chapter 2 and then to discuss those symptoms with your doctor who is obtaining your history. It is also a good idea to take summary notes with you so that you can present your story in an organized and logical manner. In addition to your symptoms, be sure to include in your history the risk factors for LD and the TBDs (such as outdoor activities like hunting or gardening) discussed in chapter 3.

There is another important piece of advice to follow when initially presenting your story to your doctor: *Start your story from when you were last well and build from there.* Tell the doctor something like this: "Doctor, I felt great until the spring of 1996 when I began having symptoms of. . . ."

The importance of giving your doctor a thorough and well-organized history cannot be overemphasized. It is likely that three-quarters of the information needed to make a medical diagnosis comes to the doctor in the form of a good patient history and physical exam. Unfortunately in these days of managed care, doctors often do not have time to obtain a thorough history and perform a careful physical examination. As a result, they are often overly dependent on other diagnostic steps (such as laboratory testing) that comprise the remaining one-quarter of the diagnostic information.

The Role of Accurate Laboratory Diagnostic Testing: The role of diagnostic tests is also critical, however, for two reasons: (1) diagnostic tests can rule out other medical causes for the symptoms (these other medical problems may actually mimic LD or TBD symptoms) and (2) diagnostic tests may be useful to confirm and/or follow a suspected case of Lyme or its co-infections. Let's discuss each of these two points.

The first reason for diagnostic testing involves doing tests to eliminate or "rule out" causes other than the tick-borne disorders as a reason for the symptoms. In chapter 3, I provided you with an extensive (but by no means complete) list of tests that are often done for the purpose of looking for hidden causes of symptoms, including endocrine diseases, chronic viral diseases, immune system disorders, neurological disorders, sleep disorders, heavy metal toxicity, chronic dental disease, and other causes. Remember, there are a number of disorders that have symptoms very similar to those of Lyme disease and the TBDs.

A Lyme-aware doctor will always be alert to the possibility that other non-Lyme medical disorders can look just like Lyme. It is also important to keep in mind that Lyme patients can get all the same diseases that people without Lyme can get. One of my patients, Alicia, illustrates this principle well.

Alicia is a 42-year-old woman who came to my office with symptoms of severe fatigue, foggy thinking, anger outbursts, various muscle and joint pains (especially of the small joints in her hands), strange rashes, and headaches that she experienced for three years. She had seen five other doctors who could find nothing significantly wrong with her. In taking her history, it was of note that she lived in the woods and had removed several ticks from her body over the years. However, there were three features of her history that sent up "red flags" of doubt in my mind as I listened to her: (1) during courses of antibiotics for sinusitis and other infections, she often would feel worse rather than better (LD and TBDs patients usually report the opposite), (2) she felt much better when the weather was dry rather than when damp (LD patients often like damp over dry), and (3) she revealed that when she left her home on vacation or business, she would often feel much better within a few days into the trip.

I completed her history and physical exam not fully con-vinced that she had Lyme disease as she suspected. I performed my usual laboratory tests, but I also asked her to see an allergist medical doctor. My suspicion was that she might be dealing with "mold" issues. Her Lyme workup came back with no evidence of Lyme or a TBD, but her allergist's evaluation came back with strong evidence of black mold (*Stachybotrys*) in her basement from previous flooding there. After appropriate treatment from the allergist and necessary home remediation, she is now improved.

The second reason for the importance of diagnostic testing involves the confirmation of a suspected diagnosis of LD or a TBD. Related to this is the usefulness of certain diagnostic tests in following the progress of Lyme treatment. In chapter 3, I discussed the laboratory tests that are done by Lyme-aware doctors for the various tick-borne illnesses. I will say more about two of those tests—the sensitive Western Blot and the CD57 lymphocyte assay—because they directly relate to treatment issues that I will be discussing in this chapter.

The sensitive Lyme Western Blot is one of the most useful Lyme tests in the office of a Lyme-aware doctor. By "sensitive," I am referring to the fact that it has a reduced number of false negative results. The reason for its increased sensitivity is that it includes the bands kDa 31 and 34. If the patient has not had the Lymerix vaccine, those bands should not be present. (An exception that we sometimes see is the situation of a false positive sensitive Western Blot due to certain viruses, syphilis, and others conditions that I discussed in chapter 3.) Unfortunately, this test is only routinely performed by a limited number of labs (such as IgeneX in California and MDL in New Jersey) and not by the usual commercial labs.

The CD57 cell test is also useful clinically, but primarily for following progress during Lyme treatment. The CD57 cell is a white blood cell of the lymphocyte classification that functions as a "natural killer cell" (NK cell). I discussed the role of NK cells extensively in chapter 4. For the sake of our discussion at this time, it is important to realize three things about the CD57 cells: (1) when they are in a healthy normal range (125-250) that is usually a sign that Lyme is under reasonably good control, (2) when very low (less than 20) that is generally a sign of poor control of Lyme, and (3) when, in addition to antibiotics, certain natural and/or non-toxic therapies (such as cat's claw, low dose naltrexone, and others) are added, often the CD57 counts rise, reflecting improvement in immune function directed against Lyme organisms.

The First "Core" Component of Lyme Therapy: Antibiotics

The proper use of antibiotics is critical to the control of LD and the TBDs. Effective antibiotic treatment depends on the following factors:

* Knowing which antibiotic drugs are most appropriate for each patient

* Knowing the most effective dosages to use

* Determining the proper duration of treatment

* Determining if combination treatment (using multiple antibiotics) is necessary.

Additionally, the antibiotic approach to Lyme disease depends on the stage at which Lyme is detected and the severity of a patient's symptoms. For example, more aggressive treatment approaches are necessary if cardiovascular and/or neurological systems are significantly involved.

Your Lyme-aware physician's clinical assessment of the likelihood of the different forms of Lyme being present is also an important factor in determining proper treatment. For example, Lyme occurs in three forms: *spirochete*, L-form, and cystic form. In general, the *spirochete* form is most effectively treated using penicillins and cephalosporins. The *L-form* responds well to the tetracycline class of antibiotics (doxycycline and minocycline) and the macrolide class of antibiotics (clarithromycin, azithromycin, and the new ketolide named telithromycin). The *cystic* form of Lyme responds to metronidazole and possibly hydroxychloroquine, tinidazole, nitazoxanide, and dapsone.

If your Lyme-aware doctor believes that all three forms are likely present, then you may need a combination of three (or more) antibiotics to treat all three forms. Many chronic LD patients, especially those who have had multiple bouts of previous antibiotics, will have multiple LD forms present and, therefore, require a combination of the antibiotic medications in order to bring LD under control. Unfortunately, there is no laboratory test that can tell your doctor which of the forms is present in your body. A Lyme-aware doctor will make that determination based on experience and clinical judgment. Again, as a general rule, the longer you have had Lyme and the greater the previous antibiotic exposure, the more likely that multiple forms will be present.

In addition to various forms of Lyme, there are other reasons that combinations of antibiotics are so vital to the effective treatment of Lyme disease. One of these reasons is that the *Bb* bacteria that cause Lyme can take root in both the body's tissues and its fluids. Generally, a single type of antibiotic cannot effectively treat Lyme when it is present in both areas of the body.

Another reason that combination antibiotic treatment may be necessary has to do with the fact that the *Bb* bacteria can burrow deep inside the body's cells, where they are able to elude the antibiotic drugs that are unable to penetrate into cells where Lyme is hiding. In such cases, combining antibiotics that can penetrate the cells with antibiotics that are effective outside the cells is usually the proper course of treatment.

A final important reason for combination antibiotic treatment concerns the fact that the *Bb* bacteria can shift from one form to another during the various cycles of their lifespan and in response to certain antibiotics. This principle directly relates to my discussion above about the three forms of Lyme. This is a very important treatment point and, therefore, I would like to further illustrate this principle.

As I pointed out above, different antibiotic drug classes work best for each of the three different forms of *Bb*. When the penicillin or cephalosporin group (affecting the cell-walled *spirochete* form) is used alone, Lyme will quickly change its form to avoid these classes of drugs. In other words, while the penicillin and cephalosporin groups of antibiotics are wonderful tools against Lyme, if used alone there is a potential problem—Lyme is induced to change its form in order to survive. Therefore, these drugs probably should not be used without concurrent use of an antibiotic that targets L-forms (such as the macrolides or tetracycline group). Otherwise, your Lyme may just be changing form from *spirochete* to L-form (or cystic form), thereby evading your treatment. To be sure of eradicating *Bb*, particularly in its later stages, the concurrent use of different classes of antibiotics is generally required

The length of time that a person has suffered with Lyme is another important factor to be considered in your Lyme treatment program. As a general rule, the longer the Lyme has been present, the longer the antibiotic treatment will last, and the more aggressive treatment may need to be for LD and TBD control. It may require six months (or more) of treatment per infection when multiple infections are present. The time length of antibiotic treatment is often able to be reduced if a person follows the self-care recommendations that I discuss in this book.

A final general principle of antibiotic use that I want to discuss is how the antibiotics are administered. Depending on the severity of a person's symptoms, the method of administration of antibiotic drugs may vary. There are three basic methods of administration: orally (PO) in the form of pills or capsules, intravenously (IV) in which antibiotics are injected into the veins, and intramuscularly (IM) in which antibiotics are injected into the muscles. In some cases, a combination of these methods may also be necessary.

Types of Antibiotic Drugs for Treating Lyme Disease

I want to discuss the specific principles of antibiotic use for Lyme disease. There are five classes of antibiotics that we commonly use for Lyme disease.

Tetracyclines. The most commonly used antibiotics in this class are doxycycline and minocycline. To be effective, tetracyclines must be administered in dosages sufficient to produce high blood levels. To achieve this, high oral daily dosages may be required, and these dosages may need to be monitored by blood levels. If these dosages are not tolerated due to side effects, the drug may need to be administered intravenously. One of the advantages of tetracyclines is that they are able to penetrate the cell walls, making them a good choice when *Bb* and other bacteria have migrated inside the cells. The usual oral dosage of oral doxycycline is 100–300 mg twice a day with food (not with dairy products or mineral supplements). The dosage for minocycline is 100 mg twice a day. (One could use higher doses, but those doses tend to cause much more side effects.) Doxycycline can also be administered intravenously. The usual dosage for IV doxycycline is 300–400 mg once a day.

Precautions: Like all antibiotic drugs (as well as drugs in general), tetracyclines can cause adverse side effects and should not be used by pregnant and breastfeeding women. They are also not recommended for children aged eight and under because they can interfere with the growth and proper development of bones and cartilage and may also discolor teeth. Other side effects that need to be monitored include nausea (they should be taken with non-dairy food for this reason), yeast infections, gastrointestinal problems, rash (usually mild), and dizziness (especially minocycline). In some instances, tetracyclines can also cause eye, kidney, and liver problems. During the course of treatment, people using tetracyclines (especially doxycycline) should avoid exposure to sunlight, as the drugs can significantly increase the risk of "sun sensitivity." This reaction can occur even through glass car windows and on overcast days and is *not* effectively prevented by sunblock. Additionally, antacids, dairy products, and iron supplements should also be avoided at the same time as tetracyclines (take an hour or more away from these substances), as these all interfere with tetracyclines' ability to be absorbed. Finally, the medications in the tetracycline family (especially minocycline) may rarely cause a condition called "pseudotumor cerebri," which is a serious complication for which the medication needs to be discontinued. The most common symptom of this condition is a severe and unrelenting headache after taking a dose of the medication. If this symptom occurs, I recommend notifying your Lyme-aware doctor promptly so that the proper evaluation may be done.

Penicillins. Antibiotic drugs in this class include oral amoxicillin and intramuscular (IM) benzathine penicillin (Bicillin LA). To be effective against Lyme, high blood and tissue levels of penicillins need to be sustained for 72 hours or more. Since blood levels of penicillins can significantly vary from patient to patient, the blood levels of amoxicillin are often measured during the course of treatment. The dose of amoxicillin commonly used for Lyme is 1,000–2,000 mg every eight hours, and it is at times combined with probenecid 500 mg, which helps to keep blood levels high. Amoxicillin combined with clavulanic acid (Augmentin) is also very effective.

Oral penicillin (such as Pen VK) is not effective. However, intramuscular penicillin, administered at a dose of 1,200,000 units two to three times a week, is highly useful. Although more painful when administered, the LA form of Bicillin is more effective than the CR form (which contains a local anesthetic.) As previously mentioned, the penicillin group should always be combined with other antibiotic classes that target the L-form (e.g., azithromycin) of Lyme and ideally the cystic form (e.g., metronidazole) of Lyme also.

Precautions: Penicillins are relatively safe. They should never be used if allergy to them is known or strongly suspected. Common side effects include fever, joint swelling, nausea, rash, and yeast overgrowth. Penicillins can also sometimes interfere with the body's production of white blood cells known as neutrophils. In rare cases, they can also be fatal if administered to people who are allergic to them.

Cephalosporins. These medications are related to the penicillin group. Drugs in this class that are most commonly used to treat Lyme include two oral preparations and two intravenous drugs. Of the oral choices, cefuroxime (Ceftin) was the first drug approved by the Food and Drug Administration (FDA) for the treatment of early-stage Lyme disease. It is given orally at a dose of 500 mg twice a day while some patients may require higher doses. The other oral cephalosporin preparation is cefdinir (Omnicef). It is very effective and can be taken as 600 mg once a day. Two other drugs in this class, ceftriaxone (Rocephin) and cefotaxime (Claforan) are usually administered intravenously.

(Other IV medicines are also used, but these two are by far the most common ones used.) The dosages for the IV preparations are 1–2 grams every eight hours in the case of cefotaxime and 2 grams once per day in the case of ceftriaxone. (Some experts prefer to use this medication twice a day, four days on and three days off, per week.) These latter two drugs are later generations of this drug class and, overall, are more effective for treating Lyme disease. During treatment, high blood levels need to be achieved. Ideally, blood levels should be measured on a regular basis throughout the course of treatment. Finally, as with the penicillins, the medications in this class should ideally be combined with the oral antibiotic classes that target the L-form of Lyme and, ideally, the cystic form also.

Precautions: Cephalosporin drugs can cause liver toxicity and may lower the white blood count, especially the cell called neutrophil. For these reasons, routine and regular testing of blood should be done to detect any adverse reactions. Ceftriaxone can also cause gallstones, which can be prevented by using the medication, ursodiol. Other possible side effects of drugs in this class include diarrhea, rash, and yeast overgrowth, which at times can be serious. Additionally, some people who are allergic to penicillins are also allergic to cephalosporins, and therefore, great caution must be used in treating a patient who is allergic to penicillin with medications in this class.

Macrolides and Ketolides: Drugs in this class include azithromycin (Zithromax), clarithormycin (Biaxin), and the ketolide, telithromycin (Ketek). All these medicines are related to erythromycin, but erythromycin itself is not an effective treatment for Lyme disease and should not be used to treat LD. Like the tetracycline drugs, macrolides and ketolides are able to penetrate cell walls and tissues. Clarithormycin is given orally at a dose of 1,000 mg per day and is very effective for treating Lyme. But it is often difficult to tolerate due to its metallic aftertaste and the various gastrointestinal problems it can cause. Azithromycin is not as effective for Lyme as clarithromycin, but is better tolerated. The dose range for oral azithromycin is 250–600 mg daily. Azithromycin produces better results when given intravenously compared to oral administration. The IV dose of azithromycin is 500 mg per day.

Some experts feel that the drug of choice in this category is telithromycin, which is both better tolerated and more effective. The usual dose of telithromycin is 800 mg per day. This drug was engineered to prevent drug resistance, a phenomenon that occurs when bacteria, after prolonged drug exposure, mutate into forms that are resistant to drug therapy. However, if telithromycin is to be used, the patient's electrocardiogram and liver function status need to be carefully evaluated, since this medication, in my experience, may have a greater chance of causing side effects involving the heart and liver than the macrolides. For this reason I rarely, if ever, use telithromycin.

Precautions: Macrolide drugs can cause cramping, diarrhea, and other gastrointestinal problems, as well as nausea, rashes, and vomiting. In some cases, they can also cause temporary hearing and vision problems (ringing in the ears, hearing loss, and blurry or double vision). They can also lead to unhealthy elevations of liver enzymes, which can be an early sign of liver damage. They may also cause reduction in white blood cell counts. Blood tests throughout the course of treatment with macrolides are necessary to monitor liver function and white blood cell (WBC) count. As mentioned, the macrolides can sometimes affect the electrical activity of the heart (called the Q-T interval), and this may need to be assessed prior to using these medications for an extended time. Additionally, macrolides can also interfere with a variety of other drugs by inhibiting the liver breakdown of other medicines. Therefore, be sure to mention to your doctor and your pharmacist any other medications you may be on prior to beginning macrolide treatment.

Metronidazole. This antibiotic drug is increasingly being used to treat Lyme disease. Originally developed to treat harmful, single-cell bacteria and parasites, metronidazole (Flagyl) has since been shown to be useful in killing off *Bb* bacteria in their cystic form. This ability to destroy Lyme cystic form is something that the other classes of antibiotic drugs cannot do. For that reason, most Lyme-aware physicians utilize metronidazole in combination with one or more of the above classes of drugs for cases of chronic Lyme where there is a high likelihood of the presence of cystic forms. The dosage is 250–500 mg two to three times a day. (Tetracyclines, such as doxycycline, are *not* used with metronidazole because they can inhibit the latter's effectiveness.)

Precautions: Common, relatively minor, side effects of metronidazole include yeast overgrowth, headache, nausea, metallic taste, and rash. More serious side effects include nerve damage that can result in numbness and tingling of the extremities and, in rare cases, seizures. Metronidazole use should be immediately discontinued if these symptoms appear. It should also not be used for anyone on blood-thinning medications, such as coumadin, since metronidazole can increase the blood-thinning effects of these drugs, potentially leading to an increased risk of internal bleeding. Pregnant women should also avoid this medication. The drug should *never* be used with alcohol or alcohol-containing products (even cough syrups), since this combination can cause severe headache, nausea, skin flushing, vomiting, and other symptoms. (This effect is similar to the anti-alcoholism medication called Antabuse.)

In summary, there are several excellent Lyme disease antibiotic choices from which your Lyme-aware doctor has to choose. Each patient's individual Lyme situation needs to be assessed to determine the precise antibiotic protocol that would be most effective. Because this type of antibiotic decision-making can be so complex, it is beyond the scope of this book to attempt to present all the possible scenarios in detail. It is advisable for a physician who is interested in becoming more Lyme-aware to visit the Web site of the International Lyme and Associated Diseases Society (www.ilads.org) for more information. On this site, one can also find excellent specific treatment guidelines for Lyme and the other TBDs by Dr. Joseph Burrascano, who truly is a pioneer in the field of Lyme medicine.

A Special Note about the "Jarish-Herxheimer" Reaction

Within a few days (usually one to three) after beginning antibiotic therapy, it is common for many patients with Lyme to suddenly begin experiencing a worsening of their symptoms. In some cases, this experience can be extremely uncomfortable. Additionally, it can also be mistaken as an allergic reaction to the antibiotic drugs that have been prescribed. In actuality, this reaction is a positive sign that the antibiotics are working and is known as the Jarish-Herxheimer reaction. Commonly this name is abbreviated to Herxheimer, or simply "Herx."

A Herxheimer occurs because the *Bb* bacteria, under attack from the antibiotics, start to break up and die, releasing toxins and other harmful debris as they do so. This, in turn, causes the body's immune system to temporarily go into overdrive in order to cope with the abrupt deluge of toxins and debris.

A Herxheimer can last from a few days to two weeks or more, depending on how disseminated the *Bb* bacteria is in the body. The greater the dissemination, generally the longer a Herxheimer will last. During this time, in addition to the temporary worsening of previous Lyme symptoms, one may also experience chills, fevers, headache, nausea, and even a drop in blood pressure levels. Don't be alarmed by this, and don't stop taking the antibiotics that have been prescribed. Do, however, contact your physician to let him know what you are experiencing, so that he can determine if your symptoms are due to Herxheimer and rule out a true allergic response to the drugs. Two "natural" ways to reduce the symptoms of Herxheimers are hydration (2 to 3 quarts of quality water a day) and the bioflavonoid quercitin (500–1500 mg per day).

Another important consideration to be aware of is that major Herxes generally occur during the *Bb* bacteria's growth phase (which phase is also known as a "Lyme cycle"). This is also the time during the *Bb* bacteria's life cycle that antibiotics are most effective in eradicating them, since they are most vulnerable during this phase. Lyme's growth phase occurs approximately every three to four weeks (up to six weeks maximum), and therefore, intermittent symptom flare-ups or Herxes usually also will occur at those same intervals. These cycle-related Herxes continue to occur over time until a sufficient quantity of *Bb* has been killed off. In most cases, symptoms of subsequent Herxheimer reactions are shorter and less severe than the initial one, indicating that treatment is progressing successfully. If your reactions continue to be of the same severity and duration, this may be a sign that there is dysregulation of your immune system that needs to be addressed or that the antibiotic regimen may need adjustment. Also, there are times when untreated co-infections need immediate attention, after which time Lyme can be successfully addressed. Whatever the cause, it is important to alert your physician if your Herxheimer symptoms continue unabated.

Types of Antibiotic Drugs for Treating Other Tick-Borne Diseases

What follows are the antibiotic treatments I have found to be most effective for treating the co-infections—the tick-borne diseases often coexisting with Lyme infection.

Bartonella/BLO

There are two antibiotics that have been found to be most useful for treating Bartonella/BLO. My choice of these two antibiotics depends on two issues: (1) the extent to which the central nervous system (CNS) is affected and (2) the presence of co-infections other than Bartonella/BLO.

Levofloxacin (Levaquin). This antibiotic is generally considered to be the antibiotic of choice for the treatment of

Bartonella/BLO. Levaquin is a member of the family of antibiotics known as fluoroquinolones, which also includes ciprofloxacin (Cipro). All the fluoroquinolones seem to have activity against Bartonella/BLO, but Levaquin seems to be the most effective. The dosage is 250-500 mg once a day. It is best to take Levaquin on an empty stomach (or with minimal food if you need to eat something due to gastrointestinal side effects). Also, it is important not to take minerals like calcium, zinc, iron, and magnesium within several hours of the dose of Levaquin, because these minerals will bind Levaquin and render it less effective. I advise that patients take levofloxacin early in the morning, or it can be taken late in the evening, but not at bedtime. Except for the tetracycline antibiotic group, the fluoroquinolones are not generally used in combination with other antibiotics. Usually the course of treatment for Bartonella/BLO is one to three months, but occasionally it may take much longer.

Precautions: Levaquin is usually very well tolerated. The major adverse reaction that may occur with use of this medication is tendonitis (inflammation of the tendons). This complication is not common, but when it occurs, the medication must be stopped for a few days to allow symptoms to resolve. It can then be restarted in a few days at a lower dose, but if the tendonitis recurs, the medication should be stopped. The mechanism for tendonitis is not clearly known, but magnesium deficiency may play a role in some patients. For this reason, I recommend that Bartonella/BLO patients ideally take 600–1,000 mg of magnesium for two weeks *before* beginning Levaquin therapy. Once Levaquin is begun, the patient should continue the magnesium, being careful to take it three (or more) hours before or after the dose of Levaquin.

Rifampin. Rifampin is a very old antibiotic that for many years has been used for the treatment of chronic infections such as tuberculosis. It is very effective against Bartonella/BLO. In particular, it is very useful for the neurological and psychiatric manifestations of Bartonella/BLO—severe anxiety and mood swings, panic, seizure-like episodes, memory loss, "spaciness," confusion, disorientation episodes, and many other symptoms. Expect a herx-like reaction during the first week or so; then significant progress often occurs during the second or third week on rifampin.

It is best used in combination with certain other antibiotics. Frequently, those combinations include rifampin with doxycycline or rifampin with clarithromycin. The combination of rifampin with doxycycline is especially helpful when a patient with Bartonella/BLO is also infected with either Ehrlichia or Lyme. The dosage of rifampin is 300 mg per day for the first week; increase to 600 mg once a day after the first week. It is advisable to use rifampin in the evening (not at bedtime) on an empty stomach, three hours or more after a meal. It may be used in the morning an hour before breakfast also.

Rifabutin is a medication in the same family as rifampin and is reportedly very effective against Bartonella also. Apparently, it can be combined effectively with azithromycin. I do not have enough experience with its use to recommend it at this time.

Precautions: Rifampin is usually very well tolerated. It will always turn a patient's urine orange. It may cause headaches and sleepiness. Liver function and blood counts should be monitored at regular intervals while using rifampin. The greatest concern about rifampin is the potential for interactions with other medications. Rifampin speeds the metabolism of certain medications, resulting in an increased breakdown of the other medications. Clinically, this drug-interaction issue often becomes a problem when certain pain medications are being used, and often a patient will require higher doses of pain medications while on rifampin.

Babesia

This parasitic organism can live inside the body's red blood cells for four months or more. It usually requires a combination antibiotic treatment for a period of two to four months to effectively control the infection. The following two medications are used in combination with a macrolide for treating Babesia.

Atovaquone (Mepron). Atovaquone may be used alone as in the product called Mepron or used in combination with proguanil as in the product called Malarone. Both preparations are effective against Babesia. Mepron is the most common form of atovaquone used against Babesia and is typically combined with azithromycin (Zithromax). Mepron is a liquid that looks similar to yellow paint and is taken as one to two teaspoons twice a day. It should *always* be taken with fatty food (such as nuts, cheese, or similar food), because it is much better absorbed by the body when it is ingested along with a fatty meal. Generally, I cycle Mepron's use as follows: three weeks *on* the medicine, and one week *off*. Azithromycin is continued for *all* four weeks.

Precautions: There are important precautions related to atovaquone. The first is that it can cause temporary liver damage, and for that reason, blood tests for liver function must be followed on a regular basis while using either of these medications. The second precaution concerns the use of supplement doses of coenzyme Q10, alpha lipoic acid, and vitamin E while on atovaquone. These should not be used while taking atovaquone because they are all fat-soluble antioxidants that tend to neutralize the pro-oxidant effects of atovaquone against Babesia.

Bactrim or Septra (trimethoprim/sulfamethoxazole). Bactrim, Septra, TMP/SMX all refer to the same medication. Like rifampin, it is a very old medication that has been used for many years to treat a host of acute and chronic infections, including parasites. It is very effective, especially when combined with a macrolide such as clarithromycin or azithromycin. The usual dosage is one Bactrim DS twice a day. At times, four or more Bactrim per day may be used, depending on the clinical situation.

Precautions: The vast majority of patients using Bactrim have no problems at all. However, as with most antibiotics, it is important to follow routine blood work (complete blood count and liver function tests) on a regular basis. In addition, Bactrim may rarely cause a severe reaction called *"Stevens-Johnson"* syndrome which can be lethal if not addressed immediately. This serious reaction is usually characterized by fever, flu-like symptoms, mouth sores, and often a skin rash. My patients are instructed to stop Bactrim immediately if any fever or mouth and/or skin sores occur. The condition usually clears in the next 24 to 72 hours. However, if it worsens, the patient needs to seek emergency care.

Ehrlichia/Anaplasma

The key to effective treatment of these organisms is early suspicion and treatment for at least 28 days. The most useful antibiotics for treating Ehrlichia/Anaplasma are doxycycline (100–200 mg twice a day) or rifampin (600 mg once a day). In difficult or resistant cases, I have used a combination of both drugs with very good success.

The Second "Core" Component of Lyme Therapy: Basic Lifestyle Health Principles and Nutritional Supplementation

I addressed antibiotics earlier in this chapter because their proper use is critical to the effective treatment of Lyme and the TBDs. In the remainder of this chapter, I will be sharing with you the core general-health principles and alternative and complementary therapies that I recommend for virtually all my Lyme/TBD patients.

Additional therapies for common specific problems and/or issues associated with Lyme—such as detoxification, lack of energy, hormonal dysfunctions, chronic inflammation, neurological factors, pain, sleep problems, and others—are discussed in chapters 7 and 8. Chapter 9 addresses additional therapies and self-care measures for achieving and maintaining overall psychological and spiritual well-being.

General Care—All Patients

What follows are the essential elements of the general care program I recommend for all patients with Lyme and TBDs. In addition to these steps, adjunctive alternative therapies, which I also discuss below, may also be advised.

1) The Lyme Inflammation Diet (LID). Since I discussed this diet and its rationale in detail in the last chapter, there is no need to go into detail about it here. Please review chapter 5 and be sure to follow the dietary recommendations you will find there for each of the stages of the diet. The reason I stress the importance of the LID is that it effectively helps to minimize and reverse the effects of chronic inflammation. Chronic inflammation is one of the main reasons so many patients with Lyme fail to improve. As I mentioned in chapter 5, once inflammation is brought under control, your body will become better able to mobilize its defenses against Lyme and other TBDs. Additionally, the Lyme Inflammation Diet is also highly effective in help your body to detoxify and rid itself of toxins. The diet will also help minimize your risk of developing candidiasis (systemic yeast infection), as well as help you to bring yeast infection under control if you already suffer from it. Of course, the LID principles would include complete abstinence from both alcohol and tobacco usage during treatment. Ongoing users of these substances generally do poorly with Lyme therapy.

2) Targeted Nutritional Supplementation. This is a very important next topic of discussion because most, if not all, patients with chronic Lyme and TBDs suffer from nutritional deficiencies. Chronic infection, along with chronic inflammation and oxidative stress (discussed in chapter five), cause this situation. In a depleted state, unfortunately, a healthy diet alone is often unable to completely address the situation. For this reason, I recommend that all patients take a general, high quality multivitamin and mineral supplement on a daily basis.

At this point, I wish to address the most common vital nutrient deficiencies that afflict many patients with Lyme and other tick-borne diseases. They are vitamins A, B-complex (especially vitamins B12 and B6), C, and D, as well as the mineral magnesium.

Vitamin A: The first vitamin ever to be discovered, vitamin A is not a single substance, but actually a complex of nutrients that include carotenoids and retinol. Vitamin A has many health functions in the body, including proper bone growth, cell differentiation, healthy eyesight, proper gastrointestinal and respiratory function, and tissue repair. For patients with Lyme and other TBDs, vitamin A is particularly important because of its significant ability to improve immune function and fight infectious disease and its role as an important antioxidant. Deficiency of vitamin A may prolong the course of Lyme arthritis. I recommend a daily intake of 3–5,000 IU of 'fat-soluble" vitamin A itself and an additional 5–10,000 units of "water-soluble" mixed carotenoids that the body can covert to vitamin A if needed. (As a precaution, vitamin A supplementation should *not* be used in pregnant women without supervision of an obstetrician.)

B-complex Vitamins: B vitamins are water soluble, meaning that they cannot be stored in the body and therefore must be obtained every day from the foods you eat and, if necessary, as a nutritional supplement. The full range of B vitamins includes B1 (thiamine), B2 (riboflavin), B3 (niacin), B5 (pantothenic acid), B6 (pyridoxine), B9 (folic acid), and B12 (methylcobalamin). B vitamins work together in the body, and therefore, when taken as a supplement, they should be part of a complete B-complex formula.

I have found that deficiencies of vitamins B12 and B6 are common in patients with Lyme and other TBDs. The reason vitamin B12 is so often deficient is that it is not found in significant amounts in plant foods. It is also easily depleted by stress, a common co-factor in chronic Lyme disease. Absorption from the intestines may be erratic, especially in the elderly. B12 plays many roles in the body, including helping to manufacture protein from amino acids and aiding in the metabolism of proteins, carbohydrates, and fats. It is also necessary for proper functioning of the nervous system and aids in the body's production of red blood cells. Additionally, B12 can boost energy levels in the body and help to counteract poor gastrointestinal problems, memory problems, and mood swings.

I recommend that virtually all patients with Lyme and related TBDs have a blood test to determine their vitamin B12 nutritional status. If a person is a vegetarian, a vegan, or on a macrobiotic diet, it is especially important that a blood test for B12 be done to assess one's B12 status. For patients with significant neurological Lyme problems, it may be important also to order two other tests: (1) homocysteine level and (2) a functional test for vitamin B12 called urinary "methylmalonic acid." If it is found that you have blood B12 levels less than 500 picograms/milliliter, elevated homocysteine, or an abnormally elevated urinary methylmalonic acid, then intramuscular injections of this important vitamin may be advised, along with supplementing with sublingual B12. I prefer the methylcobalamin or oxycobalamin preparations over cyanocobalamin. The dosage range for sublingual B12 is 1,000–2,000 mg per day. The intramuscular dose is 1,000 mg weekly.

Vitamin B6 deficiency may cause significant problems also. Among those problems are elevated homocysteine levels, carpal tunnel syndrome, anxiety (especially when combined with a deficiency of the minerals manganese and zinc in a condition called *pyroluria*—see my Web site for more information), depression (vitamin B6 is a necessary cofactor for *serotonin* production), premenstrual syndrome (PMS), migraines, kidney stones, tremors, and others.

A good diagnostic clue to B6 deficiency is an elevated blood homocysteine level. Specific blood tests for vitamin B6 can also be done. Generally, vitamin B6 is given in a dose range of 50–100 mg per day. Often vitamin B6, which is called *pyridoxine*, will be combined with an even more effective form of vitamin B6 called *pyridoxal-5-phosphate*. This is a very effective way to take vitamin B6 and highly recommended. It is also my usual practice to combine vitamin B6 with a good quality magnesium supplement, since these two nutrients work together in many biochemical processes in the body.

Remember, the standard American diet is often associated with inadequate vitamin B6 and magnesium, especially a diet that contains significant amounts of alcohol, white flour, and refined sugar, each of which tends to deplete the body of both of these essential nutrients.

Vitamin C: Another water soluble nutrient, vitamin C is perhaps the most versatile and important vitamin because of the wide range of functions it supports in the body. Its importance for patients with Lyme and other TBDs has to do with its powerful immune-boosting properties, its effectiveness in fighting infectious microorganisms, and its role as a potent antioxidant and detoxifying agent. It also acts as a natural antihistamine (especially when combined with the bioflavonoid, *quercitin*), making it an important nutrient for managing inflammation. Vitamin C is also essential for the overall health of the body's blood vessels, bones, cartilage, joint linings, ligaments, skin, and teeth, as well as for wound healing. Additionally, along with B vitamins, it is one of the most important nutrients for coping with stress and also plays important roles in the metabolism of amino acids and cholesterol and in the manufacture of hormones by the body. For patients with Lyme/TBDs, I routinely recommend a daily oral dose of vitamin C ranging from 500–2,000 mg per day in divided doses.

Vitamin D: Vitamin D is a nutrient that in recent years has become increasingly recognized for its health properties. Additionally, recent research suggests that a high percentage of people in the United States are deficient in vitamin D, especially those who usually receive little to no exposure to natural sunlight on a daily basis. Additionally, vitamin D levels in the body typically diminish after the age of 40. A study published in June 2007 in the *American Journal of Clinical Nutrition* showed that supplementation of vitamin D in older women reduced their risk of cancer by an amazing 60 percent.

Among its many important roles, vitamin D helps support the body's endocrine system, especially the adrenal and thyroid glands. Studies in recent years have shown that vitamin D plays a major role in the *regulation* (not mere suppression) of the immune system. It has been shown that low vitamin D levels are associated with increased levels of inflammatory markers such as IL-6, TNF-alpha, and CRP. As I discussed in chapter 4, vitamin D plays an important role in the reduction of autoimmunity by helping the body to control excessive Th1 responses. Its immune-regulatory function is vital to good health.

Treatment with vitamin D can reduce musculoskeletal pain in a certain percentage of Lyme patients. For this reason, I believe that Lyme patients with chronic inflammatory problems should be assessed for vitamin D deficiency with a blood test called "25-hydroxy vitamin D." Supplementation with sunlight or oral vitamin D should be done if levels are low (less than 40 ng/mL). The usual oral supplement dosage for vitamin D (D3 or cholecalciferol is the preferred form of vitamin D) is 400–5,000 IU per day, depending on the level of deficiency. The goal of vitamin D supplementation (along with sunlight) is to achieve a level of 45–60 ng/mL. I don't recommend levels over 70 ng/mL for prolonged periods of time.

Interestingly, sunlight may result in formation of 10,000–20,000 IU per day, but feedback control mechanisms in the skin prevent toxic vitamin D blood levels from occurring. Therefore, if your vitamin D level is too high, the elevated blood level must be occurring from oral intake of vitamin D and not from sunlight. Finally, there is one exception to my vitamin D recommendations above. If a person has Lyme *and* a condition called "sarcoidosis," then restriction of vitamin D may be useful.

Magnesium: Both Lyme and Bartonella significantly deplete the body's supply of magnesium. Magnesium is one of the most important mineral nutrients necessary for good health, and also one of the minerals that Americans in general are most commonly deficient in. The recommended daily intake of magnesium for healthy people is 400 mg per day, but the sad reality is that the average American gets about half that amount per day. The best nutritional sources include green foods, especially collards and chard (magnesium is to chlorophyll what iron is to hemoglobin), orange-colored foods, nuts, chocolate, figs, apricots, coconut, bran, oats, beans, and legumes.

Most widely known for its ability to support the health of the bones, heart, skeletal muscles, and teeth, magnesium also plays essential roles in the maintenance and repair of all body cells, energy production, hormone regulation, nerve transmission, and the metabolism of proteins and nucleic acids. It also helps to reverse muscular tension and is involved in the functioning of literally hundreds of the body's enzymatic reactions. A lack of magnesium can also contribute to immune system dysfunction, depression, fatigue, high blood pressure, high cholesterol, gastrointestinal problems, irregular heartbeat, memory problems, mood swings, muscle spasms and twitching, and motor skill problems.

Many chronic symptoms of Lyme/TBDs are related to magnesium deficiency, and the correction of that deficiency can be very effective in relieving those symptoms. For that reason, I routinely test nearly all patients with chronic Lyme symptoms for magnesium deficiency. The problem with blood testing is that the magnesium blood test should be done on the red bloods cells and not the serum. This is because magnesium exists primarily inside of cells (intracellular, as in red blood cells), and deficiency will not be detected in fluid outside of the cells (extracellular, as in serum or plasma) until a very profound deficiency exists. If you can afford it, the best, and also most expensive, test is the blood "ionized" magnesium (performed by most large commercial labs).

If blood testing shows low levels of magnesium *and* if kidney function is good, supplementation is highly recommended, in a dosage range of 400–1,000 mg per day. Take in divided doses because taking large amounts of magnesium may result in loose stools. There are many good products on the market, the best of which contain primarily magnesium chloride or "chelated" magnesium (such as taurate, citrate, aspartate, glycinate, and others.)

Coenzyme Q10: Coenzyme Q10 (CoQ10) is a vitamin-like substance that is found in food. It is not a true vitamin since it can also be synthesized by the body, with lessening amounts produced as we age. CoQ10 plays a variety of intricate and important roles in your body's ability to produce energy. Perhaps its most important role is that of helping the cells' mitochondria manufacture cellular fuel, known as adenosine-triphosphate, or ATP. The amount of ATP produced by the cells is directly related to energy levels. The more ATP that is produced, the more energy is available. Without an adequate supply of CoQ10, the cells are unable to produce enough ATP, resulting in energy loss and fatigue.

CoQ10 also acts as a fat-soluble antioxidant. It enhances the ability of its fellow fat-soluble antioxidant, vitamin E, to do its job. CoQ10 is a critically important nutrient for the heart, improving energy production in heart cells. Heart muscle biopsies of Lyme patients often show CoQ10 deficiency, according to Dr. Burrascano. In fact, this deficiency may be a major causative factor in the chronic fatigue of some Lyme patients. An important additional risk factor for CoQ10 deficiency is the use of cholesterol-lowering drugs called "statins." (I generally avoid the statin drugs in patients with chronic fatigue, but for those who must take the statin medications, I recommend supplementation with CoQ10 and fish oil.)

This versatile nutrient has other important functions. CoQ10 can be very helpful in the regulation of high blood pressure. Combined with L-carnitine, it can help patients with congestive heart failure. It also helps to improve immune function and has anti-cancer properties. Finally, it may act as a powerful brain anti-oxidant and "neuro-protector" (especially against neurodegenerative disorders such as Parkinson's disease).

The usual dosage range for CoQ10 is 50–200 mg per day. As a reminder, CoQ10 (and also alpha lipoic acid and vitamin E) should not be used while you are using the anti-Babesia drug atovaquone (Mepron, Malarone) because CoQ10 interferes with the action of this medication. While CoQ10 supplementation on its own can often improve energy levels, I have found that best results are achieved when CoQ10 is taken along with a full range of other essential vitamins, minerals, and other nutrients.

3) Essential Fatty Acids (EFAs). Essential fatty acids are unsaturated fats and oils that are vital for good health. They cannot be manufactured by the body and, in that sense, they are similar to vitamins. There are two main types of EFAs: omega-3 and omega-6 oils. Most Americans are out of balance in terms of their intake of these EFAs due to inadequate omega-3 food intake and excessive intake of poor quality sources of omega-6 fats and oils.

Omega-3 oils: The major usefulness of these oils in the treatment of Lyme is their potent anti-inflammatory effects. They also improve kidney function and are a major fatty acid source for the brain. They further enhance hormone production of growth hormone, thyroid, insulin, progesterone, and ACTH. Omega-3s stabilize moods and clinically have been shown to be beneficial in the treatment of depression. There are two sources of omega-3 oils.

* Plant-source—There are many good plant sources of the omega-3 oil called alpha linolenic acid, such as oils of flax seed, hemp, perilla, soya, pumpkin seed, and walnut. Green leafy vegetables also contain some of these oils. (Canola oil contains omega-3s, but I generally don't recommend the regular use of this oil for cooking.) When ingested in this alpha linolenic plant-source form, the omega-3 oil must be converted by the body to the active form by an enzyme called delta-6 desaturase. Unfortunately around 25 percent or more of the population does not make this conversion efficiently. This rate of poor conversion is even higher for people who are chronically

ill, such as with chronic Lyme disease. For this reason, I generally recommend that most of the omega-3s come from animal sources.

* Animal-source—Eating oily fish like wild-caught salmon or sardines, or using purified, mercury-free fish oil supplements at the dose range of 1,000–4,000 mg per day would comprise the most efficient methods of obtaining omega-3 oils. Additional useful sources would include animal products such as venison, free-range chicken and eggs, or beef whose diet was grass-based instead of grain-based. The advantage of the animal sources is that the animals have already converted the alpha linolenic acid in their diet to the active omega-3s called eicosapentaenoic acid (EPA) and docosahexaenoic acid (DHA).

Omega-6 oils: Two of the most common dietary sources of omega-6 oils are commercial grain-fed meats and vegetable cooking oils. It is true that omega-6 oils are essential, but each of these two common sources has a serious pro-inflammatory downside. Because of their pro-inflammatory potential, I recommend that my Lyme patients minimize their intake of the aforementioned common sources of omega-6s.

Alternatively, instead of commercial meats, use free-range and organic fish and meats (not corn-fed), which are lower in arachidonic acid (a pro-inflammatory type of omega 6).

Instead of cooking with omega-6 oils, such as corn and saf-flower oils, use monounsaturated oils such as olive oil.

The therapeutic and healthiest form of omega-6 oils that I recommend is gamma-linoleic acid (GLA). Food sources are limited and include blue green algae and oatmeal (slow cooked). Most GLA comes from the conversion of vegetable oils rich in linoleic acid (LA) by delta-6 desaturase, the same enzyme that converts the omega-3 oils to their active form. Due to chronic illness and the aging process, many people are unable to convert vegetable oils (LA) to GLA. The result is a relative deficiency of GLA despite often significant intake of the precursor vegetables oils. Combining this problem with an excessive intake of arachidonic acid, it is a setup for pro-inflammation.

For these reasons, it is usually important to supplement the diet with GLA. The most useful supplement sources of GLA originate from black currant, borage, and evening primrose oils. These oils are not pro-inflammatory. The usual supplemental GLA dosage recommendation is 240–960 mg a day. High quality supplements containing both omega-3 and omega-6 are also available.

4) Probiotics. Along with a high-quality multiple vitamin-mineral-CoQ10 supplement and an excellent supplement of essential fatty acids (EFAs), a good probiotic supplement is the third "essential" supplement that I recommend to all my Lyme patients. "Probiotics" is the term given to healthy bacteria that help to maintain the health of the gut (small and large intestines).

Antibiotics used to kill Lyme and the TBDs also, unfortunately, kill off these normal, beneficial bacteria. This unfortunate "friendly fire" kill-off makes it easier for harmful microorganisms such as *Candida albicans* (which causes yeast overgrowth) to take over the gastrointestinal tract. Therefore, the foremost purpose of probiotics is to re-establish the normal protective microflora that colonize the walls of the intestinal tract. When these healthy organisms are present in large numbers, harmful microorganisms are kept in check. (This process is called *competitive exclusion.*)

One symptom of inadequate numbers of healthy probiotic bacteria with possibly excessive growth of harmful organisms is "antibiotic-associated diarrhea" (AAD). To prevent this abnormal situation from developing, probiotics should be taken at the outset of any antibiotic usage. To correct an AAD problem that occurs while on antibiotics, it often requires large amounts of probiotics be administered, using a high quality, complete probiotic formula. For a therapeutic effect, a probiotic formula must have the right varieties of beneficial organisms and right amounts of these healthy bacteria.

In addition to the prevention of unhealthy microorganisms taking over the gut, there is another major function of the healthy probiotic bacteria—support of the immune system. Normally we do not think of the gastrointestinal tract as being important to the immune system, but it is. Fully two thirds or more of the immune system is actually located in the gastrointestinal tract, which ties *gut health and immune system health closely together.* The relationship to probiotics is this: Probiotics activate the immune tissue in the lining of the GI tract, which then in turn signals the systemic immune function to go to work producing cytokines, stimulating natural killer cells (like CD57 cells), and improving white blood cell function.

Finally, there is a very interesting connection between probiotics, fiber, and vitamin D. Probiotics break down fiber into a substance called *butyrate.* This substance in turn is an important fuel for the cells of the GI tract and probably helps in the prevention of colon cancer. Butyrate, together with vitamin D and adequate calcium, increases the action of a protein called *FoxP3.* FoxP3 protein is important for regulatory T cell (T-reg) function and the reduction of autoimmune type of immune dysregulation. Therefore, probiotics are anti-inflammatory when they are combined with adequate fiber intake and adequate sunlight exposure.

Probiotic Options: A question that I am often asked is "aren't natural probiotic sources good enough?" The answer is "yes" for normal health in the absence of antibiotics and "no" for times of antibiotic usage. Excellent natural sources of probiotics include fermented foods such as kefir, yogurt, kombucha, tempeh, and sauerkraut. These are extremely useful to include in a healthy diet and will maintain good intestinal bacterial balance unless antibiotics are used. Antibiotics virtually always disrupt normal bacterial homeostasis.

To maintain and restore the proper balance of healthy intestinal tract bacteria when disrupted by antibiotics, I recommend supplementing with a high quality probiotic formula on a daily basis. It is important to continue probiotics for several weeks (and sometimes months) after antibiotics have been discontinued in order to restore the normal balance of intestinal bacteria after antibiotic usage.

In choosing a formula, look for one that contains both acidophilus (also known as lactobacillus), which protects against yeast overgrowth in the small intestine, and bifidus (also known as bifidobacteria), which performs the same function in the large intestine. When AAD does occur, it is useful to include *Sacchromyces bulordii*, as it is the most effective probiotic in cases of AAD and other gut disorders secondary to antibiotics. The usual probiotic dosage is 5–50 billion organisms per day depending on the situation—lower doses are routine when on antibiotics, and higher doses are used when there is antibiotic-associated diarrhea or when there is yeast overgrowth. Refrigerated and acid-protected products yield the best results. Products that contain "prebiotics," which are present in order to nourish the probiotics, are better. Inulin is one of the more excellent prebiotics—natural sources include dandelion, chicory, endive, and other members of the Asteraceae family.

5) Resveratrol. This is the first of four herbal supplements that I very frequently recommend to my Lyme/TBD patients. It is particularly helpful in Lyme patients co-infected with Bartonella/BLO. Resveratrol has the unique ability to *regulate* the inflammatory process. When more inflammation is needed, resveratrol supports it; when less is needed, resveratrol supports that. This product is among the best ones to use when autoimmunity is suspected. It also has excellent brain protective properties.

There are two excellent sources of resveratrol, grape source (grapes, red wine, and grape leaves) and Japanese knotweed. The advantage of the latter product is that it contains other helpful substances that work synergistically with the resveratrol component. The dosage is 500 mg of Japanese knotweed (with 10 mg resveratrol per 500 mg tablet) three to four times a day for about six to twelve months total time of use.

6) Cat's Claw (CC). This herb, also known as "uña de gato," is from South America and has a very long history of safe medical usefulness. It is very useful in Lyme disease. Among its many functions are reduction of inflammation related to a substance called *NF-kB*, enhancement of the ability of white blood cells to ingest pathologic microorganisms, and improvement in numbers of CD57 natural killer cells. When beginning its use, it is important to *start slowly* and then to gradually increase the dosage of cat's claw to avoid inducing severe "herx" die-off side effects. It is best to cycle on and off of this herb, such as twelve days on, two days off. I recommend using CC for about six to twelve months in total, taking a two-week break every three months.

7) **Andrographis.** Used for many years in Asia, this herb likewise has a long track record of usefulness and safety. It is anti-spirochetal and anti-inflammatory. Perhaps its most important Lyme disease purpose involves its usefulness for brain protection against inflammation-induced neurodegeneration. It crosses the blood-brain barrier and concentrates well in brain tissue, the spinal cord, and cerebrospinal fluid. This makes it the most useful herb for prevention and treatment of Lyme neurological problems. For further information about this herb please consult the excellent book *Healing Lyme* by Stephen Harrod Buhner. The usual dosage of andrographis is 400 mg two to three times a day for about six months. It is important to start slowly during the first week and build up the dose gradually. *Caution:* Although generally safe, it is best to use this herb under medical supervision. It should be dis-

continued if dizziness, heart palpitations, or allergic symptoms occur. Also, this herb should not be used during pregnancy or in women trying to conceive, since it may interfere with progesterone levels.

8) Artemisinin. Derived from the herb Artemisia, this product has exceptional effectiveness against parasites such as Babesia. I use it with virtually all the Babesia patients at a dose of 100–200 mg two to three times a day. Generally, I don't start this herb until the patient has been on anti-Babesia antibiotics for at least a week. Waiting a week to begin Artemisinin seems to preserve the usefulness of it by preventing the development of resistance to it.

9) Garlic. In addition to eating garlic liberally on the LID, many patients have benefited from garlic supplements. There are many excellent products on the market. The specific product that I use is a stabilized allicin product from England and the dosage is 1200–1800 mg per day.

10) Physical Exercise. According to Dr. Joseph Burrascano, patients with Lyme disease will not return to normal unless they exercise. My clinical experience with LD and TBD patients is in agreement with that assessment. One of the main reasons I recommend regular exercise for people with Lyme and other TBDs is that it effectively boosts immune function. Research shows that consistent physical activity can also help to regulate your body's inflammation response. Exercise is also excellent for increasing endorphin production and for improving mental and emotional health, making it very useful for managing and helping to reverse the anxiety and depression that are often associated with Lyme.

It is important that you do not over-exert yourself when you begin an exercise program, especially if you have chronic Lyme disease. Ideally, it is best if you can initially work with a physical therapist under your doctor's supervision. Personal trainers generally aren't recommended, since they usually are not familiar with the special needs of chronically ill patients.

Although the thought of exercise and regular physical activity may not appeal to people struggling with the fatigue associated with Lyme and other TBDs, a *consistent and individualized exercise program is absolutely essential* for all such patients. The goal here is to gain, and then maintain, physical conditioning—especially increased strength and flexibility—while at the same time avoiding exhaustion.

Start out slowly, and work your way up to a program of sustained, strenuous non-aerobic exercises that focus on strength conditioning and improving muscle tone and flexibility. Using light weights or calisthenics training, work only one muscle group at a time, doing three sets of 12 to 15 repetitions. Then follow up with a period of extended stretching of each muscle group before moving on to exercising the next group. Also be sure to breathe fully and deeply as you exercise to further improve oxygenation.

Work up to an exercise routine of one hour at a time, not more than once every other day. Also be sure to follow the correct form for each exercise, as shown by your physical therapist. Do NOT engage in aerobic exercises, not even of the low impact variety, until your stamina improves. As you become familiar and comfortable with your exercise regimen, you can consider exercising on your own without professional assistance, but always be sure not to overdo it. Here's a tip to know if you are doing so. Take your temperature before and after you exercise. If your temperature is lower after exercising, you are pushing too hard and exhausting your adrenal glands.

Balance your exercise program with periods of rest and relaxation each day. Short naps, periods of prayer or meditation, and engaging in relaxing activities that you enjoy are all recommended. You also need to be sure that you are regularly getting enough sleep each night. The ideal time for sleep for most people is 10 P.M. to 6 A.M. Try to go to bed at the same time every night and to awaken at the same time every morning, with a goal of getting seven to nine hours sleep every night. Since Lyme/TBDs can often disrupt normal sleep patterns, you may require a sleep aid to ensure healthy sleep, especially in the early stages of your treatment. If this is the case, see my discussion of sleep in chapter 8 or consult with your physician.

11) Stress Management and Social Support. Stress, both physical and emotional, is a common problem associated with chronic illness. This is especially the case for chronic Lyme disease and other tick-borne illnesses. If not addressed, stress too can become chronic, building up to the point that it can cause anger, anxiety, depression, and feelings of being a "victim." Chronic stress can also significantly depress immune function and can trigger and exacerbate chronic inflammation. Therefore, it is very important that you learn how to properly manage stress so that it doesn't sap your strength and hope.

Chapter 9 is devoted to explaining the many steps you can take to manage stress and achieve what I call A. N.E.W. H.O.P.E. F.O.R. H.E.A.L.T.H. In addition to the stress-coping measures you will learn about in that chapter, I want to encourage you to involve your family and friends in helping you to cope with your illness. Seeking out a therapist or spiritual counselor is also advised, especially if you have been struggling with Lyme for two years or more, since by that point, neurological and psychological problems can be severe.

Please do not be turned off by the thought of seeking counseling or therapy, nor should you let the fact that you (like many Lyme patients) have been told that your problems are psychosomatic keep you from getting the help you need. A good therapist or spiritual counselor can be extremely helpful in empowering you to work through the frustrations and anger you may feel due to being sick for so long. Soothing music, relaxation techniques, and taking time away from your daily activities can be very useful in this process, as well, especially in the early stages of your treatment.

It is also important that you do not let yourself become a "Lyme cripple," with no hope of a better future. Certainly it is true that for some with Lyme it is an extremely persistent and even a life-long condition, in the sense that the *Bb* bacteria may never be completely eradicated. However, at the same time, regardless of how severe your condition may be, there is much that can be done to improve your immune system and restore its control so that, with time and continued therapy, you can return to a fully functional life.

The Third "Core" Component of Lyme Therapy: Supportive Complementary and Alternative Therapies

As I've stated more than once throughout this book, antibiotic therapy alone is often not adequate to properly and effectively treat Lyme and other TBDs. In addition to the antibiotics, dietary, nutritional, herbal, and lifestyle recommendations I've included earlier, there are other *optional* supportive treatment approaches that can also be incorporated into a comprehensive treatment protocol. While these therapies alone are not effective in directly targeting and eliminating *Bb* bacteria and other harmful microorganisms, they can help to support the immune response to Lyme and to relieve many of the associated symptoms of Lyme/TBDs. Two of the most noteworthy of these healing modalities are acupuncture and oxygen therapy.

Acupuncture: In the West, acupuncture is the most popular and most researched element of traditional Chinese medicine (TCM). According to TCM theory, health of the physical body is dependent upon the healthy flow of life-force energy known as *Qi* (pronounced as "chee"), which travels along energetic pathways in the body known as meridians. Along each of these pathways are specific sites known as acupoints. Acupuncture involves the use of needles applied to various acupoints in order to regulate the flow of *Qi* and to remove energetic blockages.

The World Health Organization (WHO) and the National Institutes of Health (NIH) are among the governmental and health organizations that have recognized the wide range of health benefits that acupuncture can provide. Among these many benefits, acupuncture has been shown to be effective for relieving gastrointestinal problems, as well as musculoskeletal and neurological disorders, all of which can be associated with Lyme disease. Acupuncture can also be of benefit to Lyme/TBD patients because of its ability to improve endorphins, boost immune function, relieve pain, and aid in the body's detoxification processes. It is especially beneficial when used in conjunction with physical therapy.

Oxygen Therapy: Oxygen therapy involves increasing the amount of oxygen that is available to the body's cells and tissues, as well as in the bloodstream. Like all harmful microorganisms, *Bb* bacteria and other tick-borne microorganisms have a difficult time surviving in oxygen-rich environments. On the other hand, when oxygen levels are low in blood, cells, and tissues, Lyme and other TBDs tend to thrive. Because of these facts, a number of Lyme-aware physicians employ various methods of elevating oxygen supply inside the body. These methods include the use of hyperbaric oxygen therapy, ozone therapy, intravenous hydrogen peroxide therapy, and intravenous vitamin C therapy. Of these four, the one that I most often recommend is hyperbaric oxygen therapy because of the clinical research and experience associated with its Lyme/TBDs usage. It also has a long safety record.

Hyperbaric oxygen therapy (HBOT) has been in use since the early twentieth century. It is primarily noted for its ability to help deep sea divers and submarine personnel adjust to the change in atmospheric pressure, and to aid burn victims. However, HBOT has also been found to have many other medical uses, including aiding in the recovery from brain injury, cerebral palsy, stroke, and other neurological conditions. It has also been demonstrated to be effective for helping patients recover from anaerobic (able to live without oxygen) infections, which is generally what Lyme and other TBDs are.

Patients receive HBOT by entering a sealed hyperbaric chamber. Once the patient is inside, the chamber is pressurized to a level up to approximately twice the pressure of the earth's atmosphere at sea level. This makes it possible for patients to breathe in oxygen at a much greater concentration than normal breathing, thus saturating the body with oxygen. HBOT sessions typically last anywhere from 30 minutes to two hours. While expensive, HBOT has been very useful, particularly in patients with neurological Lyme symptoms that do not respond to other forms of therapy. It may require twenty or more HBOT sessions to be effective.

An alternative to HBOT that some have found useful is exercise with oxygen therapy (EWOT). In this type of oxygen therapy a person wears an oxygen mask at 10 liters per minute oxygen flow while walking on a treadmill for several minutes. It has been particularly helpful for improving chronic fatigue and stamina.

Summing Up

The following questions are among those I am most commonly asked about diagnosing and treating Lyme and other TBDs.

What constitutes the most effective method of diagnosis of Lyme disease and other tick-borne illness?

As I state throughout this book, Lyme disease is often a clinical diagnosis, meaning that it can often depend on the skill your physician possesses to recognize possible symptoms and signs of Lyme and other TBDs. You can help your doctor make an accurate diagnosis by providing him or her with an accurate, well-organized, and detailed account of your medical history during the time that you undergo your medical history and physical examination. There is no one test that can reliably tell whether or not a person has Lyme disease. Rather it is the proper utilization of all three components—history, physical examination, and laboratory testing—that allows the doctor to make the diagnosis of Lyme. Various diagnostic tests that I've described in this chapter and chapter 3 should be employed in order to both confirm Lyme and/or other TBDs and to rule out any other possible health conditions.

What do I need to know when it comes to using antibiotics for Lyme disease?

While they may not be totally adequate to treat chronic cases of Lyme/TBDs, antibiotics nonetheless are an essential primary component of all treatment protocols for disseminated Lyme/TBDs. Choosing the right type of antibiotics is also highly important. The type of antibiotic drugs to use depends upon the stage at which Lyme is detected, the severity of your condition, and the presence of co-infections. Since Lyme can be present in three different forms, it is important for your doctor to know which forms are affecting you. In many complex cases of chronic Lyme, a combination of antibiotic drugs may be required. Lyme-aware physicians, in my opinion, are best qualified to make such determinations because of their experience in treating Lyme and other TBDs.

Why do you recommend lifestyle changes during the course of treatment?

Adopting a healthy lifestyle is essential for recovering from any type of chronic health condition and is especially vital for people with Lyme/TBDs so that the body's immune system has the best chance of doing its job in eliminating the bacteria and associated co-factors related to Lyme/TBDs. Many Lyme patients have stated that their Lyme disease was a wake-up call that came to them in order that they might learn to take better care of themselves.

What are the core elements of the lifestyle changes you recommend?

The primary lifestyle changes I recommend are following the Lyme Inflammation Diet (the LID), appropriate nutritional and herbal supplementation, exercise, stress management, and social support. By committing yourself to each of these lifestyle changes, you can significantly improve your body's ability to regain its health. They will also improve your ability to successfully cope with your illness while it is still uncontrolled.

Why do you recommend that alternative therapies be considered as an element of an overall treatment program for Lyme and other TBDs?

While antibiotics and the lifestyle changes I recommend can significantly improve the health of many people with Lyme/TBDs, it is often necessary to augment treatment with the therapies I mentioned above in order to ensure that patients are provided with all that they need to make a full recovery. These therapies often shorten the course of treatment for these disorders.

In the remainder of this book, Part Three, I will share with you specific strategies, conventional as well as alternative, and complementary therapies—designed to help with ten of the most common symptoms and/or problems experienced by patients with Lyme/TBDs. These problem-specific techniques are recommended for your consideration because of their effectiveness in supporting and augmenting the primary "core" approaches that I described in this chapter.

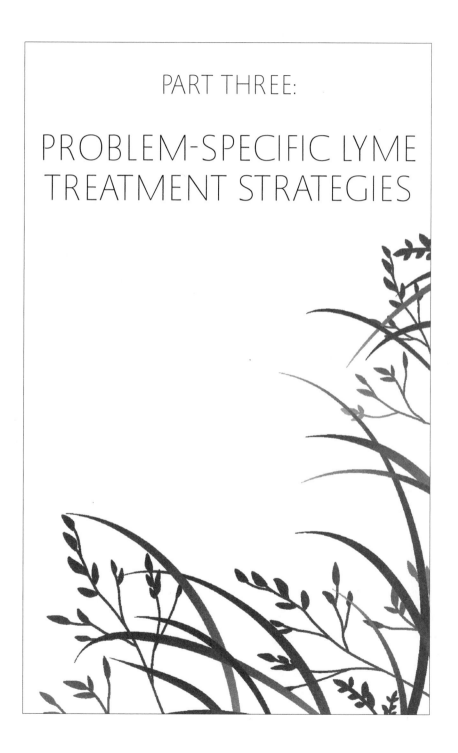

PART THREE:

PROBLEM-SPECIFIC LYME TREATMENT STRATEGIES

Chapter Seven

The Unhealthy Lyme P.I.E.E.

In this chapter, I will address the professional and self-care approaches you can use to address the first four of the most common and serious problem areas associated with Lyme and other tick-borne diseases.

Pain

Inflammation

Endocrine hormonal disruption

Energy depletion and fatigue

Together, these four elements combine to create what I call the unhealthy Lyme P.I.E.E. Addressing each of these four factors is a crucial aspect of treatment, yet all too often these are overlooked, mismanaged, or ignored.

Pain

Pain is one of the three most common symptoms of Lyme disease, along with "brain fog" (discussed in chapter 8) and lack of energy (discussed later in this chapter). It is also a major contributor to the depression and sleeplessness experienced by many patients with Lyme and other TBDs. This problem of sleep deprivation is known to worsen chronic pain, which in turn makes sleep even more difficult. This is a major vicious cycle that occurs in a large number of patients with chronic Lyme disease and the TBDs.

Pain is also closely associated with inflammation. (I discussed inflammation basics extensively in chapter 5.) However, although pain and inflammation have lots of overlapping interactions, they also are distinct from each other. For this reason, treating them properly requires specific, and often very different, approaches. There are two basic approaches for managing the pain associated with Lyme and related TBDs: (1) conventional pain medication and related therapies and (2) homeopathic, herbal, and other forms of natural and non-conventional therapies.

Conventional Pain Medication and Related Therapies

Pain management is a high priority when dealing with Lyme and TBDs. While I fully expect that infection treatment will eventually resolve pain, it is important to effectively manage pain while we are working on the core Lyme treatment program that I discussed in chapter 6. Very often, conventional pharmaceutical treatment of pain is necessary. The type of treatment depends on the cause and the severity of the pain symptoms, which can range through mild, moderate, and severe.

Mild Pain: For cases of mild pain, generally acetaminophen is effective when used properly. Most commonly sold as the brand name Tylenol, acetaminophen is an over-the-counter medicine that belongs to a class of drugs known as *analgesics* (pain relievers). It works by increasing a person's pain threshold. This means that, rather than stopping pain, it helps to prevent pain from being experienced until pain levels increase. This makes mild pain levels much more bearable.

For mild pain that is not due to inflammation (such as most cases of joint pain), low dose acetaminophen (the equivalent of two tablets three times a day) is usually both effective and safe to use. However, it should not be taken by anyone with liver problems, nor should it ever be combined with alcohol. For the best and safest results, always take acetaminophen with food. Due to the potential adverse liver side effects of acetaminophen, if you are using it on a regular basis, be sure to inform your physician. In addition you can help to protect your liver by taking the supplement N-acetyl cysteine (NAC) at a dose of 250–500 mg twice a day.

For mild pain associated with inflammation, often low doses of *non-steroidal anti-inflammatory drugs (NSAIDs)* are useful. The original NSAID is aspirin. A good modern example of this type of medication would be ibuprofen (most commonly commercially sold as Advil, Nuprin, or Motrin). Used in doses of 200–400 mg two to three times a day, this medication is safe to use for mild pain. Used in higher doses (1600–2400 mg per day) it is anti-inflammatory and there may be an increased chance of immune suppression that may limit the immune system's ability to contain the infections.

A well-known potential problem associated with use of the NSAIDs is gastrointestinal bleeding. All NSAIDs cause some microscopic bleeding. Anyone with a history of significant gastrointestinal bleeding should not use these medications unless cleared for use by their physician. Whether or not you have a bleeding history, please be aware of potential bleeding problems and vigilantly look out for signs and symptoms of bleeding. Therefore, as with acetaminophen, be sure to inform your physician that you are using NSAIDs.

Moderate Pain: For cases of moderate pain, acetaminophen and the NSAIDs should be attempted first. If not effective, however, usually prescription *mild opioid* medicines are effective. Two of the most common mild opioids are codeine and tramadol. Opioid medicines work by suppressing the body's perception of pain and reducing the number of pain signals sent by the nervous system and the brain's reaction to them. Both codeine and tramadol are generally safe to use under your doctor's supervision.

There are two main precautions related to the use of mild opioids. First of all, they are potentially habit-forming. For that reason, they have some significant abuse potential when used improperly. Proper use of these medications means taking them only as directed and for only the purpose intended, namely pain. If used for purposes other than intended, such as for fear, worry, or anxiety, they indeed have abuse potential. When used for a prolonged period of time, their discontinuation or withdrawal may require gradual tapering over a period of days to weeks. The second consideration concerns potential side effects. These would include drowsiness, making driving potentially hazardous, and a tendency for constipation.

There are four additional *non-opioid* pharmacological approaches to moderate chronic pain that I have found to be useful. The first approach is the use of certain *antidepressants*. Most commonly I have found the older tricyclic antidepressant, amitriptyline, useful. Used at bedtime in the dose of 10–50 mg, it helps with sleep and depression, as well as with pain control by reducing "nerve pain." Another useful antidepressant is the newer medication known as duloxetine (Cymbalta). This medication is used in doses from 20–120 mg and has been very valuable for controlling all manner of chronic pain from Lyme and TBDs. It works by improving the balance of the brain chemicals called norepinephrine and serotonin, thereby altering the perception of pain.

The second non-opioid approach is the use of gabapentin (also known as Neurontin). The exact mechanism by which gabapentin improves pain is not known, but it works on both inflammatory and non-inflammatory pain. It has an added benefit of improving sleep, particularly the deep sleep of "non-REM" stage 3 and 4. (I discuss sleep issues in chapter 8). The usual dose of gabapentin is 100–900 mg (or more) per day.

The third modality that is useful for pain control is the use of Lidoderm patches for up to twelve hours per day. These prescription patches contain a local anesthetic that can effectively reduce pain when placed over a localized area of discomfort.

Finally, physical therapy (PT) with all its treatment modalities is extremely useful for all types of pain—especially the moderate varieties. I highly recommend this.

Severe Pain: Lyme and other TBD patients suffering from chronic and severe pain are advised to consult with a professional *pain management specialist*. Control of severe pain may involve using strong opioid medications such as oxycodone and methadone, or fentanyl, or other strong analgesics. Management of severe chronic pain is best handled by a multidisciplinary approach involving a pain management physician, along with physical therapists, neurologists, and even psychologists. There is also a very useful role for acupuncturists, massage therapists, and chiropractors as team members. A variety of organizations can also help you locate a qualified pain management specialist. These include the American Academy of Pain Management, American Academy of Pain Medicine, American Board of Pain Medicine, and the American Pain Society. (See the resources section for contact information.)

Complementary and Alternative Natural Therapies

A number of safe, non-toxic natural treatments can also be helpful in treating pain related to Lyme and other TBDs. These include homeopathic remedies, magnet therapy, topical emu oil with glucosamine, acupuncture, and bodywork and massage therapy. (Certain herbs, as well as fish oil supplements, are also useful for pain management. These remedies, however, fall more into the category of anti-inflammatory and will therefore be discussed in the next section of this chapter under "I - Inflammation.")

Homeopathic Remedies: A number of homeopathic remedies can effectively treat pain, as was proven in a study published in the *American Journal of Pain Management* in 1998. The study involved patients suffering from pain related to osteoarthritis and determined that homeopathic treatments were "at least as effective" as acetaminophen (Tylenol) for pain relief. Additionally, the remedies posed no risk of side effects, compared to acetaminophen and other pharmaceutical pain medications.

One of the most useful homeopathic remedies for pain is *Arnica*, which is available at most health food stores. Take it according to the directions on the label in a potency of 30C. Be sure to refrain from eating or drinking for at least ten minutes after you take it. Another very helpful homeopathic pain remedy is Traumeel, an ointment that you can use to soothe painful areas of your body. Traumeel is also available at most health food stores. Some practitioners use the injectable form of Traumeel, which is apparently very effective for pain and injury.

Working with a trained homeopath can also be helpful for dealing with pain and other symptoms related to Lyme disease. To learn more about homeopathy and to locate a homeopath near you, contact the homeopathy organizations listed in the resources section.

Magnet Therapy: The use of magnets as a healing therapy dates back to the times of ancient China, Egypt, Greece, and India. Today, magnet therapy is widely used in China, Japan, and Korea, as well as in Germany, Russia, and many countries in Eastern Europe, and is gaining in popularity in the United States. The use of magnet therapy to treat pain consists of placing magnet pads or other magnetic devices over painful areas. Research shows that magnet therapy provides pain relief in a variety of ways. These include blocking pain signals to the brain, increasing endorphin levels, and increasing circulation, which in turn speeds up the delivery of healing agents to painful areas of the body. Magnet therapy has also been shown to increase the supply of oxygen in the blood and also to increase serotonin levels, leading to increased feelings of overall well-being. Magnet therapy can be effective for peripheral neuropathy.

Caution: Magnets are powerful medicine and ideally should be used under the supervision of a physician. They should not be used during pregnancy.

Topical Emu Oil with Glucosamine: Emu oil is derived from emus, birds closely related to ostriches. The oil contains high amounts of essential fatty acids (e.g., 40 percent monounsaturated fatty acids, 20 percent palmitic acid, 20 percent linoleic acid, 8 percent stearic acid, and 5 percent palmitoleic acid) and has been shown to provide relief for pain when used as an ointment. A number of emu oil products also contain glucosamine, a supplement that helps to rebuild cartilage and connective tissue and soothe aching joints. Research has shown that glucosamine also helps to halt the destruction of healthy cells that can occur when tissues become damaged. If your pain symptoms are primarily in your joints, you can also take an oral glucosamine supplement daily (2,000–4,000 mg per day).

Acupuncture: Acupuncture is based on the theory that both pain and illness are the result of blockages in the body's energy pathways, known as meridians. According to acupuncture theory, there are twelve main and eight secondary meridians and more than 2,000 "acupoints" that run along them. Acupuncturists relieve blockages and balance the flow of energy, or *Qi* ("chee"), by gently inserting needles along the meridian pathways to stimulate healing.

Practiced in China for thousands of years, acupuncture has been studied in the West since the early 1970s. Research has shown that one of acupuncture's primary mechanisms of action lies in its ability to increase production of the body's endorphin and related opioids, which act as natural painkillers. Research conducted at the National Institutes of Health (NIH) National Center for Complementary and Alternative Medicine indicates that acupuncture treatments also enhance the ability of the body to transmit electromagnetic messages throughout the body. This, in turn, can increase the transmission of other natural healing chemicals to areas of the body that are in pain or diseased.

Additional research suggests that acupuncture can also boost immune function (possibly mediated by the improved production of endorphins). It also improves the flow of neurotransmitters and neurohormones in the brain. Another commonly experienced benefit of acupuncture is an improved sense of well-being and greater relaxation, due to the increased production of endorphins. In fact, it is very rare to see a Lyme/TBD patient who does not feel better with acupuncture therapy. All these benefits can help to make a significant difference in pain and other symptoms experienced by people suffering from Lyme/TBDs.

To locate a practitioner of acupuncture in your area, contact the American Association of Oriental Medicine (AAOM), the Tai Sophia Institute, the American Academy of Medical Acupuncture (AAMA), or the National Acupuncture and Oriental Medicine Alliance (NAOMA). Contact information is provided in the resources section.

Bodywork and Massage: Regular sessions of bodywork and massage can also help to significantly reduce pain symptoms, since these therapies increase endorphin production as well. Our natural instinct to massage or rub painful areas of our bodies is a testament to the healing power of touch. There are many different varieties of bodywork and massage therapy. One of the most popular and most effective forms for pain relief is Swedish massage, which is so named because it was developed by Per Henrik Ling of Sweden in the nineteenth century after he observed massage techniques during his travels in China.

Today, Swedish massage and neuromuscular massage are popular treatments used by health practitioners throughout North America and Europe, as well as in many hospitals. They have been shown to promote relaxation, relieve muscle pain and tension, improve circulation, and enhance flexibility and range of motion. Many other types of bodywork and massage therapies provide similar excellent benefits—examples would be cranial osteopathy and Feldenkrais. To locate a certified and reputable massage therapist near you, contact the American Massage Therapy Association (AMTA). See the resources section for AMTA's complete contact information.

Inflammation

Inflammation basics were discussed in detail in chapter 5. As I stated there, chronic inflammation is directly related to the severity of symptoms that Lyme patients experience. The fact is that the greater the amount of chronic inflammation, the greater the severity of symptoms. Therefore, in order to properly treat Lyme and other TBDs, it is absolutely essential to address the problem of inflammation and to get it under control.

As chapter 5 makes clear, one of the most effective ways of achieving this goal is to follow the Lyme Inflammation Diet and it is the *cornerstone* of my Lyme anti-inflammation program. For complete information on the Lyme Inflammation Diet, please refer to chapter 5. Please keep in mind that it is important that you avoid all forms of sugar, including simple carbohydrates, as well as artificial sweeteners. Be sure to also avoid all use of alcohol, trans-fatty acids, other unhealthy fats such as arachidonic acid, and sources of advanced glycation end products (AGEs).

In this discussion I will address these three additional aspects of inflammation control.

- Conventional medications used for treating inflammation

- Nutritional, herbal, and natural anti-inflammatory therapies

- Endorphin-enhancing therapy—a novel and often very effective immune-regulatory therapy called "low dose naltrexone"

Conventional Medications for Treating Inflammation

The two categories of drugs most commonly used to treat inflammation are the NSAIDs and corticosteroids.

There are numerous NSAID drugs that work specifically on pain caused by inflammation. As we briefly discussed above, two of the most common NSAID drugs are (1) aspirin and aspirin-containing drugs, such as Anacin, Bufferin, and Excedrin, and (2) drugs that contain ibuprofen (or similar drug), such as Advil, Motrin, and Nuprin. All NSAIDs work by blocking the ability of an enzyme in the body known as *cyclooxygenase* (COX). COX enzymes produce substances known as *prostaglandins*. There are two types of COX enzymes—COX I produces helpful prostaglandins that protect the gastrointestinal tract, and COX II produces pro-inflammatory prostaglandins that lead to pain. Both types of prostaglandins are natural chemicals in your body, but *when pro-inflammatory prostaglandins produced from COX II enzymes are produced in excess, they promote both chronic inflammation and chronic pain.* The goal of NSAIDs is the reduction of COX II prostaglandins, but, unfortunately, helpful COX I prostaglandins are also inhibited. (The exception would be the medications such as rofecoxib and celecoxib, which are selective COX II inhibitors.)

Since COX I prostaglandins help to protect the stomach lining and are important for proper blood clotting, the use of NSAIDs can, over time, lead to gastric upsets and bleeding. Other side effects that can be caused by NSAIDs include constipation, diarrhea, dizziness, drowsiness, headache, loss of appetite, nausea, rashes, and vomiting. NSAIDs can also cause fluid retention, leading to edema, and lead to kidney failure, liver failure, ulcers, and prolonged bleeding after an injury or surgery. Additionally, NSAIDs can also result in diminished immune function. Therefore, they should be used with caution and only under the supervision of your physician.

Steroid medications are highly effective at reducing inflammation but can also cause serious side effects. Of particular note for Lyme patients is the fact that steroids can suppress the immune system and may also enable the *Bb* bacteria to penetrate deeper into body tissues. Therefore, systemic steroids in immunosuppressive doses should not be used, except in cases of emergencies or life-threatening situations, such as severe asthma.

I recommend that you follow the advice of your doctor if, in the doctor's opinion, steroids are essential for you. However, be aware that Lyme patients who have been given steroids for their Lyme-related symptoms prior to coming to my office often require much longer courses of antibiotic therapy for their infections. If your physician determines that the use of immunosuppressive doses of steroids is absolutely necessary, be sure to also use antibiotics throughout the course of your treatment, as well as for at least a month afterwards, in order to keep *Bb* bacteria in check.

Given the potential health risks posed by both anti-inflammatory doses of NSAIDs and steroids, I generally do not recommend them for Lyme patients unless absolutely necessary, such as for life-threatening illness. There are safer alternatives. Generally, the Lyme Inflammation Diet, pain-management strategies discussed above, and nutritional and/or herbal supplementation are the wiser and safer course of treatment.

Another potentially useful anti-inflammatory therapy is intravenous immune globulin (IVIg). Particularly helpful when gamma globulin levels are depressed, this very expensive therapy may be valuable for chronic neurological system inflammation related to Lyme. Insurance coverage is often a barrier to use of this therapy.

Nutritional and Herbal Supplementation

There are fourteen herbs and nutrients that are very effective for treating most cases of chronic inflammation, especially when used in conjunction with the Lyme Inflammation Diet. Seven of these have already been discussed as part of my "core" Lyme program in chapter 6. These include vitamin D, omega-3 oils (e.g., fish oil), omega-6 oils (e.g., GLA), probiotics, andrographis, cat's claw, and resveratrol (Japanese knotweed source). The remaining seven, which I will now discuss, include curcumin, ginger, stephania, devil's claw, white willow bark, boswellia, and systemic enzymes.

Curcumin (Turmeric): Curcumin is a primary ingredient in the spice turmeric. It offers a variety of health benefits, including acting as a natural anti-inflammatory agent. It is also a potent antioxidant and has anti-cancer properties. It supports the important immune cell called the "macrophage" as we discussed in chapter 4.

From the standpoint of inflammation and resulting pain, the reason curcumin is effective is due to its ability to inhibit pro-inflammatory eicosanoid production. Remember, eicosanoids are normal substances produced by our bodies and play a variety of important roles in the body. There are anti-inflammatory eicosanoids and pro-inflammatory eicosanoids. The body seeks a very careful balance between the two types. However, poor diet and chronic infection cause the levels of pro-inflammatory eicosanoids to become excessive. This results in triggering and prolonging inflammation. Curcumin is one of the best methods to correct this imbalance, and this correction occurs especially for the neurological system. It can be taken as a supplement

(400–700 mg two to three times a day) and, of course, may also be obtained by eating the spice, curry.

Ginger: Ginger is an herb that has been used medicinally for more than 2,000 years by traditional healers throughout Asia and the Middle East. Today, in addition to being used as a spice, ginger is widely used to prevent and treat both nausea and vomiting, especially in cases of motion sickness. It also has very powerful anti-inflammatory properties that have been extensively documented by medical research. In potency, it is similar to curcumin. I recommend that you ingest ginger regularly in your diet by adding ginger as a spice to your meals, or you can drink ginger tea. Alternatively you may take it as a supplement in either capsule or tincture (liquid) at a dose of 250–500 mg two to three times a day. Interestingly, you can also try using ginger oil as an ointment applied directly to tender areas of your body.

Caution: in higher doses by mouth, ginger may cause mild bleeding tendencies. Therefore, notify your physician if you are taking any anticoagulant medication or anti-platelet medications prior to beginning to use herbal supplement doses of ginger.

Stephania root: *Stephania* is a Chinese herb that acts as a natural anti-inflammatory and also aids the body in eliminating toxins. Practitioners of traditional Chinese medicine (TCM) commonly prescribe *Stephania* to treat both inflammation and pain. Health practitioners in Japan also use it for this purpose. The reasons *Stephania* is effective as an anti-inflammatory agent are twofold. First of all, it has the ability to reduce elevated levels of interleukin-6 (IL-6), a naturally occurring chemical in the body that is pro-inflammatory. One of the best tests of elevated IL-6 levels is your C-reactive protein (CRP). If the CRP is elevated, it is generally a reflection of high levels of IL-6.

In addition to lowering IL-6 levels, *Stephania* root also reduces brain levels of "nuclear factor kappa beta" (NF-kB). NF-kB is a protein in cells that turns on inflammation in response to certain signals. It appropriately signals the production of the inflammation process in response to invasion by microorganisms such as Lyme/TBDs. But it overproduces inflammation in response to other stimuli such as free radical and pro-oxidant excess. This latter scenario results in damaging chronic inflammation.

In the situation of a "dysregulated" (lack of normal control mechanisms) immune system, as we often encounter with chronic Lyme, it is important to provide the body with the support it needs for inflammation control. *Stephania* is very effective for brain and nervous system chronic excessive inflammation induced by Lyme, including Bell's palsy and Lyme-related eye inflammation. This herb is an important component of the comprehensive Neurological Recovery program that I will discuss in chapter 8. It can be taken in capsule form at a dose of 200-300 mg two times a day.

Devil's claw is an herb native to southern Africa, where it is traditionally used to treat fever, rheumatoid arthritis, skin conditions, and conditions involving the gallbladder, pancreas, stomach, and kidneys. It gets its name from the claw-like hooks that cover its fruit. Since its introduction to Europe and North America, research also shows that devil's claw can be very helpful in relieving pain and chronic inflammation. The exact mechanism of action is not well understood; it does not appear to work like other natural anti-inflammatory herbal products. It has performed well in medical research studies, having been shown to be particularly effective for muscle pain and tension in the neck, back, and shoulder areas. The usual dosage is 500–1,000 mg two to three times a day.

Caution: Devil's claw should not be used by pregnant women or by people with duodenal or gastric ulcers. People with diabetes, blood sugar problems, and gallbladder problems should only use devil's claw under their physician's supervision.

White willow bark is an herb that has long been prized by Native Americans for its pain-relief properties. It is also indigenous to central and southern Europe and was recommended by Hippocrates for cases of fever and inflammation. In the 1800s, researchers working for the German pharmaceutical company

Bayer, were able to derive a synthetic version of white willow bark after studying the herb's healing properties. This synthetic version is today known as aspirin. White willow bark in its natural form is nearly as potent as aspirin for relieving pain. Additionally, unlike aspirin, it does not cause gastric or intestinal bleeding or upset, making it a safer option for people who need to manage their pain symptoms on an ongoing basis. The dosage is 600–800 mg two to three times a day.

Caution: Persons who are sensitive or allergic to aspirin should avoid this herb. In addition, there is some mild increased risk of bleeding, especially when combined with other herbs and supplements that tend to "thin" the blood, such as vitamin E and ginkgo biloba. It should be avoided within two weeks prior to a surgical procedure.

Boswellia is an herb used for many years in Ayurveda. The boswellia tree is grown primarily in the hilly parts of India. The resin of the tree is used medicinally. It behaves much like the NSAIDs but without the irritation and ulceration of the stomach seen in all NSAIDs except the COX-II inhibitors like Celebrex and Vioxx (prescription products I do not prescribe or recommend due to potential cardiovascular risks). In that sense, it is like a safe and natural COX-II agent. The major way it works is to reduce the pro-inflammatory family of chemicals called *leukotrienes* by the inhibition of an enzyme called

5-lipoxygenase. In clinical studies, Boswellia is very effective in disorders such as rheumatoid arthritis, ulcerative colitis, and bronchial asthma. The usual dosage for this herb is 125 mg twice a day.

Often combination herbal products are the most convenient and cost-effective way to benefit from healing herbs. Herbal medicine experts have found that the combination of the following herbal products is particularly effective for "natural COX-II inhibition:" ginger, turmeric, oregano, green tea, rosemary, gold thread, barberry, holy basil, Japanese knotweed, and skullcap. This particular combination product is called Zyflamend and is manufactured and sold by the nutraceutical company, New Chapter.

Systemic enzymes are one of the most fascinating natural therapies for treating chronic inflammation related to Lyme, TBDs, and other causes. Basically, an enzyme is a type of protein that facilitates a chemical reaction that changes another substance. The best example that I can give you would be digestive enzymes. When we chew our food, enzymes in our mouths begin breaking down the carbohydrates in the food so that the broken up carbohydrate can be absorbed when it gets to the intestines. In our intestines, other enzymes (from the pancreas, primarily) join the mouth enzymes to further break down carbohydrates and other food stuffs such as proteins and fats. Without the action of digestive enzymes, our food could not be broken down into its absorbable components, and we would eventually die of malnutrition.

The hundreds of different types of enzymes that we produce in our bodies all have specific purposes and functions. Above, I described one type called "digestive enzymes." The truth is that enzymes are not only manufactured in our bodies, but also we are intended by our Creator to ingest enzymes in our foods. The problem is that many of the best sources of food enzymes (such as fruits and vegetables) are overly processed or overcooked and thereby have lost significant amounts of their enzyme content. The LID, fortunately, is a "high enzyme" nutrition program, which is one of the reasons for its effectiveness. Additionally, chronic illness such as Lyme increases the body's requirements for enzymes. Therefore, combining chronic Lyme illness with the standard American "enzyme-deficient" diet, Lyme patients are set up for one of the consequences of enzyme-deficiency—namely, chronic inflammation. How do Lyme disease, enzymes, and chronic inflammation relate to one another?

There are enzymes called "proteolytic enzymes" that have the function of breaking down proteins. One of the functions of these proteolytic enzymes is to break down, for the purpose of processing and elimination, substances called "circulating immune complexes" (CICs). We discussed CICs in chapter 5 as a major contributor to chronic inflammation. As a brief review, they are debris that occur as a result of the battle between the immune system and *Bb*. CICs require removal from the circulation as soon as they are formed. If not removed and digested or broken down quickly, they can trigger inflammation in joints and other places where they may circulate and deposit.

Another anti-inflammatory function of enzymes is the reduction of levels of a pro-inflammatory prostaglandin called *prostaglandin E2* (PGE2), decreasing the production of this pro-inflammatory substance. System enzymes also reduce levels of *Substance P*, which helps with diminishing chronic pain. An additional benefit, unrelated to Lyme, is that proteolytic enzymes have been shown in several studies to have potent anti-cancer effects.

Because Lyme patients are relatively deficient in these enzymes, the use of supplemental proteolytic enzymes in chronic Lyme is very helpful, and I highly encourage their use. The products used for this purpose need to be taken *between* meals and not during meals. (If used during meals, they will simply help the pancreas digest proteins better, but won't be available to help reduce CICs, PGE2, and inflammation.) The products should also be acid-protected (enteric coated), so as to bypass destruction by stomach acid, which would ruin their effectiveness. These proteolytic enzymes usually need to be used for several months, with the endpoint of use being resolution of inflammatory signs and symptoms (such as pain). Dosage recommendations depend on specific products.

Endorphin-Enhancing Therapy

In chapter 4, we discussed the fact that Lyme and the TBDs may cause the body's immune system to lose its ability to regulate itself, thereby increasing the chances of an "autoimmune-like" reaction. When this happens, the result is chronic inflammation caused by the immune system itself. The solution to this problem would include getting rid of the infection and improving the regulatory ability of the immune system.

An often-effective approach for regulating the autoimmune dysfunction associated with Lyme and other TBDs is to increase your body's ability to produce endorphins. Endorphins are chemicals manufactured by your body that act as natural painkillers. Endorphins are also associated with improved mood and enhanced feelings of well-being. An additional function of endorphins is regulation of the immune system. In fact, many of the white blood cells of the body contain receptors on their surfaces for endorphins.

Therapies, therefore, that help to improve and normalize endorphins are among the most promising and exciting of all immune regulation, inflammation management, and pain control modalities. Three of the most effective therapies in this category are acupuncture, bodywork and massage, and low dose naltrexone (LDN) therapy. I have already discussed the first two modalities. Now I would like to discuss LDN, which has excellent potential to help a dysfunctional immune system to learn to regulate itself again.

Low Dose Naltrexone (LDN) Therapy: What is naltrexone? Naltrexone is an extremely safe drug that was originally approved by the Food and Drug Administration in 1984 as a treatment for narcotic (morphine, heroin, and opium) addiction due to its effectiveness in blocking the opioid (endorphin) receptors in the brain that drive the craving for narcotics. The dose of naltrexone prescribed for this purpose is 50 mg.

Because naltrexone is able to block opioid receptors, it also is effective at blocking the reception of opioid hormones that are produced by the brain and adrenal glands, including endorphins and enkephalins (specific types of endorphins that occur at the body's nerve endings and act as transmitters). Many of your body's tissues have receptor sites for these endorphins, including, as I mentioned, many different cells in your immune system.

This makes naltrexone a potentially useful treatment for both pain management and enhancement of normal immune function. Bernard Bihari, M.D., discovered that naltrexone was able to accomplish these benefits in a low dose (4.5 mg rather than 50 mg) taken once a day at bedtime. Since Dr. Bihari's discovery in the early 1990s, low dose naltrexone has been shown to have benefit for a wide variety of illnesses related to low or unregulated (autoimmune) immune function, including many types of cancer, as well as chronic fatigue syndrome (CFS), emphysema, endometriosis, fibromyalgia, gastrointestinal disorders (celiac disease, colitis, Crohn's disease, and irritable bowel syndrome), lupus, multiple sclerosis (MS), Parkinson's disease, psoriasis, and rheumatoid arthritis. It can even be helpful for AIDS/HIV, amyotrophic lateral sclerosis (ALS or Lou Gehrig's disease), and Alzheimer's disease.

More recently, I have found low dose naltrexone to be beneficial for a number of my patients with Lyme disease. The reason for this is that LDN appears to restore the ability of the immune system to regulate itself. When the immune system regulates itself properly, there is a significant reduction in chronic inflammation of the "autoimmune" type. Taken at bedtime, LDN blocks the body's endorphin receptors for a brief amount of time (one to two hours), signaling to the body that it is time to make endorphins. It turns out that the body normally manufactures endorphins around 2:00 A.M. to 4:00 A.M. That "time to manufacture" signal by LDN trains the body to produce endorphins in its normal cyclical way again. Over time on LDN, the body no longer needs the LDN signal and is able to regulate their production without it. Dr. Don's case illustrates how dramatically this therapy is able to work in some Lyme patients.

Don is a physician whom I treated for Lyme, Babesia, and Bartonella. He was one of the sickest people that I have ever worked with, but he managed to continue to work effectively in his profession despite his illness. Over a period of nearly three years, we were able to get one infection after another under control. But it became increasingly clear that he had chronic persistent problems. It seemed that he was destined to have chronic symptoms consistent with an autoimmune disorder. When I introduced the possibility that low dose naltrexone might potentially benefit him by helping re-regulate his immune system, he was anxious to try it. Within a week he and his wife notified me that his life was changed—he had not felt this "normal" in many years. He attributed all his additional success to low dose naltrexone.

Not everyone responds as wonderfully as Dr. Don did, but many do. Because of the benefits it has shown for Lyme disease, I am currently recommending that most of my chronic Lyme and TBD patients with persistent chronic inflammation consider a therapeutic trial of LDN. Incidentally, many of those who have taken LDN have had significant improvements in their CD57 counts, indicating that natural killer function has improved. Finally, I have found that LDN works best when the following three conditions have been addressed prior to its use: (1) vitamin D deficiency has been corrected, (2) food sensitivities have been corrected by the LID, and (3) adrenal stress or adrenal fatigue has been properly corrected.

Be sure to discuss this option with your physician. You'll need a prescription to obtain it. Unlike most other medications, it's very inexpensive. (Usually it is no more than $30 to $40 for a month's supply, depending on where you purchase it. Be sure to obtain it in its unaltered, not slow-dose form, as the latter will not provide the same benefits).

Another benefit of naltrexone is that it is safe and virtually free of side effects, although occasionally it can cause sleep problems during the first week or so of its use. (Should sleep problems persist, reduce the dose from 4.5 mg to 3 mg or even 1.5 mg temporarily.) It should also be avoided by women who are pregnant and, ideally, by anyone using narcotic medications (codeine, morphine, Percocet, tramadol) until two weeks after such medicines are discontinued. For more information about low dose naltrexone, please visit www.lowdosenaltrexone.org.

Endocrine (Hormonal) Disruption

One of the major and often overlooked problems that can occur with Lyme disease is the disruption of the body's endocrine system. The endocrine system is made up of the hypothalamus, pineal, pituitary (all located in the brain), thyroid and parathyroid (located near the throat), thymus (located behind the center of the upper chest), the adrenal glands (located atop the kidneys), the pancreas, and the sex glands (ovaries and testes), as well as glandular tissues found in certain blood vessels, and in the heart, intestines, lungs, and kidneys. The primary purpose of the endocrine system is to produce and regulate hormones.

Hormones are messengers that allow your body's internal organs to effectively communicate with one another. Hormones play many vital roles in maintaining the health of the body. Some hormones also influence how we feel. Just as a good system of communication allows a large office or organization to work in harmony, the communication among your body's organs that hormones make possible helps to keep your body in a state of optimal health.

As we discussed in chapter 4, the human body maintains its health by balancing opposites in a harmonious manner. This balancing process is known as homeostasis. The endocrine system is a prime example of the ebb and flow of opposites that occur during the process of homeostasis. Just as with the immune system, where the opposites of pro-inflammatory and anti-inflammatory factors work harmoniously in a state of health, so it is with the endocrine system, where some hormones have stimulatory (sympathetic) properties and others have properties that are inhibitory/relaxing (parasympathetic). Sympathetic hormones include estrogen and thyroid hormones, while parasympathetic hormones include cortisol and progesterone.

Sympathetic and parasympathetic hormones are not always in opposition to each other. They also have complementary or synergistic functions. For example, by working together, estrogen and progesterone combine to provide women with their feminine qualities. However, just as a single out-of-place musical chord can ruin a beautiful melody, it does not take much to throw your body's "symphony of hormones" out of balance. In fact, for many people, simply life in our fast-paced modern world with its attendant stresses is enough to disrupt hormonal balance. Our bodies and hormones were not designed to live in a world of artificial indoor lighting or where our food, water, and homes are burdened with harmful chemicals and toxic heavy metals. Additionally, although the advances of modern life have allowed us to live longer than our ancestors, as we age, many of our hormones decrease to levels that interfere with and disrupt the balance of the hormonal symphony that our Creator designed.

One of the most significant causes of endocrine disruption is stress. There are many different types of stress, such as physical and emotional stress, stress caused by the presence of chemicals and heavy metals in our bodies, and stress caused by bacterial and viral infections. Obviously, Lyme disease, as well as other TBDs, causes tremendous stress on the body and consequently on the endocrine system. As a result, patients suffering from chronic Lyme and/or other TBDs typically have low energy and low or no libido, as well as insomnia and other sleeping problems, all of which are due to or exacerbated by hormonal imbalances. The major hormones most commonly disrupted by Lyme/TBDs are the thyroid hormones, adrenal hormones, and sex hormones. The hormones produced in the latter two categories can also be grouped together as steroid hormones. In order for you to fully understand why restoring hormonal balance plays such a vital role in the proper treatment of Lyme and other TBDs, let's examine each of these major hormone systems.

Thyroid Hormones

The thyroid gland is responsible for maintaining proper body temperature and regulating your body's metabolism. The thyroid also regulates how the body uses energy, as well as regulating many other organ systems and functions in the body, including cell growth and reproduction, circulation, heart rate, and sex hormones.

The thyroid accomplishes its many tasks by manufacturing the thyroid hormone *T4*. When T4 enters body tissues, it is converted to its active form, *T3*. When thyroid levels in the body decrease, the pituitary gland in the brain senses it and produces thyroid stimulating hormone, TSH. TSH, in turn, signals the *thyroid gland* to produce more T4 and, to a lesser extent, T3. Conversely, if your body has too much thyroid hormone (a condition known as hyperthyroidism), the pituitary gland produces less TSH.

Stated another way, there are three key components to thyroid hormone production: (1) the TSH from the pituitary that stimulates the thyroid gland to produce the hormones, (2) the thyroid gland that produces the hormones, and (3) the hormones, T4 and T3, themselves. A healthy thyroid gland requires a small amount of TSH to be stimulated to produce its hormones, T4 and T3. If the thyroid gland is not healthy or if there are not enough building blocks (e.g., iodine or L-tyrosine) to produce the hormones, then the TSH will be elevated. Optimal TSH is between 0.5 and

1.99. I consider an elevated TSH to be anything above 2.0 and suppressed TSH to be anything less than 0.5.

Checking the levels of thyroid hormone in patients, especially those who exhibit symptoms of fatigue, should be second nature to physicians. I recommend that a patient's levels of TSH, free T3, and free T4 all be checked. The "free" levels of thyroid hormones show the amount of thyroid hormones that are freely available to the body and, therefore, are the levels that provide the clearest indication of overall thyroid function.

There are nuances to the interpretation of the tests of thyroid function that are beyond the scope of this book. There is one thyroid function test pattern that I would like to discuss in this book—the combination of low TSH (less than .5), T4 in the lower one-third of the normal range, and T3 in the lower one-third of the normal range. This particular pattern is often seen in patients who are also suffering from a condition called "adrenal fatigue," which is frequently a major problem for chronic Lyme patients. (I discuss adrenal fatigue in more detail later in this section of the chapter.)

Thyroid dysfunction, which is common in cases of chronic Lyme and other TBDs, usually occurs due to adrenal fatigue and/or from autoimmune factors that are related to Lyme and other TBDs. It is important to address any co-existing adrenal dysfunction prior to correcting thyroid abnormalities. When thyroid function is found to be low in my Lyme/TBD patients,

I usually prescribe thyroid hormones to replace those that the body is lacking. Doing so helps the body to function better. There are three options for boosting thyroid levels: the drug Synthroid, which is a synthetic form of T4; Armour thyroid, which is derived from animal thyroid glands and contains a combination of natural T4 and T3; and long-acting T3, which in many cases is the optimal choice, since it is the most active form of thyroid replacement. No matter what approach is used, patients need to be monitored by their physicians during treatment to ensure both that the treatment is working and that it is not resulting in excessive production of thyroid hormones.

Steroid Hormones (Adrenal and Sex Hormones)

The remaining hormones that have significance for patients with Lyme and other TBDs are cortisol and DHEA (produced by the adrenal glands) and estrogen, progesterone, and testosterone (all of which are produced by the sex glands). Collectively, these hormones are called *steroid* hormones. All these hormones are very important for maintaining optimal health.

Cortisol is perhaps the most important of the naturally occurring steroid hormones because of the many functions it performs, including maintaining proper blood pressure and blood sugar levels. Cortisol is also a very powerful anti-inflammatory hormone. (For this reason, prednisone, a synthetic version of cortisol, is sometimes prescribed by *non* Lyme-aware doctors to reduce inflammation in cases of arthritis and other inflammatory conditions.) As I've previously discussed, Lyme disease is an infection and also an inflammatory disease.

If the adrenal glands of someone with Lyme disease are unable to produce enough cortisol, that person's inflammation symptoms will inevitably worsen over time. Therefore, in an attempt to reduce the pain and inflammation caused by Lyme disease, the body calls upon the adrenal glands to produce greater than normal levels of cortisol. This increased demand on the adrenals results in what is known as "adrenal stress."

Eventually, as a result of the ongoing, continuous chronic inflammation demand placed upon the adrenal glands to keep producing cortisol, the adrenals reach a point of over-exertion known as "adrenal fatigue." When adrenal fatigue occurs, cortisol is no longer produced in sufficient amounts. This, in turn, leads to the body being even less able to control inflammation. Therefore, adrenal fatigue can be considered a pro-inflammatory condition. *In that setting of cortisol depletion, it may be necessary to add low-dose, physiologic (not immunosuppressive) amounts of cortisol to your regimen.*

Compounding the pro-inflammatory problem of adrenal fatigue are other common immune stressors. In addition to chronic infection of *Bb* bacteria and other harmful microorganisms, these stressors include chronic worry and anxiety, poor sleep, and, in some cases, the presence of toxic heavy metals such as lead and mercury. A poor diet, such as the standard American diet, is another major pro-inflammatory factor that can worsen adrenal fatigue. This results in a classic vicious cycle of chronic inflammation leading to adrenal fatigue leading to more chronic inflammation, and so on.

Adrenal fatigue, if left unchecked, inevitably leads to a cascade of other hormonal disruptions and imbalances. This includes reduced thyroid function, which is confirmed by the low levels of TSH, T4 and T3 that are usually seen in people suffering from adrenal fatigue.

Another major problem caused by adrenal fatigue is a deficiency in one or more of the sex hormones—estrogen, progesterone, and testosterone. The reason for this deficiency is that, when the body becomes cortisol deficient, it will bypass the manufacture of sex hormones in an attempt to produce more cortisol. To better understand how this happens, a brief discussion of the sex hormone pathway is in order.

The sex hormone pathway has various branches. The first step in the manufacture of adrenal sex hormones is cholesterol. Cholesterol (with the help of vitamin C) is converted to pregnenolone, which is the "mother hormone" from which all other adrenal steroid hormones are formed. Pregnenolone can go in one of three directions. It can pass into the (1) progesterone branch (progesterone, aldosterone), (2) the DHEA branch (estrogen, testosterone), or (3) the cortisol branch. When adrenal fatigue forces your body to choose which branch the pre-hormones should move into, it will choose to make the cortisol branch the dominant branch since the body, in its wisdom, knows that reducing inflammation is more important to its health than maintaining sex hormones for the purpose of libido and reproduction. (You might experience this shift away from sex hormones as decreased libido or progesterone deficiency symptoms.)

Remember, *you need cortisol, not sex hormones, to stay alive.* Given the choice, the body chooses life over sex. This is the reason why very sick people usually don't have a normal sex drive. As critically important to survival as cortisol is, excessive cortisol over time can also be destructive to the body. Therefore, as we have discussed so many times in this book, the body seeks a homeostatic balance of just enough but not too much cortisol.

In men, adrenal fatigue often results in reduced levels of DHEA and testosterone. In women, the result of adrenal fatigue is often a reduction of DHEA and progesterone. Further, these hormonal reductions in women result in higher levels of estrogen relative to progesterone (i.e., higher estrogen to progesterone ratio). Estrogen is a stimulatory hormone that, when elevated relative to progesterone, can cause anxiety, poor sleep, and symptoms that mimic premenstrual syndrome (PMS). This is a possible explanation for why many women with Lyme disease feel worse just before and during their periods, since progesterone levels are at their lowest during this time.

The chemical structures of cortisol and progesterone are nearly identical to each other. This makes it easier for the body to shunt aside progesterone during times of adrenal fatigue, as compared to estrogen. As a result, most women with adrenal stress or adrenal fatigue are likely to have low progesterone (with relatively higher estrogen levels), as well as reduced levels of cortisol, DHEA, and testosterone.

Testing for Hormone Deficiencies

There are three methods physicians can use to test hormone levels: twenty-four hour urine testing (the gold standard), blood tests, and saliva tests. I recommend saliva testing as the most practical method for everyday clinical use. Unlike blood tests, which rely on a single blood sample usually taken during the day, saliva tests provide a more accurate profile of a patient's hormone levels and patterns over a twenty-four hour period. The saliva test is also very simple to perform. All a patient has to do is collect a saliva sample by placing a swab inside the mouth. Six swab samples are taken over twenty-four hours (once every four hours, taken at 8 A.M., noon, 4 P.M., 8 P.M., midnight, and 4 A.M.) Each swab sample is placed into a sealed container that indicates the time it was collected, and then all six containers are sent to a lab for testing. Saliva testing allows physicians to better detect important patterns in hormone levels—especially cortisol and DHEA—throughout the entire four-hour period.

(For a list of labs that provide saliva hormone tests, please see the resources section.) Twenty-four hour urine testing, while yielding the most reliable and accurate results, is more difficult to obtain due to the collection process.

There are two common hormone patients that I see among chronic Lyme patients. The first is a pattern of those with difficulty falling asleep at night. Such sleeping problems are often due to cortisol production not decreasing at night as it should. When this pattern exists, patients often report that they feel tired all day and more awake at night. They may also say they do their best work at night and consider themselves to be "night owls." Usually, what is really going on is that their "symphony of hormones" is out of tune.

The other very common pattern is normal or low cortisol levels at night that then spike significantly around 4 A.M. Patients who exhibit this pattern usually tell me that if they skip a meal they feel "shaky" and "horrible." Often this is because they have hypoglycemia (low blood sugar). As I mentioned above, one of cortisol's many functions is to maintain proper blood sugar levels. It does this by producing glucose from glycogen (a form of glucose stored in the body) when the body needs it. The reason that hypoglycemic patients have a spike in their cortisol levels around 4 A.M. is because by that time they have usually not eaten for eight or more hours and, therefore, they start to experience hypoglycemia symptoms. This triggers the adrenal glands to start producing more cortisol in order to supply the body with more glucose. The problem with this is that the surge of cortisol can wake patients up and make additional sleep difficult to achieve. I usually recommend that patients with this pattern follow a no-sugar, low-carbohydrate diet and suggest that they eat some protein, such as nuts or a protein drink, before they go to bed.

Treating Hormonal Disruptions and Imbalances

Hormone imbalances are most commonly treated using synthetic hormone treatments such as Provera (synthetic progesterone) and Premarin (synthetic estrogen). Some Lyme-aware physicians, like myself, avoid such treatments because they don't act in the body the same way that the body's own hormones do, and they also carry the risk of side effects, including an increased incidence of heart disease and cancer. Additionally, oral estrogen drugs are also pro-inflammatory, a fact that is documented by increased levels of C-reactive protein (CRP) and interleukin-6 (IL-6) that are common in women who use such medications.

As a healthy alternative to synthetic hormones, I recommend the use of natural, or "bio-identical" hormones that are derived from natural sources such as soy and yam and which have chemical structures that are identical to the hormones in our bodies. Bio-identical hormones are much better tolerated by the body and have a much lower risk of dangerous side effects. The preferred method of application of bio-identical hormones is transdermal hormone creams that are absorbed through the skin. Like all other forms of hormone treatments, bio-identical hormone therapy should only be employed under a physician's supervision.

Energy Depletion and Fatigue

As I mentioned at the beginning of this chapter, lack of energy is one of the most common health complaints among people with Lyme and/or other tick-borne diseases. Additionally, in most cases of chronic Lyme disease, energy depletion is usually the last symptom to improve, unfortunately.

To improve energy levels, exercise and an overall healthy lifestyle are absolutely critical. Please review my exercise/activity recommendations from chapter 6. A healthy diet, such as the Lyme Inflammation Diet, is also extremely important. In addition to these factors, energy levels can also be improved using various conventional medications and nutritional and herbal supplements. In some cases, imbalances in the endocrine system (discussed above) may also need to be addressed, particularly with regard to the functioning of the adrenal and thyroid glands. I'll be dividing my discussion of energy depletion and fatigue as follows:

* Conventional Medications for Improving Energy Levels

* Complementary and Alternative Therapy with Glutathione

* Nutritional Supplementation

Conventional Medications for Improving Energy Levels

One of the most useful prescription medications for improving energy levels in patients with Lyme/TBDs is a drug called Provigil (modafinil). Provigil is approved by the Food and Drug Administration (FDA) to improve wakefulness in people who suffer from daytime drowsiness and an excessive need to sleep during the day. Provigil can also help to improve mood and mental alertness, helping to relieve the symptoms of "brain fog" that are also common among Lyme patients. It does *not* act by the same mechanism as brain stimulants such as Ritalin or Adderal. While Provigil is very effective, it is also very expensive. Insurance coverage is, unfortunately, a common problem with this medication. Effective dosage is from 100–400 mg per day.

Caution: As with most drugs, Provigil is not without the risk of side effects, so its use needs to be monitored by your physician. Additionally, Provigil should not be combined with alcohol and is not recommended for women who are pregnant.

Another prescription drug that can help with improving energy and reducing fatigue is Wellbutrin (bupropion), a commonly prescribed antidepressant. Wellbutrin is an excellent choice for Lyme patients who are fatigued and also depressed. Like Provigil and all prescription medications, it too carries the risk of side effects. The usual dosage is 150–300 mg per day.

Complementary and Alternative Therapy with Glutathione

In previous chapters I have mentioned the importance of glutathione (GSH). It is one of the most vital substances that our bodies manufacture. It serves multiple roles as:

* Powerful antioxidant (e.g., lungs and brain)

* Detoxifier (e.g., liver, brain, heavy metals)

* Immune system support and regulation (e.g., NK cells like the CD57)

Glutathione is manufactured from the amino acid methionine, which is converted to cysteine. Cysteine then, along with glutamine (in the form of L-glutamate) and glycine, combines to form GSH. Along the pathway to the final GSH product, many cofactors are required in its production, including vitamins B2, B6, B12, folic acid, and the mineral, selenium. Therefore, when nutritional B-complex vitamin deficiencies occur, as in Lyme infection, GSH production is almost certainly affected. Other causes of glutathione deficiency include smoking, alcohol or acetaminophen misuse, diabetes, HIV infection, and cancer. GSH is found in several foods, particularly avocado, asparagus, walnuts, fruits and vegetables, fish, and some meats; however, it is not significantly absorbed through the gastrointestinal tract, and many believe that dietary GSH is utilized by the gut itself.

I have found that supporting glutathione levels in the Lyme patient is very helpful for many reasons, particularly chronic fatigue and neurological dysfunction related to Lyme. There are two major ways to support GSH body levels: nutritional supplementation and intravenous administration.

GSH Oral Supplementation Support: As mentioned, oral glutathione is not significantly absorbed. There is an absorbable form of GSH available now called "acetylglutathione" that is effective when used as a dose of 100 mg two to three times a day. In addition, other supplements that are absorbed are very useful for supporting GSH production by the body itself. These include the following.

* N-acetyl cysteine (NAC) in doses of 500–1,500 mg per day

* Alpha lipoic acid in doses of 200–300 mg per day

* Undenatured whey protein at a dose of about 10 grams per day

* Vitamin C in doses of 500–2,000 mg per day

* L-glutamine 1,000–3,000 mg a day on an empty stomach

* Herbal products such as turmeric, milk thistle, garlic, cumin, black cumin, ginger, holy basil, poppyseed, and pomegranate

Use of the above supplements has been helpful, not only in improving energy levels related to GSH depletion, but also in supporting liver and immune system function. Most of my

Lyme/TBD patients are taking at least one or two of those supplements regularly.

Intravenous Glutathione Infusion: There are many occasions where a Lyme patient with severe fatigue or severe neurological dysfunction will require much higher doses of GSH than can be achieved by supplementing with the GSH enhancers alone. In those cases, intravenous glutathione has been close to a life-saver for them. It is very safe to use and is administered in an IV dosage of 500–2,000 mg.

Energy-Enhancing Nutritional Supplementation

There are a number of useful nutrients and herbs that can help to improve energy levels and reduce fatigue. Nutrients in this category include carnitine, coenzyme Q10 (CoQ10), D-Ribose, SAM-e, NADH, and tyrosine. Alpha glycan, which is derived from rice that comes from Thailand, can also be helpful.

Carnitine: Carnitine, also known as L-carnitine, is an amino acid substance synthesized by the body from the amino acids lysine and methionine. L-carnitine helps to produce energy in the body by aiding in the transport of fatty acids to the mitochondria, which are the energy factories in all your body's cells. It is also involved in the stabilization of blood sugar.

Foods that are excellent sources of L-carnitine include red meat (particularly beef—free range preferred) and dairy products. As an aside, I have often wondered whether red meat craving may be a symptom of inadequate L-carnitine in the diet, because people often feel so much better once that craving is satisfied.

L-carnitine is available in most health food stores as a supplement under the names acetyl-L-carnitine and L-carnitine. Acetyl-L-carnitine is particularly helpful for brain fatigue and has been shown to improve brain function, such as memory. L-carnitine is effective for general fatigue in Lyme patients and should be used at the dosage of 500–1,000 mg per day.

Coenzyme Q10: CoQ10 plays a variety of intricate and important roles in your body's ability to produce energy. Perhaps its most important role is that of helping the cells' mitochondria manufacture cellular fuel, known as adenosine-triphosphate, or ATP. I discussed CoQ10 extensively in chapter 6 and refer you back to that discussion.

While CoQ10 supplementation on its own can often improve energy levels, I have found that best results are achieved when CoQ10 is combined with L-carnitine. It is also best taken along with a full range of other essential vitamins, minerals (especially magnesium), and other nutrients.

D-Ribose: D-ribose is a naturally occurring carbon sugar that is found in all living cells. Like CoQ10, it too plays an important role in the production of ATP. D-ribose is actually the structural backbone of ATP and the first step in ATP formation. It is also important for the health of ribonucleic acid (RNA) and plays a role in the formation of DNA. Supplementing with D-ribose can help your body to produce greater levels of ATP, leading to greater and more sustained energy. Additionally, D-ribose can also act as a natural anti-stress and anti-anxiety agent, thereby helping to improve feelings of overall well-being. Most effective when combined with magnesium and CoQ10, the usual dosage of D-ribose is 2–5 grams two to three times a day.

SAM-e: SAM-e, which stands for S-adenosyl-L-methionine, is another amino acid that can help improve energy levels. Like D-ribose, SAM-e is also present in all the cells of the body. In addition to its ability to help maintain proper functioning of the mitochondria, one of the primary ways in which SAM-e helps to boost energy lies with its ability to enhance liver function and liver detoxification. Your liver is one of your body's most important organs, performing more than 1,500 functions each and every day. When liver function becomes sluggish or impaired due to the buildup of toxins, overall health suffers, as does energy production.

One of SAM-e's other important benefits is the role it can play in helping to relieve depression, making it an excellent choice for Lyme patients who are both chronically fatigued and depressed. Research has shown that SAM-e works as fast, or faster, than most FDA-approved antidepressant drugs, without their risk of side-effects. SAM-e also helps the body to produce the hormone melatonin, which is essential for healthy sleep, as well as for feelings of well-being.

Dosage recommendations for SAM-e are 200–1,200 mg in divided doses per day. I usually ask a patient to start with 200 mg in the morning on an empty stomach and in a few days add 200 mg in the afternoon. A few days later increase the dose by 200 mg more in the morning again, then the afternoon in a few days, and so on. Also I generally have my Lyme patients taking SAM-e to also supplement with vitamin B12.

NADH: This supplement is a derivative of the vitamin, niacin. It has been shown to be helpful for chronic fatigue and often can be helpful for neurodegenerative disorders like Parkinson's disease. The dose is 5–10 mg two to three times a day.

Tyrosine: Tyrosine, also known as L-tyrosine, is another amino acid that can help to improve energy. Additionally, tyrosine can improve concentration and mental alertness, making it useful for Lyme/TBD patients who suffer from fatigue and "brain fog." It also acts as a mood-enhancer and improves neurotransmitter function, which is something most Lyme patients require. It is also a necessary precursor of all the thyroid hormones (along with iodine) and sympathetic nervous system hormones (dopamine, epinephrine, and norepinephrine). The usual dose is 500–1,000 mg per day.

Caution: Tyrosine should be used cautiously for patients with Bartonella because it may increase anxiety in Bartonella patients. (These patients already tend to be anxious.)

Summing Up

What follow are answers to the most commonly asked questions about Lyme disease and P.I.E.E.

What does P.I.E.E. stand for?

P.I.E.E. stands for pain, inflammation, endocrine disruption, and energy depletion, four of the most significant symptoms associated with chronic cases of Lyme and other tick-borne diseases. Until each of these four factors is properly addressed, recovery from Lyme and other TBDs is usually much more difficult and, in many cases, impossible to achieve.

What are the most effective methods of treating the pain associated with Lyme and other TBDs?

Pain treatments fall into three categories: pain medication and conventional therapy, endorphin-enhancing therapies, and herbal and other therapies. Additionally, treatment approaches vary depending on the degree of pain symptoms (mild, moderate, and severe).

One of the inflammation treatments you recommend is low-dose naltrexone? Why?

Because naltrexone is able to block opioid receptors, it also is effective at blocking the reception of opioid hormones that are produced by the brain and adrenal glands, including endorphins. Many of your body's tissues have receptor sites for these endorphins, including nearly every cell in your immune system. The way naltrexone works is that it helps to "reset" the endorphin production cycle. When the endorphin cycle is properly restored, the result is better regulation of the immune system, resulting in reduced autoimmune inflammation. This benefit makes naltrexone an ideal treatment for helping to re-regulate a dysregulated immune system. In my opinion, low-dose naltrexone is one of the most important and exciting newer treatments for Lyme disease, as well as for many other health conditions where chronic inflammation plays a major role.

What are the most effective methods of treating inflammation associated with Lyme and other TBDs?

Adopting the Lyme Inflammation Diet, which is discussed in chapter 5, is perhaps the single most important step for reducing chronic inflammation in the body. In addition to the Lyme Inflammation Diet, various pharmaceutical drugs, as well as nutritional and herbal supplements, can also be effective. Such treatment choices are best undertaken under the guidance and supervision of your doctor.

Why is proper hormone function important for Lyme disease and other TBDs?

Hormones, which are produced and regulated by the glands that make up your body's endocrine system, are absolutely essential for good health. Hormones act as chemical messengers in your body that allow cells and organs to communicate with each other. When the endocrine system is disrupted and your body's hormone levels become imbalanced, this communication process is also disrupted, leading to a host of potential health problems.

Lyme disease, as well as other TBDs, causes tremendous stress on the body and, consequently, on the endocrine system. When this happens, the endocrine system is unable to effectively regulate other body systems, including the immune system, leading to an overall worsening of Lyme/TBD symptoms. This sets up a vicious circle. As a result, patients suffering from chronic Lyme and/or other TBDs typically have low energy and low libido, as well as a host of other problems, all of which are due to or exacerbated by hormonal imbalances.

How can patients with Lyme/TBDs determine if endocrine disruption is contributing to their health problems?

This can easily be achieved by testing patients' hormone levels. Thyroid is evaluated by blood testing. One of the most effective method for assessing adrenal function is a saliva hormone test that collects saliva samples throughout the day and night over a twenty-four hour period, enabling physicians not only to assess hormone levels, but also to determine patterns of hormone imbalances.

Which hormones are most commonly involved in Lyme disease and other TBDs?

All your body's hormones are important for good health. In cases of Lyme and other TBDs, the hormones that are most typically disrupted or imbalanced are thyroid hormones (TSH, T4, and T4), adrenal hormones (cortisol and DHEA), and the sex hormones (estrogen, progesterone, and testosterone).

What do you recommend to bring hormone levels back into balance?

Thyroid hormone imbalances can be treated using Synthroid, Armour thyroid, or long-active T3, which is often the best choice, since T3 is the most active form of thyroid hormone.

Imbalances in the class of steroid sex hormones (those produced by the adrenal and sex glands) are best treated using natural, or bio-identical, hormone therapy under a doctor's supervision.

What are the most effective methods of treating energy-depletion associated with Lyme and other TBDs?

To improve energy levels, a healthy diet, exercise, and an overall healthy lifestyle are essential. Additionally, certain conventional drug medications can help to improve energy levels, as can various nutritional supplements (especially D-ribose and CoQ10). Neither of these approaches is an effective substitute for eating right, exercising regularly, and following a healthy lifestyle.

This concludes my discussion of the approach to the first four of the serious and common "specific" difficulties that I deal with in working with Lyme and TBD patients. In the next chapter, I will deal with the other six specific common issues and problems encountered by Lyme and TBDs.

Chapter Eight

Improving Your Lyme
G.L.A.N.D.S.

✳

In this chapter I will deal with the next six common specific problems areas encountered by Lyme and tick-borne disease (TBD) patients. G.L.A.N.D.S. is another acronym I use to refer to these six factors that are often associated with chronic Lyme and other tick-borne diseases (TBDs). G.L.A.N.D.S. stands for the following:

> **G**astrointestinal tract function and related gastrointestinal problems
>
> **L**iver health
>
> **A**nxiety and depression
>
> **N**eurological function and related problems
>
> **D**etoxification
>
> **S**leep and sleeping problems

Like the elements of the unhealthy Lyme P.I.E.E. discussed in chapter 7, in order to most effectively treat chronic Lyme and other TBDs, each of these six factors must be properly addressed. In this chapter, I will provide my recommendations for accomplishing this goal.

Gastrointestinal Tract Function and Related Gastrointestinal Problems

The gastrointestinal (GI) tract is vitally important to your health. Restoring optimal GI function is also essential in order to successfully treat Lyme and other tick-borne diseases. An interesting fact about the GI tract is that it is where 70 percent of your body's immune system is located. Since the immune system is critical for controlling Lyme and other TBDs, the necessity of a healthy GI tract should be obvious. Additionally, your body's ability to properly digest and absorb nutrients and medications depends on a healthy GI tract. Your ability to overcome Lyme and other TBDs is significantly reduced when GI tract function is impaired and/or when gastrointestinal problems are also present. My discussion of the GI tract is divided into three parts:

* Overview of Normal GI Tract Function

* Common Problems Encountered in the GI Tract

* Treatment of GI Tract Problems

Overview of Normal GI Tract Function

The GI tract begins at the mouth, travels down through the esophagus, into the stomach, and then into the small and large intestines. The mouth, of course, is where the process of digestion begins. To help with this process, it's important that you adequately chew your food. Usually, this means chewing (up to thirty or more times) every bite of food. Properly chewing your food is important for two reasons. Doing so greatly reduces the size of food particles, making it much easier for them to be digested and assimilated. It also ensures that enough saliva is produced and mixed with your food. Saliva contains enzymes that further help to break down food.

Once food is properly chewed, it is swallowed and passes through the esophagus into the stomach, where it is mixed with further enzymes, as well as hydrochloric acid, which is essential for the proper breakdown and digestion of proteins. After the stomach does its job, food then enters the small intestine, where most of the digestion and assimilation occurs as further enzymes, along with bile, are mixed with it. Depending on the types of meals you eat, food remains in your small intestine for an average of four to six hours, as many of the nutrients it contains are assimilated and absorbed into the body, passing through the intestinal walls. Finally, what foodstuff remains enters into the large intestine, which absorbs water and minerals and eliminates waste products as stool.

Problems can occur at every step of this digestive process, starting in the mouth in cases of insufficient production of saliva by the salivary glands. In the esophagus, irritation can occur due to an influx of stomach acid if the sphincter (the valve that separates the esophagus from the stomach) is not tight enough. This can also lead to "acid reflux." In addition to excessive acid, problems in the stomach can also be due to a lack of hydrochloric acid production, a condition that is particularly common among people who regularly use antacid and acid blocking medications. Interestingly, a lack of stomach acid can lead to more acid reflux because the normal function of the sphincter separating the esophagus and stomach depends on the presence of adequate stomach acid.

Among the most common GI problems are those associated with the small and large intestines. In the small intestine, these problems can include insufficient bile and/or enzyme production. Either of these problems leads to poor digestion. In the large intestine, irritable bowel and antibiotic-related diarrhea are common. In either, overgrowth of unhealthy yeast (especially Candida) and/or unhealthy bacteria is a fairly frequent occurrence, especially among people who use antibiotics without the replacement of friendly bacteria called "probiotics." (See my discussion in chapter 6.)

Here are some important points to remember when it comes to maintaining the health of your gastrointestinal tract:

1) Nothing in the GI tract functions well unless there is adequate hydration. To ensure this, drink plenty of pure water, from eight to ten glasses, throughout the day. The goal is to drink enough water so that the urine is a pale yellow color.

2) As we grow older, the aging process tends to make the gastrointestinal tract less efficient at performing its functions. Although this is a natural consequence of life, it can be minimized with proper diet (especially the Lyme Inflammation Diet discussed in chapter 5), along with the use of natural digestive aids that we will discuss further in this chapter.

3) Adequate stomach acid is essential for healthy digestion, especially with regard to protein-rich foods. As I mentioned above, the use of antacid or acid-blocking medicine is a common cause of stomach acid deficiencies, particularly in people who suffer from acid reflux. If needed, stomach acid can be increased by taking betaine hydrochloride (betaine HCl) supplements *with meals*. A useful dosage range is between 300–600 mg, depending on need. Sipping apple cider vinegar mixed in water can also help to improve stomach acid deficiencies. Both betaine and apple cider vinegar may also help to tighten and improve the function of the sphincter valve that is designed to keep acid from entering the esophagus from the stomach.

4) For proper digestion of food as it enters the small intestine, adequate amounts of bile (produced by the liver) and pancre-

atic enzymes (produced by the pancreas) are necessary. To help stimulate bile and pancreatic enzyme production, I recommend the liberal use of various spices with your meals. Useful spices for this purpose include cinnamon, coriander, curry, fennel, garlic, and ginger.

5) Fiber and the amino acid "glutamine" are also essential for healthy gastrointestinal tract function. Glutamine acts as a direct fuel for the GI tract. It also is necessary for the production of glutathione (GSH), the powerful antioxidant that protects the cells of the GI tract from free-radical (oxidative) damage. (I discussed GSH in chapter 7.) Fiber is also important because it is converted by friendly GI tract bacteria into small chain fatty acids that form butyrate. Butyrate is then converted into acetate, which the intestinal cells use for energy. Unfortunately, today many people are deficient in fiber due to poor eating habits.

6) The health of the GI tract also depends on an adequate supply of the "friendly" bacteria that naturally reside in the intestines. Friendly bacteria are essential for many reasons, especially for the breakdown of fiber in order to produce butyrate fuel and for preventing the overgrowth of yeast, unhealthy bacteria, and other harmful microorganisms. The two most common and beneficial types of friendly bacteria are lactobacillus, which accounts for approximately 25 percent of the GI tract's healthy bacteria and is found mainly in the small intestine, and bifidobacteria (also

known as bifidus), which accounts for about 50 percent of all healthy bacteria and is found primarily in the large intestine. (For more information, see chapter 6.)

7) Another beneficial microorganism necessary for healthy GI tract function is a type of healthy yeast called *Saccharomyces*. It is very useful in keeping unhealthy yeast, including candida, under control.

Common Problems Encountered in the GI Tract

Two of the most common problems or imbalances that occur in the gastrointestinal tract are yeast overgrowth (candidiasis) and, less frequently, overgrowth of a toxic bacterium called *Clostridium difficile* (pseudomembranous colitis).

Candidiasis frequently occurs as a result of combining excessive sugar intake (which *Candida albicans* and other unhealthy yeast feed upon) and the kill-off of healthy, friendly bacteria by antibiotic drugs. Overly acidic pH levels due to poor diet, hormone imbalances, stress, exposure to environmental toxins, and the use of other drugs, such as steroids and oral contraceptives, can also cause yeast overgrowth.

All patients with Lyme and other TBDs are at risk for developing candidiasis due to the need for antibiotics as part of their treatment. Candidiasis not only weakens the GI tract and immune system, but its symptoms often mimic those of Lyme and TBDs. For example, people with candidiasis frequently experience anxiety and depression, brain fog, chronic fatigue, dizziness, and joint pain, all of which are also very common symptoms of Lyme and TBDs. When candidiasis symptoms and Lyme symptoms exist at the same time, it can be very confusing to your Lyme-aware doctor. For this reason, it is important that you do everything you can do to prevent candida infection.

Overgrowth of *Clostridium difficile* is also primarily due to the use of antibiotics. When overgrowth occurs, *Clostridium difficile* primarily spreads in the large intestine. Symptoms of *Clostridium difficile* overgrowth can include abdominal cramping, diarrhea, foul-smelling flatulence, and excessive buildup of mucous within the GI tract that can show up in stool. This treatable problem can be very serious and may require treatment with a medication called *metronidazole* (which is also used for the cystic form of Lyme).

There is another problem that needs to be mentioned. This problem, *celiac disease*, afflicts some patients with Lyme/TBD. Symptoms of celiac disease can be similar to those of Lyme and can be confused with Lyme (and vice versa). For this reason, this condition should be considered in patients with chronic Lyme/TBD. Celiac disease is caused by sensitivity of the GI tract to *gluten*, a component of grains such as wheat, rye, and barley. Corn does not contain the actual gluten substance, but rather a substance called "zein," which does not cause problems in celiac patients. (Additionally, gluten is an ingredient in certain medications and vitamin supplements, as well as in common household products, including the adhesive in envelopes and stamps.)

When people with celiac disease eat or use gluten-containing foods or products, gluten triggers an immune response that damages or destroys *villi*, which are tiny protrusions that line the small intestine. Villi help nutrients from food and antibiotic medications taken by mouth to be absorbed into the bloodstream so that they can be delivered to the body's cells, tissues, and organs. As a result of the damage and destruction to villi caused by gluten, people with celiac disease become malnourished no matter how much food they eat because their bodies are unable to properly absorb nutrition.

Most cases of celiac disease are genetic, meaning that it runs in families. In some cases, it can also be triggered by viral infections, severe stress, and life events such as childbirth, pregnancy, and surgery.

Treating GI Tract Problems

The following guidelines can help you to maintain the health of your GI tract, as well as correct any problems that may be present:

* Follow a healthy diet, preferably the Lyme Inflammation Diet, which is low in sugar and simple carbohydrates and is rich in enzymes and fiber.

* To help maintain a healthy balance of friendly bacteria, use probiotics daily, especially during and after antibiotic treatments and for several weeks after taking antibiotics. During the course of antibiotic treatment, take probiotic supplements between doses of antibiotics. For best results, open at least one of your probiotic capsules daily and swish its contents in your mouth before swallowing. Acidophilus and bifidus are the most common types of probiotic supplements, but other helpful varieties are also available. Recent research shows that probiotics may have profound balancing effects on the immune system, even helping reduce autoimmunity and allergy problems. Good quality, sugarless cultured yogurt that is rich in lactobacillus can also be helpful. (See chapter 6.)

* Be sure to chew each mouthful thoroughly, and during the day, drink lots of pure filtered water (ideally away from meals, since excess water with meals can interfere with the digestive process by diluting stomach acid).

* The use of spices with your meals can also aid digestion, as can supplementing with digestive enzymes (taken with meals), such as apple cider vinegar, Swedish bitters, and betaine HCl. Discuss use of these with your Lyme-aware doctor.

* To further help protect the health of the GI tract and aid in its healing, take glutamine supplements (2,000 mg two to three times daily).

* If you suffer from candidiasis (yeast overgrowth), you may need to consult with a physician experienced in

its treatment. (Most Lyme-aware physicians are.) Be sure to avoid all sugar and simple carbohydrate foods and take probiotic supplements several times a day. In some cases, the use of the anti-yeast antibiotic, Nystatin (500,000 to 3,000,000 units a day) may be necessary. Unlike most antibiotics, Nystatin is not absorbed into the blood stream and has a gentle effect on friendly bacteria in the GI tract. More difficult cases may require a stronger antibiotic known as fluconazole (Diflucan) 100–200 mg per day for up to a month.

* To treat *Clostridium difficile*, daily frequent probiotic supplementation is also called for. Specifially, *Saccharomyces* may be very helpful. More serious cases may need to be treated with metronidazole (Flagyl) 500–2,000 mg per day for several days to several weeks.

Liver Health

Your liver is one of your body's most important organs, and healthy liver function is absolutely essential for good health. In this section, I will cover the following subjects:

* Basic Liver Functions

* Tests of Liver Function

* Preventing and Reversing Liver Damage

Basic Liver Functions

Located primarily on the right side of your body, behind the lower ribs, the liver is equal in size to a football, making it the second largest organ in your body. (Your skin is the largest.) The liver performs literally thousands of different functions each and every day. The following are some of the more important liver functions:

* Aiding in digestion and regulating overall metabolism

* Regulating the transport of fat stores in the body

* Manufacturing new proteins, including proteins necessary for healthy immune function

* Producing energy quickly whenever the body requires it

* Storing vitamins, minerals, and glucose and other sugars

* Regulating blood clotting ability

* Maintaining proper hormone balance

* Eliminating bacteria and toxins from the bloodstream

* Metabolizing alcohol and toxic chemicals

* Processing pharmaceutical drugs and then eliminating them from the bloodstream

Based on these and the many other functions the liver performs, it is accurate to say that the liver provides one of the most significant lines of defense against disease, compared to many of your body's other organs. Therefore, when liver function becomes impaired, your body's disease-fighting ability diminishes as well. Additionally, without a healthy liver, your body is unable to adequately digest (or process) food and obtain the nutrients they contain. Nor is it able to minimize the burdens of toxins that all of us are exposed to in our polluted world. Needless to say, impaired liver function also makes it much more difficult for your body to successfully recover from Lyme disease and other TBDs. Therefore, I recommend that all patients with Lyme/TBDs do all they can to protect their livers and have their liver function closely followed by their doctors.

Tests of Liver Function

Despite the many important roles that the liver plays in maintaining your body's health, unlike most other organs, when its function becomes impaired, the liver does not provide obvious warning signs of what is happening. If warning signs appear at all, usually it is only after liver function has deteriorated to dangerous levels. Fortunately, your physician can easily and accurately determine how well your liver is functioning using various blood tests. There are many, many tests of liver function that can be done by your doctor. However, the most useful tests for basic screening of liver health include:

ALT—This test measures blood levels of ALT (alanine aminotranferase), an enzyme that is found mainly in the liver. (ALT also occurs in smaller amounts in the heart, kidneys, pancreas, and your body's muscles.) Small levels of ALT in the blood are normal, but when the liver becomes damaged or diseased, blood levels of ALT rise. Because the ALT test screens for ALT blood levels, it is one of the most accurate indicators of liver damage.

AST—Like the ALT, the AST (aspartate aminotransferase) is another liver enzyme. Some level of AST is always normally present in the bloodstream. However, when the liver becomes damaged or diseased, AST blood levels increase. The amount of AST in the blood is directly related to the degree that the liver is diseased or damaged, making the AST test a very reliable indicator of the severity of liver damage or disease.

Hepatitis A, B, and C Panel—Hepatitis is a disease that causes inflammation in the liver. It is caused by three main strains of hepatitis virus: A, B, and C. Because of the increased occurrence of hepatitis in recent years, I generally recommend that a hepatitis B and C test be included among the initial liver blood tests your physician conducts. (Hepatitis B and C can become chronic.)

Preventing and Reversing Liver Damage

To help support the health of your liver I recommend the following lifestyle and self-care approaches, all of which can also help to reverse liver damage:

* Avoid liver toxins that deplete the liver of glutathione (GSH). Glutathione is critical for healthy liver function. The most common and important liver toxin is alcohol, which should be eliminated from your diet for at least as long as you are being treated for Lyme/TBDs. Improper use of acetaminophen may cause glutathione depletion also.

* To increase the supply of glutathione in the liver, supplement your diet with the nutrients vitamin C, N-acetyl cysteine (NAC), or alpha lipoic acid. A once daily dose of 300–600 mg of each nutrient is appropriate for this purpose.

* Drink green tea two to three times a day. Green tea is a rich source of substances called *catechins*, which protect against liver toxins. Green tea has also been shown to have strong antioxidant properties.

* Milk thistle is an herb with a long history of use for liver problems. As the most helpful natural liver protector, it stimulates the production of liver glutathione. Take 300–600 mg of milk thistle in capsule form a day. Often I will ask my Lyme patients on antibiotics to take this herb for liver protection even if liver functions tests are normal. If they are not using the herb, they are instructed to start milk thistle immediately if any abnormality of liver function testing occurs.

* Also supplement with a good multivitamin/mineral formula that contains the antioxidants beta carotene, vitamin C, vitamin E, selenium, and zinc. Another excellent antioxidant for the liver is grape seed extract in the dosage of 60–120 mg twice a day.

In cases of Lyme disease, in addition to its usual detoxification functions, the liver also needs to detoxify the body of Lyme toxins and antibiotic residues. To assist in this process, the following guidelines can be extremely helpful:

* Make foods high in omega-3 oils a regular part of your diet. Sardines and wild-caught salmon are excellent food choices for this purpose. Also take purified fish oil supplements on a daily basis (2,000–3,000 mg per day).

* Eat plenty of raw foods, especially fresh fruits and vegetables. Plant-based foods (except beans, potatoes, and tomatoes) better help the processes of liver detoxification when consumed raw or juiced rather than cooked. Artichokes and dandelion leaves are two particularly liver-helpful vegetables. Phases One and Two of the Lyme Inflammation Diet (LID) are designed to help jumpstart this cleansing and detoxification process. I highly recommend that the LID be followed according to the guidelines I provided in chapter 5.

* Eat only organic foods if possible. Nonorganic foods contain herbicides and pesticides and other substances that add to the burden of liver detoxification. Organic foods, by contrast, help to reduce the toxin burden placed on the liver.

* Make nuts a regular part of your diet, as they assist both liver and gallbladder function. They are an excellent source of healthy oils and quality protein. Nuts also make an ideal snack food between meals.

* Use only healthy omega-6 oils, such as borage, black currant seed, and evening primrose oils. Avoid unhealthy sources of omega-6 oils like some vegetable cooking oils that may help increase the deposit of fats in the liver, thus adding to its burden. Cooking with olive oil will assure you that you have adequate omega-9 oil intake.

Anxiety and Depression

Everyone experiences anxiety and depression at some point in their lives, yet for some people these can become serious problems, significantly affecting their overall health. These disorders rank as the most common psychological problems in the United States and affect an estimated 27 million Americans at some point in time. In this section I will discuss both topics:

(1) Anxiety in Lyme/TBD Patients

* The Spectrum of Chronic Anxiety

* Factors That Can Cause Anxiety

* Treating Anxiety

(2) Depression in Lyme/TBDs Patients

* The Spectrum of Depression

* Factors That Can Cause Depression

* Treating Depression

The Spectrum of Chronic Anxiety

Chronic anxiety is a very common problem among people with Lyme and other TBDs. Approximately 50 percent of chronic Lyme/TBD patients experience serious psychological problems, with anxiety being chief among them. Frequent symptoms of chronic anxiety include impaired ability to relax, exaggerated or excessive worry, unusual fears, feelings of panic and impending doom, and poor sleep. Other common symptoms include shortness of breath, headaches, irritability, lightheadedness, muscle tension, nausea, sweating, and shakiness and trembling.

Many patients with Lyme/TBDs who suffer from serious anxiety are referred to psychologists or psychiatrists because of their disorder. In many cases, they are also prescribed medications, such as Xanax and other drugs known as benzodiazepines. Proper treatment can be problematic, however, unless care is given to answering the question: What came first, the anxiety or the Lyme/TBDs? In other words, physicians need to know whether their patients were suffering with anxiety disorders prior to becoming infected with Lyme/TBDs, or whether the anxiety they are experiencing is a result of Lyme/TBDs. Knowing the answer to this question can make a big difference in terms of effective patient care.

Fortunately, there are a number of clues physicians can look for in order to determine whether Lyme/TBDs is the cause of their patients' anxiety.

* Anxiety symptoms occurred at or around the same time as the onset of other symptoms associated with systemic Lyme/TBDs.

* Anxiety symptoms do not correlate with any typical life stressors that might otherwise explain anxiety, such as job loss, family crisis, relationship issues, death of a loved one, or other kinds of common stressors.

* There is only partial and incomplete improvement of anxiety symptoms despite treatment with usual anxiety therapies, such as counseling, medications, or other treatment modalities.

Factors That Can Cause Anxiety

Some infections are more likely to cause anxiety than others. In general, Lyme and Bartonella/BLO are the tick-borne diseases that cause the most severe levels of anxiety. Bartonella is especially anxiety-causing.

A major contributing factor to anxiety in Lyme/TBD patients is the *chronic stress* caused by infection with *Bb* and other tick-borne bacteria. As I discussed in chapter 7, chronic stress can lead to hormonal disturbances that result in excessive levels of "stress hormones," cortisol and norepinephrine, being produced in the body. These hormones themselves cause psychological effects. Over time this increased adrenal demand can cause adrenal stress and fatigue. This, in turn, can result in other hormonal abnormalities, especially progesterone deficiency in women and testosterone deficiency in men. Among the most common symptoms associated with progesterone and testosterone deficiencies are fatigue, anxiety, and sleep disturbances.

Magnesium deficiency is another contributor to anxiety. Most Americans have a magnesium-deficient diet. The body's magnesium stores are further depleted by Lyme disease and Bartonella/BLO. Common symptoms caused by magnesium deficiency are dizziness, headache, heart palpitations, muscle cramps and twitches, nervousness, and sensitivity to noise. These are all also symptoms of anxiety. To determine if you suffer from magnesium deficiency, have your physician order either an "ionized" magnesium blood level or a red blood cell (RBC) magnesium blood test. As I have told you previously, magnesium levels in the red blood cells are a much more reliable indicator of magnesium levels in the body than serum magnesium levels.

Poor diet in general is another factor that must be addressed in order to relieve symptoms. Dietary stimulants in the form of caffeine, glutamates (such as monosodium glutamate, or MSG), and artificial sweeteners such as aspartame (Nutrasweet) can also contribute to anxiety in Lyme/TBD patients. These products need to be avoided.

Treating Anxiety

Anxiety is one of the major presenting complaints of my new patients with Lyme/TBDs. The following treatment approaches can be very helpful in relieving anxiety disorders in Lyme/TBD patients:

* The antibiotic drug rifampin can often be extremely effective in treating severe anxiety symptoms that are due to Lyme/TBDs. *Severe anxiety is often a clue to the presence of Bartonella/BLO*, and rifampin is one of the most useful antibiotics against Bartonella/BLO (and also happens to treat Ehrlichia, Anaplasma, Lyme, and several other organisms). Please refer to chapter 6 for my complete recommendations related to this extremely valuable antibiotic.

* Follow the Lyme Inflammation Diet, which includes eliminating your caffeine, aspartame, MSG, and other stimulant intake. Interestingly, in some patients onions and garlic may have a stimulatory effect also and, though very healthy food choices, may need to be curtailed.

* To increase magnesium levels if the RBC magnesium level is in the lower half of the normal range (or less), take a *magnesium supplement* daily (400–1,000 mg, in divided doses). *Caution:* If you have kidney disease, consult with your physician concerning supplementation with magnesium.

* To support adrenal function and, therefore, help to relieve/reverse hormonal imbalances, vitamin B complex (especially vitamin B5), vitamin C, and the herbs eleuthrococcus (Siberian ginseng) and rhodiola (goldenroot) can be helpful. (See my discussion of these adrenal supporting products in chapter four.)

* Consider receiving acupuncture and/or Swedish massage on a regular basis. Both of these therapies are effective for relieving anxiety symptoms and also provide a host of other health benefits.

* Emotional and spiritual support in the form of counseling can also be very helpful, along with the recommendations provided in chapter 9.

In addition to the nutrients and herbs mentioned above, the nutritional and herbal supplements listed below can also help to relieve anxiety symptoms.

* Inositol is a member of the B complex family that is found in beans, peas, lentils, cantaloupe, cereals, and nuts. Take 500 mg two to three times per day. (Inositol is especially good for anxiety characterized by obsessive worries and/or obsessive-compulsive tendencies.)

* GABA (500 mg two to three times per day) with pyridoxal-5-phosphate, a derivative of vitamin B6. GABA is a neurotransmitter known for its relaxing effects. Chinese foxglove is an excellent natural source of GABA.

* L-theanine, an amino acid, can also be helpful. Take 100–200 mg once a day. Green tea is an excellent source.

* Passion flower (350 mg two to three times per day).

* Valerian root, taken as a tea or tincture. Valerian root is related to the benzodiazepine group of drugs and is best taken near bedtime.

* Kava kava and St. John's wort. Though both of these herbs can relieve anxiety symptoms, I don't recommend them very often because *they cannot be safely combined with antidepressant medications.*

The Spectrum of Depression

Like anxiety, depression is a very common symptom in persons with Lyme and other TBDs. Lyme and Babesia patients seem to be especially prone to depression in my observation, as opposed to Lyme and Bartonella patients, who are more disposed to develop anxiety.

One of the main problems many people with depression face is their inability to admit they suffer from it. Usually, this is due to fear that they will somehow be judged negatively. But not admitting to depression can be dangerous. Left untreated, depression can become severe, leading to a number of other health problems. It can even lead to thoughts of suicide. Therefore, I recommend that anyone suffering from ongoing depression admit that they have a problem and seek professional help. Many physicians have some level of training in depression care, as well as for other psychological problems. Depending on the severity of symptoms, your physician may refer you to other health care professionals who specialize in mental and emotional problems. These include psychiatrists and psychologists, as well as counselors and practitioners in the field of mind/body medicine.

The short-term use of prescription medications and/or natural therapies can be very helpful in treating depression and should not be overlooked as part of a comprehensive treatment approach for Lyme and other TBD patients. Additionally, depression is a major suppressor of the immune system and, as I explained in chapter 4, unless immune function is fully restored, healing Lyme/TBD patients is extremely difficult, if not impossible.

Factors That Can Cause Depression

Like anxiety in relation to Lyme/TBD patients, treating depression effectively requires determining its cause. In people with chronic Lyme/TBDs, obviously the infection and its symptoms can be a direct contributing factor. Lyme and Babesia particularly cause profound depression in my experience. However, depression can also be caused by a variety of other factors, both mental/emotional and physical. These factors when combined with Lyme/TBDs make management of depression very challenging for a Lyme-aware doctor.

Mental/Emotional Factors: Causes of depression in this category include marital and other relationship issues, unresolved issues from the past, financial worries, job loss or difficulties at work, major life changes, and chronic stress related to emotions. Ironically, sometimes major positive changes in one's life can also result in depression. These can include marriage, the addition of a child, a job promotion, and a sudden financial windfall, to name just a few.

Physical Factors: Common physical triggers of depression include allergies (both food and environmental), chronic inflammation, chronic pain, hormonal imbalances, nutritional imbalances, poor diet, and stress. Depression can be caused by certain medications and can also be a warning symptom of underlying disease, including candidiasis (systemic yeast overgrowth), certain types of cancer, diabetes, hypoglycemia (low blood sugar), sleeping problems (full discussion to follow later in this chapter), toxic states such as heavy metal overload (such as mercury), and thyroid problems (both hyper- and hypothyroidism).

Because depression can be caused by so many potential factors, it is important to first determine the specific causes at work in each individual before a proper treatment plan can be implemented.

Treating Depression

Although chronic depression needs to be treated by a health care professional, the following self-care guidelines can also be helpful in minimizing symptoms.

Diet: Follow the Lyme Inflammation Diet, which is low in sugar and refined carbohydrates. Consider eating frequent nutritious snacks to keep blood sugar levels balanced. If possible, make sure all meals and snacks are combined with a protein food (nuts, eggs, yogurt, meat, and so forth). Avoid all junk food (especially foods sweetened with aspartame, which depletes serotonin), sweets, and alcohol. Also be tested for food allergies and sensitivities, if suspected, and avoid all foods to which you are found to be allergic or sensitive.

Nutritional Supplements: Take a B complex vitamin supplement along with additional B6, folic acid, and B12. Vitamin C can also be helpful, as can magnesium (400–1,000 mg per day if kidneys are normal), omega-3 (up to 10,000 mg of fish oil per day), and the amino acid 5-HTP (50–100 mg at bedtime), choline (250 mg per day which also helps with liver and brain health), SAM-e (200–1200 mg per day), or tryptophan (500–1000 mg at bedtime—under the supervision of your Lyme-aware doctor, naturopathic physician, or psychiatrist). It is important that your vitamin D level be checked and that you use sunlight and supplementation to keep your 25-OH vitamin D level in the ideal range (45–60 ng/mL). This is especially important in the winter when sunlight exposure is more limited. Studies have linked vitamin D deficiency and seasonal affective disorder (SAD), although the mechanism is not totally clear.

Herbal Supplements: Both ginkgo biloba and St. John's wort can help relieve mild depression. I don't recommend St. John's wort very often, however, because it can interfere with antidepressant and other medications.

Exercise: Exercise is *one of the best natural antidepressant lifestyle choices you can make.* Try to exercise regularly each week, following the recommendations in chapter 6. I cannot overemphasize this point and I strongly recommend that you go back to that chapter and review my recommendations.

Lifestyle: In chapter 9, I will go into greater detail concerning these and other self-help emotional and spiritual practices that will improve mood and well-being. Try practicing *deep breathing exercises* for five to ten minutes for a few times each day. For best results, sit comfortably in a chair and breathe deeply with your eyes closed, inhaling slowly through your nose and breathing deeply into your belly.

Another helpful lifestyle choice is to *focus on enjoying something each day.* Consciously seek out opportunities to engage in activities that give you pleasure and that are relaxing. Try to engage in at least one such activity at least once a day. Spending time in nature can also be helpful.

Try not to dwell on negative thoughts and seek out experiences that make you laugh, since laughter provides a wealth of healthy benefits, and try to get adequate sunlight exposure for at least a half hour every day. During overcast days and during winter, consider using a "sun box" device, which mimics natural sunlight. For more on healthy lifestyle choices, see chapter 9.

Sleep: Try to go to sleep at the same time each night and to awaken at the same time each morning, and sleep for at least 7.5 hours. (See section on sleep later in this chapter.)

If needed there are conventional medical approaches to depression that really do work. I strongly recommend that you consider them as temporary ways to deal with the biochemical imbalances in your brain that can be caused by Lyme and the TBDs. The following prescription medications, taken as directed under your doctor's supervision, can also be helpful in relieving depression:

* Amitriptyline (10–100 mg at bedtime). This is an effective drug for treating depression associated with chronic pain and/or depression. However, it can frequently cause significant dry mouth, urine retention, and excessive morning drowsiness. Two other drugs that have similar properties (and fewer side effects) are nortriptyline (25–75 mg per day) and trazedone (50–150 mg per day).

* Cymbalta (up to 120 mg per day). Cymbalta is an excellent choice if chronic pain is also an issue.

* Lexapro (10–20 mg once per day). Lexapro is especially useful when chronic anxiety is also present.

* Paxil (20–50 mg). Paxil is a good choice when depression is accompanied by panic and/or social anxiety. Weight gain may be a chronic problem with this antidepressant.

* Wellbutrin (150–300 mg once per day). Wellbutrin is especially helpful in cases of depression accompanied by chronic fatigue. Another advantage is that it does not interfere with REM (dream) sleep. It has the added advantages of helping with smoking cessation and does not cause weight gain, unlike many of the other recently introduced antidepressants.

* Zoloft (25–100 mg once per day). This is the overall best-tolerated antidepressant drug in my practice and is the one that I most commonly prescribe. Most people prefer taking this medication at night.

Neurological Function and Related Problems

One of the more challenging aspects of treating chronic Lyme and other TBD patients is that of effectively dealing with problems related to neurological function. Several factors, often occurring simultaneously during Lyme/TBDs, contribute to this challenge. The six factors that I will address individually include the following:

* Infection, ongoing and not yet controlled by antibiotics and the immune system

* Chronic inflammation, especially due to poor diet and unhealthy lifestyle

* Oxidative stress, particularly due to a deficiency of glutathione (GSH) and other crucial antioxidants

* Neurotoxin accumulation

* Brain metabolism problems, involving abnormalities in the way the brain and neurological tissue handle glucose and other energy sources

* Neurotransmitter, hormonal, and miscellaneous other items

Let's examine each of these factors.

1) Infection: First and foremost, in any approach to helping a patient with neurological problems related to Lyme or the other TBDs, is to deal effectively with the ongoing infections themselves. This is done by a combination of antibiotics (particularly intravenous ceftriaxone or oral rifampin), lifestyle changes (including diet, exercise, and stress management), nutritional supplements, and alternative therapies. All these areas, which are the "core" elements of my Lyme/TBD treatment strategy, are covered in chapter 6. I place infection control first on my list in this section because it is critical that it be the first priority; otherwise, nothing else will be very effective.

2) Chronic Inflammation: The role of chronic inflammation in chronic neurological conditions has been extensively addressed in medical research. According to neurologist David Perlmutter, M.D., an expert on neurodegenerative diseases and the author of *Brain Recovery* and of *The Better Brain Book*, chronic inflammation (especially when combined with glutathione deficiency) is the primary cause of chronic degenerative brain diseases, including Alzheimer's and Parkinson's. Interestingly, the increased incidence of such diseases in recent decades has been accompanied by a parallel rise in poor eating habits (a major cause of chronic inflammation) and nutrient-deficient foods. Our diets fail to adequately provide the body with all the nutrients it needs. The current standard American diet encourages a pro-inflammatory state instead of a balanced homeostatic state that was our Creator's original design. The topic of chronic inflammation has been discussed extensively in chapters 5 and 7 of this book. I refer you to those chapters for further details. However, I would like to re-emphasize the fact that most (if not all) chronic Lyme and TBD patients do suffer from chronic inflammation. One of the most useful blood tests for chronic inflammation is the C-reactive protein (CRP) that I discussed in chapter 5. Also in that chapter, I provided you with a self-assessment questionnaire that you can use to determine if you are at risk for chronic inflammation.

Finally, in chapter 7, I reviewed the most useful approaches to controlling chronic inflammation. In terms of the specific control of neurological chronic inflammation, the following nine therapies stand out as being extremely useful and effective for brain and neurological inflammation:

* **The Lyme Inflammation Diet.** This is the most powerful action you can take to reduce, as well as prevent, chronic inflammation. Be sure to emphasize fish and other seafood that are rich in essential fatty acids. Herring, sardines, and wild-caught salmon are excellent choices. Additional healthy "brain foods" include avocados, beans, blueberries, nuts and seeds, pomegranate (as well as pomegranate juice), and whole grains.

* **Essential fatty acids** (omega-3 and healthy omega-6). Aim for 2,000–5,000 mg of purified fish oil per day. Flax and other omega-3 sources are good, but may not be effective in a chronically ill person. Supplemental omega-6 oils, such as borage oil at 240–960 mg per day, are highly useful also.

* **Vitamin D3.** Take vitamin D3, which is a better source than vitamin D2 (commonly used in nutritional supplement products). It helps with immune-regulation and the reduction of NF-kB levels. The dose is 400–5,000 IU per day with the goal of bringing the "25-OH vitamin D" blood level to 45–60 ng/mL.

* **Green tea.** Freshly brewed green tea provides a variety of health benefits, including protection against inflammation by reducing levels of NF-kB. Be sure the tea is freshly brewed and avoid bottled and powdered green

tea products, because these do not provide the same benefits. Drink two to four cups per day.

* **Curcumin.** One of the most versatile anti-inflammatory herbal products, it has been shown to improve immune function as well as reduce levels of NF-kB. It also helps increase glutathione levels. The dosage is 800–2,100 mg per day.

* **Stephania root.** This herb is very effective for reducing neurological inflammation, including Bell's palsy and Lyme-related eye inflammation. It has been shown to reduce IL-6 and NF-kB. The dosage is 300–600 mg per day.

* **Resveratrol.** This important phytochemical substance should be a mainstay for most Lyme/TBD patients. It has the unique ability to modulate and regulate inflammation so that the body gets what it needs. Excellent sources include Japanese knotweed, grape leaves, and grapeseed. The Japanese knotweed dosage is 500–1,500 mg per day.

* **Andrographis.** This herb, like Japanese knotweed, is a mainstay herb useful for most Lyme/TBD patients. It has excellent anti-spirochetal properties, as well as exceptional abilities to reduce levels of NF-kB and to increase activity of *PPAR gamma*. (I will discuss this important topic later in this section.) The standardized herb dosage is 400–1,200 mg per day. See the chapter 6 discussion of andrographis for precautions and side effects of andrographis.

* **Low dose naltrexone** (LDN). For certain patients, the immune-regulatory action of low dose naltrexone is nearly miraculous. In cases of chronic neurological inflammation, a trial of LDN is safe and potentially very effective. The dosage is 4.5 mg per night.

In some cases of severe chronic inflammation, some patients may also require the short-term use of anti-inflammatory drugs. Aspirin and certain non-steroidal anti-inflammatory drugs (NSAIDs) such as ibuprofen have been shown to both reverse and protect against chronic inflammation. More recently, they have also been shown to have benefit for people with brain diseases, including Alzheimer's and Parkinson's. Such drugs should only be used under your doctor's supervision, however. Acetaminophen should be avoided because it can deplete glutathione.

3) Oxidative Stress: Oxidative stress refers to the situation where the body is overloaded with free radicals and pro-oxidant chemicals that are unneutralized by sufficient antioxidants. It is important to remember that the body needs free radicals and pro-oxidant chemicals (like hydrogen peroxide) in order to kill foreign invaders like *Bb*. However, when the body is in a constant state of pro-oxidant excess, the result is an unbalanced, abnormal, and unhealthy state called oxidative stress. Remember, for proper balance and homeostasis, pro-oxidants must be balanced with sufficient antioxidants.

Like the unhealthy pro-inflammatory state, the condition of pro-oxidant excess (oxidative stress) is potentially very damaging to the body. In fact, the pro-oxidant and the pro-inflammatory states are related—oxidative stress increases inflammation by inducing the production of the pro-inflammatory chemical NF-kB (see chapter 7). Additionally, along with chronic infection, our poor diets and unhealthy lifestyles are major contributors to oxidative stress. Thankfully, the Lyme Inflammatory Diet (LID) is an extremely useful tool for balancing the oxidative stress state because it provides an abundance of antioxidants. Often it is important to combine the LID with the use of supplemental antioxidants (oral supplements and even intravenous glutathione) when fighting Lyme and the TBDs. In this section I will discuss the critical importance of specific antioxidant support related to Lyme neurological damage.

Below are five oral antioxidants and one intravenous antioxidant that I have found to be very useful in working with my neurologically challenged Lyme/TBD patients:

* **Vitamin C.** This antioxidant is the most important antioxidant not manufactured inside the body itself. It is critical that Lyme/TBD patients get adequate vitamin C both from diet and in supplement form. Vitamin C comes in two forms—naturally occurring water-soluble (*ascorbic acid*) and human-engineered fat-soluble (*ascorbyl palmitate*). The fat-soluble vitamin C has eight times the effectiveness of the water soluble type, especially for

regenerating vitamin E and other antioxidants. There are areas of the brain—especially the *nucleus accumbens* (vital to movement control) and *hippocampus* (vital to memory)—that contain very high concentrations of vitamin C. In addition to the aging process, oxidative stress related to Lyme depletes these areas of vitamin C. The brain and other neurological tissues have a high amount of fatty tissue; therefore, fat-soluble vitamin C in the form of ascorbyl palmitate should ideally be included as part of the daily vitamin C intake. For that reason, I recommend 500–2,000 mg of vitamin C routinely, with a portion (200–500 mg per day) coming from ascorbyl palmitate.

* **Vitamin E.** In the form of *mixed tocopherols* it is very important. Be sure to avoid synthetic "dl-alpha tocopherol" which, in my opinion, is ineffective. It is critical that your vitamin E supplement contain an adequate amount of *gamma tocopherol*, which is the type of vitamin E most useful for neurological healing and protection. The dose is 200–800 IU of mixed tocopherols, ideally with one-third or more from gamma sources. *It is always necessary to use vitamin C while using vitamin E, because vitamin C regenerates vitamin E, preventing it from becoming toxic.*

* **CoQ10.** This is a fat-soluble antioxidant, and high doses of CoQ10 have been shown to be effective against neurodegenerative disorders such as Parkinson's disease. Routinely, Lyme patients should be taking CoQ10 on a regular basis (see chapter 6), but when serious neuro-

logical symptoms persist, the amount of CoQ10 needs to increase to 200 mg three or four times a day.

* **Grapeseed extract (GSE).** Due to its content of a very powerful antioxidant called proanthrocyanidin, GSE is exceptionally useful as a brain antioxidant. The usual dosage is 60–200 mg twice a day.

* **Alpha lipoic acid (ALA).** This is another powerful fat-soluble antioxidant that is crucial to regeneration of other antioxidants like vitamins C and E. It is one of the best antioxidants for the production and regeneration of the brain's most important antioxidant, glutathione. ALA helps with peripheral nerve symptoms, as well as with central nervous system and brain problems. It also lowers NF-kB and is therefore also an anti-inflammatory. The usual dosage is 200–300 mg per day.

* **Glutathione (GSH).** This is the most important anti-oxidant produced by the body itself. When GSH levels are depleted in neurological tissue, damage can occur. Dr. Perlmutter, whom I mentioned earlier, believes that, along with chronic inflammation, GSH depletion accounts for most of the damage of neurodegenerative disorders like multiple sclerosis and dementia. For this reason, I commonly prescribe intravenous (IV) GSH to my Lyme patients with moderate to severe neurological symptoms. IV GSH (500–2,000 mg per dose) is always coupled with a complete array of oral antioxidants, particularly alpha lipoic acid and often N-acetyl cysteine,

which both help in the production of GSH. And, as I mentioned in chapter 7, there is an orally absorbable form of glutathione called acetylglutathione that is currently available for use without a prescription. For more information on GSH usage visit my Web site, www.lymedoctor.com.

4) Neurotoxins: By definition, *neurotoxins* are chemical products that are toxic to the neurological system. Many of these substances can seriously impair neurological function. Like certain other harmful microorganisms, such as mold and fungi, *Bb* and the TBDs produce these toxic substances during infection. This helps to explain why many people who suffer from chronic Lyme and other TBDs frequently experience "brain fog" and other cognitive problems. The problem is that these toxins can persist even after the microorganisms themselves have been eliminated. There are two sources for the neurotoxins: (1) those toxins directly produced in the area of infected neurological tissue (e.g., Lyme brain infection) and (2) those toxins originating from infection elsewhere in the body but are circulated in the blood and end up being stored in the body's fatty tissues, instead of the bloodstream. Among the fatty tissues in which these toxins embed themselves are, unfortunately, brain and nerve tissues.

When it comes to detecting neurotoxins, standard medical diagnostic tests (blood, urine, DNA) are usually inaccurate. All too often, they show normal readings even when neurotoxins are present. Fortunately, there is a test that is effective for determining whether neurotoxins are present. Known as the *visual contrast sensitivity* (VCS) test, it is also inexpensive (less than $20) and non-invasive and can be performed online in as little as five minutes, according to Ritchie C. Shoemaker, M.D., a leading proponent of its use for patients with various types of infections, including Lyme.

The VCS test is a reliable indicator of neurotoxins because these harmful substances predictably interfere with the brain's ability to distinguish contrasts of black, white, and gray. The greater the level of impairment of this distinguishing ability, the greater the likelihood that neurotoxins are present. More information about the VCS (including taking it online) is provided on Dr. Shoemaker's Web site: www.chronicneurotoxins.com.

A positive VCS test means that the viewer had difficulty distinguishing the contrast between light and dark bars. A positive score, along with exposure to likely sources of neurotoxins such as *Bb*, when combined with typical symptoms, is a reliable indicator of neurotoxins. Follow-up VCS tests can also be used to monitor the effectiveness of the treatments chosen to eliminate the neurotoxins.

The drug cholestyramine (CSM) is effective for eliminating neurotoxins. Welchol may also be used and is much easier to take, according to patient feedback. These therapies work by binding neurotoxins in the bile (small intestine) and then filtering them out of the body through the stool. Like all other drug therapies, CSM, a prescription medication, should only be used under a physician's supervision. During the course of treatment, the VCS test discussed above should be used to determine how well the treatment is working.

Prior to and during treatment with anti-neurotoxin therapy (such as CSM), steps to reduce inflammation in the body should also be taken. Otherwise, CSM commonly will initially trigger an unpleasant intensification of neurotoxin symptoms (like a "herx") as it goes to work. For this reason it must be started very slowly and the dosage built up gradually. CSM can deplete the body's stores of fat soluble vitamins (A,D,E,K), and these must be supplemented while using CSM.

Natural (non-pharmacologic) neurotoxin detoxification may also be considered, especially for those intolerant of CSM or Welchol. These involve the following substances:

* **Zinc** (If deficient, supplement 15–50 mg per day, always balanced with copper.) Signs of zinc deficiency include white spots on the fingernails and low blood alkaline phosphatase level.

* **Chlorella** (Take one gram two to three times a day thirty minutes before largest meals, but as far away from your vitamin C supplements as possible.)

* **Resveratrol** (See my discussion in chapter 6.)

* **Modified Citrus Pectin**

* **Activated Charcoal**

* **Phospholipid** exchange (recommended for deep tissue neurotoxin removal by Lyme expert, Dr. Dietrich Klinghardt; dosage is one tablespoon a day)

5) Brain Metabolism: There is another very important factor that requires discussion—how the brain and neurological tissues handle the energy fuel, glucose. As you recall, glucose is the major energy fuel for the body, and a very high percentage of that fuel is utilized by the neurological system on a daily basis. A significant amount of scientific research has linked abnormalities in the way the brain handles insulin and glucose with neurodegenerative disorders such as Alzheimer's disease. It turns out that insulin action is necessary for proper absorption of glucose by the neurological tissues and for sending certain signals into the cells. It is an abnormal response by these tissues to insulin that often is a problem. This abnormal response is termed "insulin resistance." As insulin resistance worsens, it leads to increased oxidative stress, chronic inflammation, neurotoxin buildup, and eventually neurological cell death. I believe that this neurodegenerative mechanism plays a major role in the brain and nerve symptoms of Lyme/TBDs patients.

Fortunately, there are ways to normalize insulin resistance. At the same time, it is possible to help open the brain cell wall channels for detoxification, which is a function of insulin signaling. Those ways involve the stimulation and activation of nuclear receptors in nervous tissue called *peroxisome-proliferator activated receptors* (PPAR). Let me explain. The peroxisome is a small structure within the cells that functions to do what the cell was intended to do by our Creator's design—for example, peroxisomes in the pineal gland produce melatonin. They are also responsible for helping the nervous tissues eliminate substances such as neurotoxins and toxic heavy metals (e.g., mercury). When insulin signaling is working properly, the PPARs function and cellular glucose fuel together help the cells to perform their intended roles. When PPARs are poorly functional due to insulin resistance, the cell functions poorly and the degenerative process is allowed to proceed. As nerve cell degeneration occurs, it results in memory loss, poor learning capacity, inadequate neurotransmitter production (acetylcholine, dopamine, norepinephrine, serotonin, and so forth), and eventually cell death.

There are several natural and pharmacological methods that can be used to bypass insulin signaling and enhance (stimulate, or "agonize") PPAR function. The natural methods should be *combined with good sources of omega-3 oils and omega-6 oils* and include the following substances.

* **Conjugated linoleic acid (CLA).** Although not an "essential" fatty acid, CLA is a very important poly unsaturated fat found in many animal foods, such as beef, lamb, and cheese. Higher levels are found in free-range meat products, which are low in arachidonic acid and higher in omega-3s. CLA is an antioxidant, is anti-cancer, and is a potent stimulator of PPARs. The usual dosage is 1–5,000 mg per day depending on symptom severity.

* **Curcumin.** This amazing herb/spice has been discussed in chapter 7 because of its anti-inflammatory effects. It has positive PPAR functions in addition to its role in reducing NF-kB and pro-inflammatory IL-12. Recent research has documented its usefulness in preventing neurodegenerative diseases such as Alzheimer's. See chapter 7 for dosages.

* **Chlorella.** In addition to helping rid the body of neuro-toxins by binding them in the intestines, chlorella also helps detoxification by stimulating PPARs, thereby aiding the nervous tissue cells in eliminating their stored toxins. Dosages were discussed earlier in this chapter.

* **Alpha lipoic acid (ALA).** This antioxidant helps the brain and nervous system tissues in so many different ways, such as through stimulation of PPAR receptors and enhancing insulin sensitivity. Dosages were discussed earlier in this chapter.

* **Andrographis.** Along with resveratrol and stephania root, this is one of the best herbal resources for brain

health in Lyme patients. It has PPAR-activating effects. Dosages were previously discussed in chapter 6.

* **Green tea.** Like other products mentioned in this section, it has many uses in Lyme treatment including PPAR stimulation. Two to four cups per day are recommended.

* **Alpha glycans.** This substance was discussed in chapter 4. Unlike every other product that I have mentioned, I do not have scientific documentation of its mechanism of action. However, based on extensive clinical use, I believe alpha glycan products most likely work as powerful PPAR agonists. Though expensive, they possibly should be considered for this purpose.

The pharmacological PPAR agonists include:

* **NSAIDs.** These are mild PPAR stimulators, which along with their anti-inflammatory role, may explain their usefulness in neurodegenerative disorders.

* **Anti-diabetic medications.** These are mentioned for the sake of completeness. While they have been useful for improving insulin sensitivity and PPAR stimulation, their cardiovascular side effects make them less than ideal for use in Lyme and TBD patients, and, therefore, I do not recommend their usage. Their names are Actos (pioglitazone) and Avandia (rosiglitazone).

6) Neurotransmitter, Neuropeptides, Hormonal, and Miscellaneous Other Neurological Issues: In concluding this section of chapter 8, I would like to cover a few other issues that have significant impact upon Lyme/TBD patients and their neuro-logical function.

Neurotransmitters. There are numerous biochemicals in the human nervous system. Neurotransmitters are bio-chemicals that are used for signaling between cells in the nervous system. There are four basic classes of neurotrans-mitters: (1) serotonin, (2) acetylcholine, (3) dopamine/norepinephrine, and (4) GABA.

Problems that occur during Lyme/TBDs include inad-equate manufacture and imbalances of these neurotrans-mitter levels. For example, *Bb* is known to adversely affect tryptophan and serotonin metabolism, thereby predisposing Lyme patients to serotonin-related depression. The follow-ing general non-pharmacologic recommendations may be helpful in improving key neurotransmitters. For a more detailed discussion see my Web site.

* Increase intake of soy lecithin and brazil nuts, which serve as a source of choline used to manufacture the important neurotransmitter, *acetylcholine.*

* Increase intake of tryptophan (e.g., in turkey) and serotonin (e.g., in walnuts, Biblical nettles) to help with serotonin production and reduce depression; one could also take sup-plemental tryptophan or 5HTP (50–100 mg at bedtime.)

* Increase tyrosine intake (e.g., from fish, meat) or take sup-plemental tyrosine for improved production of *dopamine,*

epinephrine, and *norepinephrine. Caution*: Tyrosine supplementation may worsen anxiety in some patients, especially those with incompletely treated Bartonella/BLO.

* Use green tea to increase theanine, which improves *GABA* levels.

* Use low doses of melatonin (1–3 mg) at bedtime if you are having trouble falling asleep.

Neuropeptides: The most important neuropeptides are the endogenous opiate-like substances such as endorphins and enkephlins. I have discussed this group of neuropeptides extensively throughout several chapters of this book and refer you to those chapters for further information

Hormones: There are several key recommendations that I previously discussed in other chapters that I wish to reinforce here. Each is important for helping to reduce neurological and psychiatric symptoms in Lyme/TBD patients.

* Thyroid and adrenal functions usually need to be evaluated when Lyme symptoms have become chronic. Treatment of low thyroid function with thyroid replacement hormones is common in Lyme treatment. Likewise, treatment of adrenal stress (or fatigue) can result in dramatic improvement in neurological symptoms. This may include DHEA in appropriate doses based on lab testing and often *physiologic* doses of cortisol when treating adrenal fatigue.

* Sex hormone deficiencies or imbalances may also play a major role in neurological and psychiatric Lyme symptoms. Pregnenolone levels should be checked and, if low, supplementation with pregnenolone can have a profound effect on brain function. For women with sleep difficulties and/or anxiety, progesterone levels should be assessed and supplemented to optimal levels. Additionally, women should avoid *oral* estrogen products (e.g., birth control pills, hormone replacement) due to their pro-inflammatory side effects. Topical estrogen and oral or topical progesterone are acceptable. For men, assessment for testosterone status is useful. Supplementation to optimal levels is very helpful.

Miscellaneous Other Items: There are several other potential recommendations that I want to discuss in relation to Lyme/TBD neurological functioning. Some of these may be appropriate for you, but, as with all recommendations in this book, it is best to discuss each with your Lyme-aware physician.

* Consider taking acetyl L-carnitine, which helps reduce oxidative stress, improves brain energy stores by fatty acid mobilization, and facilitates growth of healthy neurological tissue. Dosage is 250 mg daily.

* Consider taking phosphatidylserine (PS), which attenuates several neuronal effects of aging and degeneration and improves memory. Dosage is 100–300 mg per day (in evening near bedtime is best).

* Consider taking phosphatidylcholine (PC), which is an important source of choline (for making acetylcholine) derived from lecithin. It is a key component of the normal membrane structure of cells. It also aids in detoxification of the brain (improving memory) and of the liver. Dosage is 400–500 mg twice a day. At times it may be helpful to administer PC in higher doses intravenously as a technique called "phospholipid exchange."

* Consider taking ginkgo biloba, which is a powerful brain antioxidant. It also improves blood flow to the brain. Dosage is 60–120 mg twice a day.

* Consider high dose intramuscular vitamin B12, which may help with regeneration of damaged neurological tissue. Although it is advocated by some Lyme experts, I have not found it to be consistently useful. It is very expensive to use the special methylcobalamin that is imported from Europe.

* Consider using vinpocetine supplements, which may increase brain blood flow and improve brain oxygenation. The dose is 5–20 mg per day.

* Consider concentrating your LID choices on "brain foods," including *water*, egg yolks, peanuts, wheat germ, liver, meat, fish, cruciferous vegetables, beans, other nuts, turkey, milk, potatoes, whole grains, antioxidant fruits, avocado and healthy omega-3 and -6 foods, green vegetables.

- Consider practicing brain-exercising activities such as Sudoku (see www.websudoku.com), crossword puzzles, reading, and Jeopardy.

- Consider neurofeedback, which is a very useful technique to help retrain and rewire the brain by using computers and EEG biofeedback, principles. (See www.eegspectrum.com for further details and explanation.)

Detoxification

A sad but inescapable fact of life today is that all of us live in a far more toxic world than our ancestors did. Our modern lifestyle includes the widespread use of literally tens of thousands of chemical compounds that were nonexistent one hundred years ago, which, if not properly managed, pollute our soil and air and water supplies. Toxic heavy metals such as lead and mercury are also common in today's environment. It is not surprising then that researchers have identified more than four hundred toxic chemicals in human tissue.

Compounding the problem of toxicity are the toxins that can accumulate in the human body as a result of eating junk foods, which are laced with a wide variety of artificial and unhealthy chemicals. Another set of problems arises from medical sources—overuse (or misuse) of pharmaceutical drugs and mercury contained in dental amalgam fillings. The fact that most Americans spend 90 percent of their day indoors doesn't help either. According to the Environmental Protection Agency (EPA), indoor air in the United States can be as much as one hundred times more polluted than outdoor air.

As a result of this ongoing assault of environmental toxins that we all face, our bodies are under an ever-increasing burden to accomplish the normal processes of detoxification that our Creator built into them. When the organs of detoxification, such as the liver and skin, are unable to keep up with this toxic assault, toxins become lodged in the cells and tissues (particularly fat cells and tissues) and start to wreak havoc on a variety of body processes. This, in turn, can result in impaired immune function, impaired metabolism, hormonal imbalances, increased inflammation, diminished cognitive function, chronic lack of energy, unhealthy weight gain, and many other health problems, including cancer.

Of particular significance to people infected with Lyme and other tick-borne diseases is the role that toxins can play in helping such harmful microorganisms escape elimination by the immune system. Research indicates that toxins make it more difficult for the immune system to identify and target harmful bacteria, fungi, and viruses, making it easier for such microorganisms to take deeper root in the body and cause more serious symptoms. Lessening the body's toxic burden is therefore vitally important in all cases of chronic infection, including Lyme disease and other TBDs.

Steps to Prevent Toxic Buildup in Your Body

As with all other health issues, when it comes to dealing with toxins, prevention is key. While there may not be much you can do individually to clean up our toxic world, there are many simple and effective steps you can take to minimize environmental pollution in your home and workplace.

* **Improve Indoor Air Quality.** To help clean the indoor air you breathe at home and at work, place plants throughout your residence and workplace. Plants help to add moisture and increase oxygen levels in indoor air, and also act as natural filters for carbon dioxide and certain other organic chemicals. Investing in a humidifier and negative ion generator can also improve indoor air quality.

* **Let Fresh Air Circulate.** You can easily accomplish this by opening your windows to let fresh air into your home. Sleeping with your bedroom windows open is also recommended.

* **Eat Healthily.** By eating healthy foods, you help to supply your body with the nutrients it requires to aid in its processes of detoxification. The Lyme Inflammation Diet is an excellent way to accomplish this goal, since it provides for a healthy balance of nutrients, healthy fats, fiber, and quality proteins, all of which the body needs to detoxify efficiently.

* **Drink Plenty of Pure, Filtered Water.** Regularly drinking water throughout the day helps your body to flush

out toxins. To ensure the quality of the water you drink, consider purchasing a quality water filtration product. Be sure to drink enough water so that your urine is pale yellow. For most people this means about eight to ten glasses of water per day.

* **Use Environmentally Friendly Products.** Most common household products today contain potentially harmful chemicals. These include synthetic materials such as those found in carpets, fiberboard, insulation materials, particle board, plastics, and polyester, as well as a variety of chemicals in common household cleaning and other products. Fortunately, healthy, nontoxic alternatives to such products are becoming more widely available nationwide.

* **Avoid Secondhand Smoke.** In addition to nicotine, cigarettes contain hundreds of other harmful chemicals, which can harm both smokers and people regularly exposed to secondhand smoke. (If you smoke, seek professional help in order to quit.)

* **Clean Carpets and Rugs Regularly.** Carpets and rugs can be a breeding ground for toxic molds, bacteria, and other harmful agents. To minimize this problem, clean carpets and rugs on a regular basis with nontoxic cleaners.

* **Make It a Habit to Spend Time in Nature.** Spending time outdoors in a natural, unpolluted setting is a healthy habit that everyone should cultivate. Obviously, though, you will want to avoid or take precautions in outdoor

areas that are known to have a high concentration of ticks, fleas, and other insects that can transmit Lyme and other TBDs.

Steps to Aid Detoxification

To best determine whether or not you suffer from excessive toxicity, I recommend that you consult with a health professional experienced in this area, which includes many Lyme-aware physicians. You can also locate physicians who specialize in the use of professional detoxification therapies by contacting the American Academy of Environmental Medicine (AAEM), the American and International Boards of Environmental Medicine (ABEM/IBEM), or the American College of Advancement in Medicine (ACAM). (See the resources section for contact information for each of these organizations.)

In addition to working with your doctor to detoxify, you can also take the following self-care steps to help reduce the level of toxins in your body:

* **Eating Healthily.** Once again, the Lyme Inflammation Diet is excellent in this regard. Be sure to include foods with known detoxification properties, such as organic fruits (apples, blueberries, cherries, grapes, lemons, and pineapple), beet greens, celery, garlic, green leafy vegetables, and onions. Fresh juices made from organic fruits and vegetables can also be helpful. Also be sure to drink plenty of pure, filtered water to help flush out toxins.

* **Detox Baths.** Regularly bathing in hot water to which Epsom salts have been added can help draw out toxins from the skin. For best results, make your bath as hot as you can tolerate, add two pounds of Epsom salts, and bathe for at least 20 minutes or until bath water cools. Do this once or twice a week. As alternatives to Epsom salts, you can also use two pounds of baking soda, or one pound each of baking soda and sea salt.

* **Dry Skin Brushing.** Vigorously brushing your skin with a dry skin brush helps to discard dead skin and open up skin pores, making it easier for toxins to pass out of the body. Additionally, dry skin brushing also stimulates lymphatic function. (The lymphatic system is an important component of your body's detoxification system, acting as a filtration system for carrying away toxins and waste by-products from cells and tissues so that they can be eliminated through urination.) For best results, do this once a day, ideally before bathing or showering.

* **Breathing Deeply.** Breathing deeply from your abdomen also helps to eliminate toxins. Do this for ten to twenty minutes once or twice a day.

* **Exercising.** Although in the initial stages of treatment, aerobic exercise is not recommended for most people with chronic Lyme/TBDs, once you and your physician feel that you are up for it, aerobic activities can improve your body's ability to get rid of toxins. Brisk walking, exercising on a treadmill, and jumping on a mini-trampoline (rebounder) are all excellent types of

aerobic exercise that can aid detoxification.

* **Getting a Massage.** Receiving a Swedish or lymphatic drainage massage on a regular basis (once a month or more) can further improve lymphatic function.

* **Taking a Sauna.** Saunas are another excellent way of helping to flush out toxins from your body. This is especially true of far-infrared saunas, which emit dry heat that can penetrate to a depth of up to three inches into the body, triggering the expulsion of toxins from fat cells. Whichever type of sauna you choose, be sure to drink adequate amounts of water during the sauna to avoid dehydration.

Certain nutritional and herbal supplements can also aid the body in ridding itself of toxins. These include the antioxidant glutathione which supports brain and liver function; vitamin C, which aids in the overall process of detoxification and provides many other health benefits, including improved immunity; and niacin (vitamin B3), which can be taken in doses up to 500 mg per day for short periods to help fat cells and tissues expel toxins—but it will cause severe flushing. Garlic capsules can also be helpful, as can chlorella (a type of blue-green algae), and the spice cilantro. Chlorella and cilantro act as natural detoxifying "magnets" that pull toxins, including heavy metals, from the body. Review these suggestions with your Lyme-aware doctor before embarking on them to make sure you have the correct protocol for your situation.

The Problem of Heavy Metals

One of the most common and serious types of toxicity today is exposure to heavy metals, which include lead and mercury, as well as a variety of other heavy metals that can significantly impair overall health. Heavy metal exposure can occur as a result of eating too much of the wrong kind of seafood, breathing polluted air, drinking unfiltered water, eating food laced with pesticides, vaccination (a number of vaccines contain thimerasol, a mercury derivative), and dental amalgam fillings.

Treating heavy metals effectively requires the help of a physician trained in this area. Since common dental amalgam fillings are one of the most significant sources of mercury in the body, you may also need to work with a holistic or "biological" dentist who is skilled at safely removing such fillings and replacing them with fillings made from non-toxic materials. (To locate a biological dentist in your area, see the resources section.)

If you suspect you are affected by heavy metals, your first step should be to have yourself tested for them. This can be accomplished by working with your physician, who can order various lab tests, such as a packed red blood cell analysis (which screens for the presence of heavy metals in red and white blood cells) and provocation tests (which involve the use of agents such as DMSA, DMPS, or EDTA that bind or "chelate" to heavy metals and pull them out of the body so that they pass into the urine for measurement). Some physicians also use a hair analysis test, which involves cutting a small amount of hair from the body and sending it to a lab for testing. I have not found hair analysis to be accurate enough to depend on, and therefore, I do not perform that test. I completely rely on red blood cell analysis and urine provocation testing for the diagnosis and follow up of heavy metal overload.

Should it be determined that heavy metal toxicity exists, the next step is a proper course of treatment. One of the most effective treatments for heavy metals is known as *chelation therapy*. Most commonly, this may involve the use of chelating agents such as DMSA, which is taken by mouth. Or it may, in severe cases, require DMPS or EDTA, which are administered intravenously, usually over a series of twenty to thirty treatments. As the chelating agents enter the bloodstream, they start to attract and bind to heavy metals so that they can pass out of the body during urination. Prior to or during this time of chelation therapy, people with dental amalgam fillings may also need to have them replaced.

Far-infrared sauna therapy is another useful method for aiding in the elimination of heavy metals, as well as other toxins. *Clay baths* can also be helpful. This form of therapy consists of covering the body with healing clays, which help to draw out toxins through the skin.

Whichever form of therapy you and your doctor use to reduce the load of heavy metals in your body, for best results you should continue using it under his or her supervision until additional provocation tests show that your heavy metal load has been effectively reduced. If, during this process, you start to feel worse, be sure to let your doctor know, as this could be a sign that your kidneys and or liver need to be supported and/or that you are detoxifying too quickly. For best results a "slow but steady" pace is recommended, which may require patience on your part.

Sleep and Sleep-Related Problems

Sleep problems are nearly universal among persons with Lyme and most other tick-borne diseases. Such problems are a major contributor to symptoms such as "brain fog," chronic fatigue, depression, and impaired immune function that are associated with Lyme and other TBDs. Restoring adequate quality sleep for Lyme/TBD patients is therefore one of the highest priorities, even if it involves the temporary use of sleep medications.

To understand why restful sleep is so important to health, let's take a moment to discuss sleep in more detail. Most adults spend one-third of their lives sleeping, during which time a variety of self-repair mechanisms take place in the body. Unless proper sleep is attained (at least 7.5 hours each night, and for some people as much as 9 hours), we inevitably wake up to start the day feeling fatigued. Lack of sleep also makes it impossible for your body to properly manufacture hormones, including cortisol, endorphins, and growth hormone. Restful sleep has also been shown to provide many psychological benefits, all of which diminish when sleeping problems occur. Recent research shows that both memory and our ability to learn are greatly influenced by the amount and quality of our sleep. Sleep experts divide sleep into two types, rapid eye movement (REM) sleep and non-rapid eye movement (NREM) sleep.

REM sleep comprises approximately 20 percent of sleep and is where dreaming occurs. For most people, NREM sleep comprises approximately 80 percent of the total amount of sleep they get each night, assuming they are sleeping properly. NREM sleep is further divided into two stages, stages 1 and 2 (light sleep) and stages 3 and 4 (deep sleep). Deep sleep is also known as slow wave sleep (SWS). These most important deep sleep stages of NREM sleep (stages 3 and 4) actually begin soon after you retire.

Slow wave sleep is the deepest and most refreshing type of sleep and accounts for between 10 percent and 20 percent of the total amount of sleep people get each night. It is essential for proper cell and musculoskeletal tissue regeneration, optimum performance of the cardiovascular system, normalized blood pressure, hormonal balance (including growth hormone production), and proper maintenance of the metabolic system. Slow wave sleep is most prominent in youth and declines with normal aging. Alcohol consumption can also diminish slow wave sleep. The decline in levels of slow wave sleep in proportion to overall sleep that occurs as a result of aging is likely related to the increase in sleeping problems that are more common among older people.

Primary Causes for Sleeping Problems

In addition to infections of *Bb* and other tick-borne bacteria, all of which can disturb healthy sleep patterns, the primary causes of sleep disturbances include the following:

* **Normal aging** (especially with regard to slow wave sleep)

* **Poor sleep planning.** People with Lyme/TBDs need to go to bed at the same time every night and wake up at the same time every morning. This is critical for Lyme sleep recovery.

* **Shift work.** Working late shifts and/or alternating between day and night shifts can significantly disrupt normal sleep patterns. If at all possible, patients with Lyme/TBDs need to avoid shift and evening work until they get their illness under control.

* **Caffeine and other stimulants.** People with Lyme/TBDs need to avoid coffee, black tea, and other stimulants until their illness is under control. Care should also be taken when eating dark chocolate and/or drinking green tea, both of which should be avoided after noon or so.

* **Alcohol and nicotine.** Both alcohol and nicotine can significantly interfere with healthy sleep and should be avoided altogether.

* **Eating too close to bedtime.** Doing so can lead to fitful sleep as the digestive process takes place.

* **Exercising too close to bedtime.** Although for some

people, exercising in the evening helps to promote restful sleep, for many others late evening exercise produces
stimulating effects that make falling asleep difficult.

* **Lack of darkness.** Prior to sleep, your body starts producing the hormone melatonin. Melatonin is essential for
restful sleep. Melatonin then continues to be produced
while you are sleeping, with peak production usually
occurring between 2 A.M. and 4 A.M. For the full effects
of melatonin to occur, however, sleep experts say that you
should attempt to sleep in a room of total darkness.

* **Electronic devices in the bedroom.** Electric alarm
clocks, computers, televisions, and other electronic
devices located too close to your bed can disrupt sleep
because of the electromagnetic frequencies they emit.
Known as LEFs, these frequencies have been shown by
researchers to disrupt the body's own electromagnetic
field. Ideally, you should avoid placing electronic devices
in your bedroom. If you must keep them located there,
be sure they are placed at least eight feet away from your
bed.

* **Nutritional deficiencies/imbalances.** A lack or imbalance of various nutrients is quite common among many
people with sleeping problems. Magnesium deficiency
is especially common, resulting in muscle cramping
and twitching, increased nervousness, and other sleep
disruptions. Other nutrients that are necessary for restful sleep are calcium and various B vitamins, especially
vitamins B6 and B12, folic acid, and inositol. However,

B vitamins taken just before bedtime can also disrupt sleep due to their ability to cause vivid dreams.

* **Hormonal changes.** This is another common factor in sleep disorders, especially in men and women forty and older. In men, reduced levels of testosterone can disrupt sleep and cause problems such as sleep apnea. Higher than normal levels of testosterone can also interfere with healthy sleep. In women, reduced progesterone levels is the most common hormonal issue associated with sleeping problems. Progesterone levels can fall during the week before a woman's menstrual period and also when a woman enters perimenopause. Women on estrogen replacement therapy that is unbalanced with progesterone can also experience sleeping problems, although this scenario is much less common today than it was in the past. Estrogen-progesterone imbalances can also be caused by foods containing estrogen-like chemicals and pesticides. Another common hormonal imbalance related to sleeping problems is increased cortisol production due to stress. (For more on hormonal imbalances and how to correct them please see chapter 7.)

* **Low blood sugar (hypoglycemia).** People with low blood sugar problems often experience a steep drop in blood sugar levels during the night, causing them to awaken due to hunger pangs and feelings of shakiness. Blood sugar levels will usually improve by following the Lyme Inflammation Diet discussed in chapter 5.

* **Medications.** Many commonly used medications can also interfere with sleep, especially among the elderly. Such medications include those that produce daytime drowsiness, along with anticonvulsants, antidepressants, antihistamines, blood pressure medications, pain relief drugs, muscle relaxants, and drugs for treating Parkinson's disease. Ironically, many sleeping medications can also cause sleep problems if they are used for long periods of time or abused.

* **Anxiety and depression.** Both anxiety and depression (see above) are common in patients suffering with chronic Lyme disease, as well as other tick-borne conditions, especially Bartonella. The fears, worries, and racing thoughts associated with anxiety and depression can significantly disrupt and prevent healthy sleep.

* **Stress.** Chronic stress causes your body to produce elevated amounts of epinephrine and noreinephrine, both of which stimulate the sympathetic nervous system, creating a "fight or flight" state that is not conducive to restful sleep. Stress also results in higher than normal cortisol levels, which also interferes with sleep.

* **Other medical problems.** Various other health problems can also prevent and interrupt restful sleep. These include anemia and iron deficiency, arthritis (especially rheumatoid), back and/or chronic pain, fibroids, gastrointestinal disorders (see above), kidney disease, neuromuscular disease, obesity, peripheral neuropathy, Parkinson's disease, prostate problems (enlarged prostate, prostatitis), respiratory conditions, and thyroid problems.

Treating Sleeping Problems

When it comes to treating sleeping problems there are a variety of options from which to choose, ranging from natural approaches to conventional medications. Effective treatment choices depend on the nature of the problem, as well as its severity.

Here is a recap of tips that can help ensure a good night's sleep.

* Plan to go to sleep at the same time each night and to wake up at the same time each morning. Doing so helps condition your body to sleep and awaken at the same time each night and day, making it easier to fall asleep and awaken more refreshed.

* Avoid alcohol, caffeine, and other stimulants.

* Avoid eating late in the evening. However, also avoid going to sleep feeling hungry, as this can interfere with a restful sleep and cause a sharp drop in blood sugar, awakening you during the night.

* Sleep in darkness to ensure adequate melatonin production.

* Eliminate electronic devices from your bedroom or, at the very least, make sure they are placed at least eight feet away from your bed.

* Exercise regularly but avoid late-evening exercise, as this can be too stimulating.

* A warm bath before bedtime can be conducive for sleep, as well.

One of the most common sleeping problems is insomnia, or the *inability to fall asleep* once you've gone to bed. To help cope with insomnia, consider the following approaches:

Mild Insomnia: Take 1.5 mg of melatonin an hour before bedtime. Dr. Binyamin Rothstein, author of *Brain Fog*, suggests using melatonin in the following way: (1) open a capsule and put 1.5 mg of the powder under your tongue; take a small sip of water, swish in the mouth for a minute, and swallow; (2) then lie down in a quiet, dark room, and you will probably fall asleep within 20 minutes; (3) be sure that you don't do any stimulating activity after taking the melatonin, because if you do something (e.g., read or watch TV), then it will backfire and it will keep you up for hours. If melatonin does not help, a warm cup of valerian tea can also be helpful. Acupuncture can be very helpful for this problem.

Moderate Insomnia: Take a glycine supplement (2,000–3,000 mg) before retiring. (Glycine is an amino acid.) Valerian tea can also help.

Severe Insomnia: In cases of severe insomnia, a sleep medication is often necessary short-term and possibly longer. Most of the time, the benzodiazepine medications (relatives of valerian) are helpful, such as Ambien or Klonopin. At times, it is necessary to use short-acting barbiturate medications, with caution, because they are potentially very habit-forming.

Another common sleeping problem is *difficulty staying asleep.* If you suffer from this problem, consider the following approaches:

Mild Symptoms: The amino acids L-tryptophan (500–1,000 mg) or 5-HTP (50–100 mg) taken before bedtime can help promote lasting sleep because of their ability to increase serotonin production. Serotonin is a neurotransmitter that is associated with calm, restful sleep, as well as improved mood. Supplementing with glycine (2,000–3,000 mg) can also help with this type of sleep problem in addition to insomnia.

Moderate Symptoms: For moderate difficulties staying asleep, a sleep medication may be required. Helpful drugs to choose from include Rozerem (8 mg), Ambien (10 mg), Lunesta (2–3 mg), or Sonata (10 mg), all of which are common, effective sleep medications.

Neurontin (100–900 mg), an anticonvulsant drug originally developed to treat seizures, has also been shown to help sleeping problems, including difficulty staying asleep at night. Neurontin (gabapentin) has the added benefit of helping with pain control. Certain tricyclic antidepressant drugs, such as amitriptyline (10–25 mg), can also help with both pain control and sleep. All these prescription drugs have certain precautions and can cause potential side effects. They are also contraindicated in certain circumstances, such as specific health conditions, allergies, and the use of certain other medications. Your Lyme-aware physician is in the best position to evaluate this for you.

Severe Symptoms: In the situation where other aforementioned sleep remedies are not effective, I recommend considering the controlled prescription drug, Xyrem. Because of its potency and potential to cause harmful side-effects and abuse, its use and dosage must be determined by your physician, and its usage carefully monitored. Despite its downside, Xyrem is a very effective sleep medication and deserves consideration.

Improving Slow Wave Sleep

As I mentioned above, slow wave sleep is the deepest, most restful phase of sleep and one that promotes a wide variety of health benefits. Many patients with Lyme/TBDs have decreased levels of slow wave sleep, compounding the many other problems caused by their illness. Therefore, increasing the amount of slow wave sleep you get during the night should be a high priority so that your body will become better able to heal.

Supplementing with glycine (2,000–3,000 mg just before bedtime) is a safe and often effective way to increase slow wave sleep. In addition, glycine helps to increase REM activity (dream sleep). Researchers believe that having adequate amounts of REM sleep also plays a vital role in our overall health, especially with regard to our mental and emotional health.

Conventional sleep medications can also be used to increase slow wave sleep. These include tricyclic antidepressants, gabapentin, and Xyrem. Gabitril, like gabapentin, was originally developed as an anticonvulsant drug for the treatment of seizures. It can also help increase slow wave sleep. To learn more about these drugs, consult with your physician and only use them under his or her supervision.

Summing Up

What follow are answers to the most commonly asked questions about Lyme disease and the G.L.A.N.D.S.

Why is it important to consider the gastrointestinal tract when treating Lyme and other TBDs?

Ensuring healthy gastrointestinal (GI) tract function in people with Lyme/TBDs is important for a number of reasons, beginning with the fact that the GI tract makes up 70 percent of your body's immune system. When immune function is impaired, your body's ability to deal with Lyme/TBDs is severely compromised.

Additionally, various GI conditions, including celiac disease and candidiasis (systemic yeast overgrowth), can significantly impair the ability of people to recover from Lyme/TBDs and also increase the severity of their symptoms. The overgrowth of a toxic bacterium called *Clostridium difficile* can pose similar problems, as well.

Why is the liver so important when it comes to Lyme/TBDs?

The health of the liver is important for *all* diseases, not just Lyme/TBDs. When liver function becomes impaired, your body's disease-fighting ability is greatly diminished. Additionally, a healthy liver is essential for adequately digesting food and efficiently providing your body with nutrients that foods contain. And the liver is perhaps the most important organ in the body when it comes to eliminating toxins.

Why are anxiety and depression so often associated with Lyme/TBDs?

Because of the many debilitating and persistent symptoms that can be caused by Lyme and other TBDs, it's only natural that at least half of all people with chronic Lyme/TBDs are susceptible to anxiety and/or depression, simply due to the poor quality of life Lyme/TBDs can cause. Additionally, both anxiety and depression in people with Lyme/TBDs can have a physical basis, due to how the microorganisms that cause these diseases can interfere with the delicate homeostatic balance in the body. As I pointed out above, one of the keys to effectively treating anxiety and depression in people with Lyme/TBDs lies in first determining whether it is Lyme/TBDs that are causing them, or whether anxiety and depression were present before infection with Lyme/TBDs began. Knowing the answer to this question is vitally important.

What is the relationship between Lyme/TBDs and neurological problems?

Lyme and other TBDs can cause neurological problems in three primary ways. Once the bacteria that cause Lyme/ TBDs take root in the body, they start to manufacture toxic substances that can continue to wreak havoc in the body even after the bacteria themselves have been eliminated. Certain of these substances can affect the brain and nervous system and are therefore known as neurotoxins.

Neurological problems can be further compounded by many factors, including how the microorganisms that cause Lyme/ TBDs can trigger and worsen chronic inflammation, deplete the body's supply of glutathione, and add to the toxic burden of the neurological system by way of neurotoxins. Lyme-aware physicians seek to address all these and other factors as part of a comprehensive Lyme/TBD treatment program.

Why is detoxification so important when it comes to Lyme/TBDs?

When toxins build up in the body's cells and tissues, they can significantly impair the functioning of many of your body's systems. This can lead to impaired immunity, poor metabolism, hormonal imbalances, increased inflammation, diminished cognitive function, chronic lack of energy, unhealthy weight gain, and many other health problems, including cancer. Additionally, toxins can help the microorganisms that cause Lyme and other TBDs to escape detection by the body's immune cells. This makes it easier for the microorganisms to take deeper root in the body and cause more serious symptoms. Lessening the body's toxic burden is therefore vitally important in all cases of chronic Lyme/TBDs.

Why are sleeping problems so common among people with Lyme/TBDs?

The fact that sleeping problems are present in nearly all people who suffer with chronic Lyme/TBDs is primarily due to the various symptoms that are caused by these diseases, such as pain, heightened stress, and so forth. Additionally, since sleeping problems are already prevalent in our society, due to a variety of factors, infection with Lyme/TBDs can set up a vicious circle in which sleeping problems are made worse and, as a result, the body becomes further unable to cope with Lyme/TBD infection. As part of the overall Lyme/TBD patient care, restoring healthy and adequate sleep is a high priority.

Our final chapter of this book is the last but certainly not the least. In that chapter, we will deal with one of the oft-ignored major keys to all health and healing—the mind-body-spirit connection.

Chapter Nine

Keeping Hope Alive: Psychological and Spiritual Considerations for Lyme Disease

❋

Because of the difficult challenges inherent in treating chronic Lyme disease, it is all too easy for people who suffer with it to lose hope that they will ever be well again. Often, this sense of hopelessness can lead to feelings of depression, sorrow, and even anger. As a result of these frustrating things, you can feel as if all the doors of your life have been closed to you. It is not at all hard to understand why so many Lyme patients feel helpless and even hopeless at times.

If the responses that I just described apply to you, please be assured that they are normal human responses to your situation. However, given the potential severity of Lyme disease symptoms, it's important that they not be allowed to dominate your life experience on an ongoing basis. The most important reason is that you want a life that involves purpose, enjoyment, peace, health, and happiness. What is there to look forward to when life is mainly about frustration and hopelessness and fear? When those emotions dominate your thinking, life feels like a waste of time. You want your life back.

Another reason that you don't want these negative emotions to dominate your life is that it is now well-established that such emotions can significantly depress immune function and negatively impact your body's ability to heal. Additionally, such emotions can obscure the many lessons that Lyme disease can impart if you are willing to look and learn from them.

In this chapter, I am sharing with you a variety of self-care healing strategies that you can use to improve your psychological and spiritual health. Taken together, these strategies will empower you to have A. H.O.P.E. F.O.R. H.E.A.L.T.H. This is an acronym I have chosen because of how important true hope, along with a positive psychological and spiritual outlook, is in the healing process. The acronym stands for the following aspects of psychological and spiritual health:

Appreciation

Higher Power

Optimism

Prayer and Positive Vision

Eating Right

Forgiveness

Oxygen/Breathing

Relationships

Humor

Enjoy Today

Alternative Resources

Light

Trust

Helping Others

Each of these aspects can make a powerful difference in how well and quickly you heal.

As a holistic, integrative physician, I cannot over-emphasize the importance that psychological (both mental and emotional) and spiritual issues have to overall health. Yet this relationship between health and "body, mind, and Spirit" is poorly understood by many in our society. Most of us are accustomed to thinking about health and disease only in physical terms. As we begin to view health and illness from a holistic perspective, we can start to better appreciate the interconnectedness of our thoughts, beliefs, attitudes, and emotions to our overall health. Adopting this perspective also enables us to discover the enormous healing resources that are available to us through prayer, meditation, and other spiritual practices that deepen our connection to our Creator, or God.

The following case history of one of my patients clearly illustrates how taking time to address our psychological and spiritual well-being can also improve our physical health. Susan came to see me because of chronic Lyme disease. She appeared pale and depressed, as many of my Lyme patients often appear. The diagnosis of Lyme was straightforward, and we were quickly able to get her onto the correct therapeutic antibiotics, diet and lifestyle changes, and supplements. However, as Susan's general physical status improved, I remember noting that she still seemed depressed and even somewhat angry.

Upon more close analysis of her life situation, it became very clear that Susan had isolated herself from virtually everyone—from her children, her church family, and her friends. She admitted that despite feeling better in general, she still felt angry about having lost years of productivity due to Lyme. She was also still angry at doctors who had not been able to help her in the past—especially those who told her that her problems were mostly psychologically based. At this point, I knew that Susan was not going to be able to fully recover without intensive psychospiritual work.

The first step was to prescribe (I actually wrote this on a prescription pad) two simple, easily doable things for her: She was to watch America's Funniest Videos daily, and she was to make a list every morning of ten things for which she felt she could be grateful today. One month later, she was feeling better. She was actually amazed at how much better she felt. The next step was to recommend that she regularly return to her church and also begin to reconnect with her spiritual roots through prayer and Bible reading. She did this also, just as I had instructed. As a result of going back to her church, she also initiated counseling with one of the female counselors at the church.

The final step was to begin to do something to help others who might be struggling with the same issues as she—chronic undiagnosed Lyme disease. She thought about starting a support group, but I discouraged that because I didn't think she was ready to take on such a major responsibility. Instead, I recommended that she help another support group leader who I knew needed help. That idea worked out very well for both my patient and the support group leader.

Susan is now doing very well and is off all Lyme treatments. She feels that Lyme has actually been beneficial in helping her find her life's purpose. This new perspective on her life has contributed not only to her healing, but also to the healing of many others that have now been helped by her efforts. Many Lyme patients struggle with the exact same issues that Susan struggled with. If you are one of those patients, there is hope for you also.

Now let's examine each of the factors involved in creating A NEW HOPE FOR HEALTH in more detail.

Appreciation

When we become ill, especially with a condition as serious as Lyme disease, it is easy to lose sight of appreciation. In fact, the most common response to illness is anything but appreciation. You may ask yourself at this point, what is there to appreciate about Lyme beyond the fact that it's ruining my life? This is certainly an understandable response. However, if you find yourself continuously dwelling on all the negatives associated with Lyme disease (and chronic illness in general), you are actually impeding your ability to heal.

You may find this statement difficult to believe, but it's backed up by numerous studies in the relatively new scientific field of psychoneuroimmunology (PNI), more commonly known to the public as mind/body medicine. Research shows that our bodies' immune system is directly influenced by our thoughts, emotions, and beliefs. During the times in which we experience appreciation for our life and circumstances, emotions such as happiness, joy, and peace are commonly experienced. Such emotions have been shown to directly and powerfully enhance immune function, as well as the functioning of many other body systems. On the other hand, emotions of fear, anger, sorrow, and frustration, all of which are common when we fail to appreciate the blessings of our daily lives, act to suppress immune function. Therefore, taking time each day to notice all that there is to appreciate about your life can be a very effective self-care health strategy.

Another word for appreciation is gratitude. The Law of Attraction says that if you express gratitude, you will attract and be sent more things to be grateful for. Perhaps this was why the Christian mystic Meister Eckhardt said, "If the only prayer you ever pray is 'Thank you,' it would suffice." A grateful spirit keeps you positive and hopeful in the midst of difficulty. This is true even if the difficulty is Lyme disease or other serious illnesses.

My own experience, both personally as someone formerly with active, chronic Lyme disease and clinically with my patients, bears this out. I believe that my bout with Lyme disease (and the various associated health problems I experienced) turned out to be an opportunity in disguise. Had I not gone through that challenge and—with the help of God and of the wonderful people placed by God in my pathway—found the solution I needed to reclaim my health, I would not now have the opportunity to make a difference for others with Lyme disease. Lyme was in fact a blessing to me because it taught me so much about the important things in life.

I understand that when you are in the midst of very difficult pain or other symptoms you may not feel there is much to appreciate. However, I encourage you, no matter how sick you may be, to commit yourself to taking time to appreciate the blessings and lessons that come your way each day. Also begin to be appreciative in advance of your blessings because you trust that whatever happens is going to ultimately be used for your benefit. By doing so, you will be surprised how much there is for you to be grateful for, despite your illness. The added benefit is that you'll also help to mobilize and strengthen your immune system, thereby improving your health.

Initially, the benefits you receive by practicing appreciation may not seem noticeable to you. However, with time, the benefits will start to become more obvious and build upon each other to enhance your well-being. Additionally, you'll begin to regularly experience greater feelings of happiness and acceptance. The more you take time to notice and appreciate all that you have to be grateful for, the more positive things will start to happen for you.

Here are two simple yet powerful ways in which you can cultivate appreciation.

Begin Your Day with Appreciation: Each morning, before you get out of bed, close your eyes and take a few minutes to think about someone or something in your life that brings you happiness and makes you grateful for being alive. Allow yourself to become immersed in the happiness you feel and acknowledge to yourself how much you appreciate that person or experience. By getting in the habit of performing this simple exercise on a daily basis, you will soon find yourself noticing many other experiences throughout the day for which you can be grateful. As you do so, take a moment each time to truly acknowledge your appreciation.

Keep an Appreciation Journal: This is another easy way to become more aware of all the people and experiences you appreciate in your life. Each night before going to bed, review your day and write down everything that you experienced that you are grateful for. Once your list is complete, take a moment to give thanks for everything that you wrote down.

Higher Power

The vast majority of Americans (95 percent) believe in God or a Higher Power. This is hardly surprising, since nearly everyone, at some point in their lives, has at least one incident where they experience "a connection with the Divine." Yet, when people develop chronic and debilitating health conditions like Lyme disease, sometimes they forget to call on God to help them as they struggle with their health challenges. When they remember to do so, they very often find that their lives improve. This fact is borne out by a variety of scientific studies that have examined the relationship between spirituality and health and disease.

Researchers have discovered that patients who believe in God, or a Higher Power, and regularly engage in religious or spiritual practices derive significant health benefits compared to patients who are not religiously or spiritually oriented. Among their findings, they discovered that religious and spiritual factors resulted in improved psychological factors (reduced anxiety, reduced depression, reduced anger and hostility), improved general health, improved blood pressure levels, and increased survival time among patients with life-threatening diseases such as heart attack and cancer. Patients who regularly pray or meditate are more likely to experience what is called the *relaxation response*, compared to other patients. The relaxation response is a term coined by Dr. Herbert Benson. It is characterized by improvements in metabolic and heart rate, blood pressure levels, and respiration. Research has also shown that people who regularly (at least once a week) attend services at their church, mosque, synagogue, or other place of worship are generally healthier and happier than other people.

For all the above reasons, I encourage my patients to engage in religious or spiritual practices that they are comfortable with. I also encourage them to actively call upon God to aid them in their healing journey. I find that those who heed this advice are better able to cope with Lyme disease, as well as any other illnesses they may have. I am confident that by turning your life over to God, you will derive similar benefits.

Optimism

Optimism is another important factor when it comes to dealing with and recovering from Lyme disease. Another word closely related to optimism is *hope*. Typically, when it comes to optimism and hope, people who become chronically ill fall into one of three categories: 1) those with *true hope*, 2) those with *false hope*, 3) and those with *no hope* (hopelessness). Obviously, only true hope has real value in relationship to healing.

True hope means precisely that—hope or optimism that is grounded in reality. Once people tap into true hope to cultivate an ongoing state of optimism, the result is what I call "the arousal of passion for the possible." In other words, they become motivated to achieve the healing results they know to be within their reach based on fact. And the reality is that many people with chronic, debilitating Lyme disease, including myself, have fully recovered from it. And many others have experienced significantly improved health, even if a portion of their symptoms remain. Knowing and, more importantly, *accepting* that you too can triumph over Lyme disease provides you with the hope and confidence you need in order to make the right decisions and take the proper actions to improve your health. When you decide to patiently persist in performing these health-enhancing actions, it is possible that you can achieve the results you desire.

The powerful positive healing energy that is generated from true hope and optimism are crucial for your Lyme-recovery journey. When you are empowered with this potent energy called hope you will have an attitude that says, "It is possible that I *can* get well." As a result of that attitude, you can make a commitment to the *journey* of the healing process—journey that is one of hopeful determination to battle this problem with everything God has empowered you with, realizing that the journey is one of enlightenment and learning as part of your healing.

False hope, on the other hand, can be an impediment to the healing process. In some cases, people with false hope have expectations of positive outcomes or results that are not based in reality. Such patients tend to be passive in their approach to healing, expecting that "everything will be all right" and that their doctors will "fix it for me." This is in stark contrast to patients with true hope, who actively participate in their own healing. Unlike truly optimistic patients, people with false hope also tend to lose patience when they don't get the results they expect, or when they don't heal quickly. They have an attitude that says, "I *will* get well," coupled with an attachment to a specific outcome. As a result, should that outcome not occur, they are more likely to give up on themselves and to stop following the guidance and direction of their physicians.

Patients with *no* hope often fail to make an effort to get well in the first place. Their underlying attitude tells them, "I cannot and will not get well." As a result, they tend to resign themselves to a life of pain and suffering. They also often view themselves as victims of circumstance and feel powerless to change their fate. Ironically, an attitude of hopelessness can often turn into a self-fulfilling prophecy. As we have seen, disempowering negative emotions can dramatically suppress immune function, making it far more difficult for your body to heal.

Now that you understand what true optimism means, ask yourself which of the above-mentioned categories you currently are in. If you aren't already among those who have true hope, perhaps you need to better educate yourself about what is possible when it comes to recovering from Lyme disease. The case histories in this book, along with my own recovery, illustrate that Lyme disease does not have to be a life sentence of pain, suffering, and emotional distress. If my patients and I can heal, it is likely that you can too. But to do so, you have to be willing to take the necessary steps that I am sharing with you in this book.

Most patients with chronic Lyme disease have spent many frustrating years alternating between "no hope" and "false hope." The goal of healthy Lyme treatment should be realistic true hope that says, "With good medical care, my full commitment to do all that I can do, and God's help, it *is possible* that I can get well." In other words, when you develop a Lyme Battle Plan that includes your Lyme-aware health care team, your hopeful and confident commitment to do all you are empowered to do, and your trust in God to do what is in your best interest, you have assembled a winning team and can expect an excellent journey to your recovery. Such an attitude and plan allow the healing journey to be a full and rich experience of learning and growing, no matter the final outcome.

Prayer and Positive Vision

Both prayer and positive vision build on what I shared with you in the sections on *Higher Power* and *Optimism* above. Prayer is a powerful tool for healing that many people overlook. When we pray and keep our focus on a positive vision of victory, instead of resigning ourselves to feelings of being a victim of our health challenges, it is possible for true miracles of healing to occur.

There are many ways to pray. I find that the most effective ways are those that combine prayer with gratitude for the blessings you already have in your life, and a positive expectation that what you pray for is already becoming a reality. In the Bible, Jesus counsels us in the ways of prayer, telling us, "Ask and it will be given unto you; seek and you will find; knock and the door will be opened to you." (Matthew 7:7) By praying in this manner, you will start to receive answers to your problems. Many times, the answers may come in ways that you didn't expect, such as a sudden hunch or intuition, or an unexpected suggestion from someone that leads you to discover a better way of dealing with your problems. By praying regularly, you will become better aware of such responses from the Higher Power (God) that oversees all of our lives.

There are occasions when a patient will say that they have prayed and prayed and prayed, yet nothing happens. How does one deal with what seems to be unanswered prayer? I have found that prayer requires patiently waiting, but not inaction. In other words, the answer may not come immediately, but if a person keeps doing what God is telling them to do the answer *will* eventually come. Remember, if you are in a rowboat in the middle of a lake and a severe storm is coming, you should pray as hard as you can, while you row as hard as you can. Therefore pray, obediently do what you can, and trust that God will do what is best in God's time.

Extensive research documented by Dr. Larry Dossey in his book *Healing Words* demonstrates that prayer really does work. For example, in a well-designed study at a teaching hospital in San Francisco, it was shown that a group of cardiac intensive-care-unit patients who were prayed for (without knowing it) recovered much better than a group of matched patients who were not prayed for. Dr. Dossey further says that the evidence suggests that the prayer most likely to get results is "let the best thing that can happen, happen." This is the same prayer that Jesus prayed when he said, "Nevertheless, not my will but thine be done."

Maintaining a positive vision as you pray is also very important. It is helpful to see yourself as you want to be—whole, healthy, and happy. Your body has an amazing desire and capacity to try to recreate whatever the mind's image projects to it. In fact, there is evidence suggesting that your immune cells will even attack tumors if you visualize them doing so. If that can happen against tumor cells, I believe it can also happen against

Lyme organisms. Try the following exercise twice a day after a time of prayer and thanksgiving: Sit in a comfortable and relaxed state, take a few very deep breaths, and picture your white blood cells (such as the CD57 NK cells) hunting down and finding Lyme germs and then injecting them with lethal chemicals.

It is vital that you keep positive healing images in your mind, especially when you are tempted to feel discouraged. The truth of the matter is that whatever you think about happens to you. Dwelling on positive images of yourself and your future helps positive things come to you by the law of attraction. Positive thinking also helps you to avoid victim thinking, which is characterized by helplessness, negativity, complaining, anger, self-pity, and depression. Remember: *Victims don't heal.* By choosing not to be a victim and actively putting your trust in God, you make it possible for what you ask for to be "given unto you."

Eating Properly

I covered the importance of eating healthy in Chapter Five. In that chapter, you learned how to eat in a way that both supports your immune system and significantly reverses chronic low-grade inflammation. Another important benefit of healthy eating is improvement in your emotions and cognitive abilities. People who habitually eat well are more likely to experience feelings of well-being characterized by happiness, contentment, enthusiasm, and other positive emotions. This is in contrast to people who eat in an unbalanced fashion, who experience more feelings of fatigue, mood swings, easy frustration, and depression. The reason for this is that a healthy diet provides us with more energy with which we can carry out our daily tasks with less resulting fatigue.

Eating right also provides your brain with the nutrients it requires to function most effectively. As a result, muddled thinking or "brain fog" is less likely to occur. Memory also typically improves, as do problem-solving abilities. If you want to truly feel well in "body, mind and Spirit," eating properly is essential. Often when changing something as basic as our eating habits, we need assistance in the form of a structured plan. In order to stay on target for your nutrition goals, I recommend that you regularly review and apply the healthy eating guidelines that I provided for you in chapter 5.

Forgiveness

Forgiveness is another important yet often overlooked aspect of the healing process. Mark Twain described forgiveness as "the fragrance left by the flower on the heel of the shoe that has just crushed it." Practicing forgiveness does not mean that you say that a wrong or an injustice was not done. Rather, when you practice forgiveness, you are simply deciding to turn the responsibility for righting that wrong over to a different authority while you go on with your life. When you forgive, you release your healing energies to help your Garden (body) recover its immune function.

By holding on to feelings of unforgiveness, bitterness, and resentment, you are literally dragging around a heavy weight from your past. However, once you start to forgive, you immediately begin to detach yourself from the hurts of the past and let go of their burdens. This frees you up to use your life energy much more productively for healing. Even though it may not feel like it, forgiveness is actually enlightened self-interest—you are the one who benefits the most from the act of letting go that we call forgiveness. It is as the saying goes, "Let go and let God."

I find that people who commit themselves to doing whatever is necessary for healing invariably discover that there is someone or some event from their past that is in need of their forgiveness. In many cases, it is themselves that the patients need to forgive. Sometimes, forgiving ourselves can be the most difficult challenge we face in our journey back to health. Yet, when we make the effort, the positive difference it makes is well worth it.

To get in the habit of forgiveness, I recommend that you regularly keep the following in mind: "I must completely forgive _____. Until I forgive _____ I will be in chains. When I set _____ free, I will be free also." Practice this for all those whom you need to forgive, even the tick that bit you. Doing so can make a huge difference in how well and soon you heal.

Finally, it is important to remember that forgiveness is a process similar to peeling off layers of an onion. The process takes time, as layer after layer of what you need to forgive is revealed to you. Don't feel bad because the feelings of anger come back. And don't get impatient. This is all a very normal process, which is part of the grieving that must occur for you to be able to say "goodbye" to that which you have lost as a result of the injustice that happened to you. Just stay with the process, don't rush it, and do what you can do today. And tomorrow is another day with its own challenges, for which God will give you the strength you need.

Oxygen/Breathing

Oxygen is one of Lyme disease's worst enemies. The reason for this is that the *Bb* bacteria that cause Lyme, like most other harmful microorganisms, cannot survive in an oxygen-rich environment. (Activities that deplete your body's oxygen supply, especially smoking cigarettes, are Lyme's best friends.)

The easiest way to increase the amount of oxygen in your blood is by practicing deep breathing. I recommend that you try to do this by taking deep, abdominal breaths. Do this at least three times a day (morning, after lunch, and evening), breathing deeply for at least thirty times each session. Ideally, perform this exercise outdoors to get the additional benefits of breathing fresh air.

In addition to bringing more oxygen into your body, regular practice of deep abdominal breathing will also help you to release stored stress and tension. It can also help to improve your mood. Once you begin to experience the many benefits that deep abdominal breathing offers, you will find it easy to make it a part of your daily health practice. The book *Conscious Breathing* by Dr. Gay Hendricks is an excellent resource that I frequently recommend to my patients for learning more about this wonderful healing discipline called breathwork.

Relationships

The importance of healthy relationships to good health is also well-documented by medical researchers. A lack of healthy relationships has been shown to increase the likelihood of illness, as well as of stress. Additionally, good relationships with others can make a significant positive difference in how well patients cope with chronic and debilitating conditions such as Lyme disease.

I encourage my patients to turn to their families and friends when they feel they need support, and I recommend that you do the same. I also recommend that you take time to reciprocate, and to do your best to "be there" for your loved ones when they need you. Doing so helps to take your attention off your own problems. In fact, many patients report that their pain, fatigue, and various other symptoms of Lyme disease tend to be forgotten or diminished when they are enjoying themselves with those they love.

Another important type of relationship for Lyme patients is the one they can develop by contacting a local support group. Because of the increasingly widespread incidence of Lyme disease, Lyme support groups can now be found in many cities and towns throughout the country. You can also find support groups online by searching for them on the Internet. (See the resources section for more information about this.) Since these support groups primarily consist of current and former Lyme patients, they can be extremely helpful to you in a variety of ways. Not only are support group members able to appreciate your own experiences with Lyme disease, they are also apt to provide you with useful information and a perspective that can only come from others with direct experience of what you are going through.

One word of caution about support groups, however. Most groups are very healing places where you can learn from others who have been in Lyme recovery for a long time and where you can receive a supportive ear as you tell your story. But some support groups may be a negative for you. Pay close attention to whether the goal of the group is to facilitate healing rather than to enable the members to indulge in ongoing victim mentality behaviors. That is to say, if the purpose of the group is to have a regular "pity party," then that's one party I suggest you skip.

If the members are not growing and progressing, but staying angry and feeling victimized, then the energy of that group will not be a healing experience for you.

One other important, yet often under-appreciated, relationship that I encourage you to cultivate is the one you have with your physician and other health care providers. As I stated earlier in this book, the ideal relationship between patient and doctor should be a partnership, not a dictatorship. Be an active participant in your professional health care treatment, and be willing to share what you are going through in your health journey so that your doctor can best meet your needs.

As the famous saying goes, "No man is an island." This is especially true during times of illness. The more that you can surround yourself with understanding loved ones and support group members as you deal with Lyme disease, the easier your struggles will be.

Humor

The Bible tells us that "a merry heart doeth good like a medicine." (Proverbs 17:22) Today, scientific researchers are confirming this. In the past few decades, medical research, such as that performed at Loma Linda University, shows conclusively that humor has very beneficial effects on our immune system. From our previous discussions earlier in this book, you know that part of that benefit is mediated by the endorphin system.

Laughter is also a good form of exercise. When we laugh, the muscles of the face, shoulders, diaphragm, and abdomen get a good workout. Laughing also increases the supply of oxygen in the blood and even burns up calories. When we laugh, we also tend to experience a lessening of any pains we may have.

One of the most famous examples of this fact was documented by Norman Cousins in his book *Anatomy of an Illness*. Prior to writing it, Cousins suffered from ankylosing spondylitis, a potentially crippling disease. As part of his self-healing program, Cousins decided to spend as much time as possible doing things that made him laugh. He especially enjoyed watching Marx Brothers movies and reruns of the TV show *Candid Camera*. He found that the more that he laughed, the more his pain diminished. Eventually, his condition completely improved, never to return. Another famous proponent of humor as a healing tool is Dr. Patch Adams, who has made it a primary focus of his medical practice, doing all he can to make his patients laugh.

I, too, find that laughter is powerful medicine and an antidote to just about every problem we may encounter. I also find that patients who laugh a lot are better able to see the optimistic side of life and to deal with their challenges more easily. So I encourage you to also look for the humor in your day-to-day experiences and to take time to enjoy them. Additionally, make it your goal to enjoy at least three hearty belly laughs each and every day. You may be surprised by how much of a positive difference doing this can make in your life.

Enjoy Today

There is another important self-help practice that you should consider adopting—learning to live in the here and now. As obvious as that principle seems, in reality, most of the time we don't practice it. The truth is that so many of the gifts given to us by our Creator are provided for our daily pure enjoyment, but we are often too busy and too preoccupied about tomorrow to stop and enjoy them. We really have forgotten how to "stop and smell the roses." The following exercises may be helpful to you in re-learning how to enjoy today as we did when we were children. Do as many as you can each day for a month.

* Stop and enjoy either a sunrise or a sunset every day.

* Identify at least two objects in nature every day of different shapes and colors, and focus on those objects for a minute each—for example, a flower, a tree, a bird.

* Spend ten minutes a day with a pet and just enjoy the relationship—dogs and cats work best, but even watching fish in an aquarium serves the purpose.

* Play with a young child ten minutes a day, by going for a walk, reading, playing catch, wrestling, and other creative "fun" things to do.

* Listen to relaxing music daily.

* Read from an inspiring book daily.

* Take a "Sabbath" rest day each week where you don't

work and you don't worry—just take a full day to enjoy life and contemplate the Creator's beautiful gifts.

There is a related useful technique that has recently become popular called "mindfulness." It is an activity that can be done at any time of the day. It is done by bringing the mind to concentrate and focus on what is happening in the present moment, while at the same time simply noticing the mind's usual chatter and judgmental commentary about the events of life. For example, you can be mindful of the sensation in your painful knee while walking, of the sound of the rain on the roof, or the feeling of soapy water while bathing the dog. You can also be mindful of the mind's commentary: "I wish I didn't have to walk any further. I like the sound of the pitter-patter of rain. I wish bathing the dog wasn't so boring and the soap wasn't drying out my skin." Now, once you have noticed the mind's running commentary of judgment on the events, you have the choice to release those judgments: "bathing dog: boring" may become "bathing dog; bathing dog." In this example, you can see that dog bathing does not have to be judged "boring"; dog bathing is only a process of coordinating the dog with soap and water. Therefore, any activity done "mindfully" in this way is a way to change our focus from the "head" evaluation mode with its negativity and judgment to the "heart" awareness mode with acceptance and even appreciation. With some practice it is possible to enjoy each day this way all the time.

Alternative Resources

The best medicine embraces all possible treatment options—both conventional and alternative. Alternative resources, therefore, include both conventional medicine (such as antibiotics) and all the alternative and holistic treatment choices that I shared with you in chapters 6 through 8. Working with an integrative, Lyme-aware physician can help you discover which of these alternative options are best suited for your specific needs. Your physician can also best advise you on how you should employ these treatment options or refer you to experts in their use.

Remember, in order to get well, you must be willing to consider all possible treatment approaches. This is particularly true of Lyme disease, because of how difficult it can be to treat the *Bb* bacteria once they spread through the body, stubbornly taking root in your body's tissues. At the same time, however, be careful not to believe everything you hear or read. Be discriminating about sources of information, and be sure to work with a licensed health practitioner in order to safely and cost-effectively use alternative therapies.

Light

This aspect of psychological and spiritual health can be attained in a number of ways. The most obvious is the light we receive from the sun. Just as plants needs sunlight to thrive, our bodies also benefit from sunlight. In this age of skin cancer fears, due to depletion of the ozone layer, it's easy to forget that some exposure to the sun is actually good for us. Sunlight has many healing properties and is essential for vitamin D production by our bodies. Recently, a number of medical studies have shown that most of us are deficient in vitamin D, in part because of a lack of regular exposure to natural sunlight.

I recommend that you try to expose yourself to sunlight on a daily basis if possible. If your diet is rich in the Rainbow Foods I discussed in chapter 5, you should be obtaining sufficient antioxidants to protect you from harmful ultraviolet (UV) rays. It's not necessary to stay outside for a long time, since sunlight's benefits can be obtained in a few minutes. For fair-skinned people, all that is required is about 10 to 15 minutes of sunlight per day.

Caution: If your doctor has prescribed an antibiotic that causes sensitivity to sunlight, you should avoid even small amounts of sunshine for the entire course of your treatment. The most common antibiotics that cause this type of sensitivity are the tetracyclines (e.g., doxycycline) and the quinolones (e.g., Levaquin).

Another form of healing light is known as far-infrared radiation, or FIR. Originally developed in Japan, a number of far-infrared devices are now available in the United States and other countries, including far-infrared saunas that, unlike regular saunas, emit dry heat. These saunas and other devices work by sending healing FIR rays penetrating into the skin, where they cause fat cells to release stored toxins. Additionally, as body temperature is raised, harmful microorganisms, including the Bb bacteria, are weakened while, simultaneously, immune function is enhanced. For a list of companies that provide FIR saunas and other devices, see the resources section.

I believe that the most important source of light for all of us is the Divine Light that is found by listening to the Word of God. As I discussed above, developing a connection to God or a Higher Power and regularly engaging in prayer or meditation can make a dramatic difference in your health, as well as in your ability to tolerate any present health symptoms.

Trust

Most Lyme patients have seen at least seven or eight doctors before finally finding a doctor who can correctly diagnose and treat them. One of the most frightening things that they are asked to do once they meet a Lyme-aware doctor is to trust again. For many, this is difficult. It requires believing that this practitioner can help them despite their negative experiences of the past.

Trust is a crucial component of the healing process. To a certain extent, trust in and of itself can result in powerful healing reactions in the body. Take, for example, the placebo effect. A few years ago a study was done in which a dental extraction was performed on two groups of patients—one group received the usual anesthesia for pain control and the other group received a placebo. Approximately 25 percent of people having a tooth extracted using placebo claimed that it worked. The logical explanation is that somehow their trust in the dentist and in the injected material generated something (likely endorphins) that resulted in pain relief.

However, trust goes a lot deeper than the placebo effect. Trust embodies many of the concepts we have discussed earlier in this chapter—God, hope, optimism, prayer, positive vision, positive relationships, and forgiveness. Trust always involves action based on a decision to believe in something. Many times chronically ill patients will have lost the ability to trust because they have been disappointed so many times before.

How do you reestablish the ability to trust? Humans are blessed with an inner wisdom that I call "heart wisdom" that will lead us correctly if we allow it. Heart wisdom is nurtured by our relationship with God and by our healthy relationships with other people. It is also fed by knowledge coming from reliable information. Very often a skilled counselor, such as a psychologist, can be extremely helpful in assisting us on the ⁊ing to listen to our inner heart wisdom. The help- ⁊ counselor is especially helpful when we have ⁊s children.

⁊s to learn as much as we can, pray diligently, cultivate healthy relationships (and let go of unhealthy relationships), including therapeutic psychological and/or spiritual relationships, and listen to the direction in which our heart is pointing us. Notice that I said heart and not emotions. Too often emotions lead us in the direction that our woundedness would take us—the direction of fear, anger, shame, and other negative directions.

There are seven steps that I have found useful in determining whether we are correctly tuning into heart wisdom, which I believe comes as a gift from God, or from some other, unreliable, source:

(1) Pray for direction and then put our will in "neutral." That is to say, we are willing to say, "Not my will but thine be done." This does not mean that we do not have a desire for the direction; it simply means that we are willing to surrender that will to a Higher Authority to direct us to the best pathway.

(2) Listen to the inner voice of our impressions. We put that inner voice information in the portfolio, but realize that it might be tainted by unhealthy emotions like vengeance and fear.

(3) Gather as much reliable information as possible. It is my belief that a major source should be books of spiritual wisdom, such as the Bible. The heart wisdom direction needs to be consistent with the wisdom information that we have learned.

(4) Discuss the issues in question with at least two healthy friends, acquaintances, or counselors. We put their counsel and

advice in the portfolio with the results of the previous steps.

(5) Look at the overall circumstances. Often, as we step back and look at the big picture, we can see a jigsaw puzzle being put together. The next puzzle piece to go in place may be apparent from the view from this perspective.

(6) Make a decision based on the previous steps as to what heart wisdom is saying. Based on the understanding of heart wisdom, we now have trust, or if you prefer, faith. The evidence of that condition of trust is that we enter into a mental state of "rest." From that state of rest, we confidently walk according to the direction of heart wisdom without fear or doubt.

(7) Realize that if doors are closing on our chosen pathway, we may have missed the heart's wisdom. Usually when that happens, we need to go back to step one, because we haven't yet really surrendered our agenda to God.

Helping Others

Altruism is the unselfish act of helping others who are in need. Research shows that this activity may have a powerful and positive effect on our health. One interesting study reported in early 2007 was performed at Duke University. The results of the study showed that students who engaged in selfless, altruistic behavior had a detectable change in their brain scan, with activation of the "posterior superior temporal cortex" of the brain. Without going into scientific detail, it is believed that the health effects result in reduced stress responses. This health-enhancing outcome is probably due to the activation of the relaxation response that I mentioned above—heart rate and blood pressure are reduced and stress hormones are normalized.

Positive immune system effects and pain relief occur with altruistic behavior and are likely mediated through the endorphin system that we have referred to so often in this book. Mental health improvements associated with altruism include a reduction in anxiety and depression and improved feelings of well-being. Finally, altruism results in improved social and spiritual health. As with my patient, Susan, giving back to others through selfless behavior helps the recovery process.

Summing Up

Once again, let's review the key points of this chapter by answering some of the most commonly asked questions about psychological and spiritual health in relation to Lyme disease.

Why are addressing psychological and spiritual health concerns important for people with Lyme disease?

Addressing such concerns is important for all patients, not just those with Lyme disease, since the most effective health care approaches are those that address the "whole person."

The effects of Lyme disease can be very challenging, not only physically, but also mentally and emotionally. For this reason a "whole person" treatment approach is especially important. In fact, I've found in many cases that engendering A. N.E.W. H.O.P.E. F.O.R. H.E.A.L.T.H. is the single most important element in determining how well patients with chronic Lyme are able to cope with their condition.

If addressing these psychological and spiritual aspects of health is so important, why do so many doctors fail to do so?

In actuality, a growing number of physicians, as well as many other types of health care providers, are now paying more attention to their patients' mental, emotional, and spiritual concerns. This is especially true of Lyme-aware physicians, most of whom offer a holistic, "whole person" treatment approach. This is a trend that I expect to continue, due to the ever-increasing amount of research that is occurring in the field of mind/body medicine, as well as research into the health benefits of prayer, meditation, and other spiritual practices.

On the other hand, many doctors still continue to only symptom-care for Lyme and other patients. In cases of early stage Lyme disease, this may be all that is necessary for patients to get well. In my experience, however, treating symptoms alone is never enough when it comes to dealing with Lyme disease once it has spread and become chronic. That is why I recommend that Lyme patients do all they can to locate and work with a Lyme-aware physician if at all possible.

What if patients cannot locate such physicians?

Providing a solution for that problem is the main reason that I wrote this book, since there are many things that all Lyme patients can do on their own to improve their likelihood of recovery. This is particularly true of many of the recommendations in this chapter. While I feel the ideal situation for all Lyme patients is to partner with a Lyme-aware physician, most of the elements that make up A. N.E.W. H.O.P.E. F.O.R. H.E.A.L.T.H. are of a self-care nature that anyone can apply. All it takes is a willingness to do so.

Conclusion

*

At the beginning of this book I told you that there is hope for patients with chronic Lyme and the other tick-borne diseases (TBDs). Now that you have read this far, you understand why I can make this statement with confidence. More importantly, you now know what you can do to begin reclaiming your health and recovering from Lyme and other TBDs. By working with a Lyme-aware physician and applying the recommendations I have shared with you, you too can begin to triumph over your health challenges and return to the life you knew before they began.

It's important for you to realize and accept that your journey towards full recovery from Lyme/TBDs will not happen overnight. Weeks and perhaps months may go by before you start to notice significant improvement. During that time, do not be discouraged, for when it comes to Lyme and other TBDs, patience is indeed a virtue. If you commit yourself to following the guidelines I've presented, the improved health you seek will increasingly become reality.

As your healing journey unfolds, here are some points I recommend that you keep in mind:

1) Your health is ultimately your responsibility. Although I strongly advise you to seek out and work with a Lyme-aware physician, don't overlook the fact that there is much that you can accomplish on your own. That is why many of the guidelines and recommendations I've shared, beginning with the Lyme Inflammation Diet, are of a self-care nature. Begin applying them today, and be willing to put in the time and effort that they require. Doing so will make a big difference in how quickly and fully you heal.

2) Remember that every experience in our lives brings with it important lessons. This is true even of Lyme and other diseases. Therefore, I encourage you to take time to reflect on the lessons your illness may be presenting you. Many people afflicted with chronic illness, when they take the time to look for such lessons, discover a need to make changes in other areas of their lives, beyond simply a change in diet or more exercise. Are you being called upon to make such changes, as well? Be willing to ask yourself such questions and see where they may lead you.

3) Realize that you are not alone. In addition to your physician and other health care practitioners with whom you may choose to work, be willing to ask for support as you need it from your family and friends. Turning to support groups can also be helpful, so long as they don't turn into "pity parties." Also be sure to ask for help and guidance from God. Doing so can make all the difference in how well you heal.

4) Recognize that health is a journey without end. Many people, once they recover from illness, cease to follow the principles that allowed them to get well. This is a mistake. My hope for you is that you not only will recover from Lyme/TBDs, but that you will then continue to apply the principles you've learned by reading this book for the rest of your life. By doing so, you will discover that there are really no limits to how healthy you can be, not only physically, but also mentally, emotionally, and spiritually.

I also encourage you to stay informed about Lyme and other TBDs, since there is still much that remains to be discovered about these increasingly common conditions. To this end, I recommend that you visit my Web site, www.lymedoctor.com, where you can sign up to receive ongoing news about Lyme/TBDs as I become aware of it. My commitment to helping others recover from Lyme/TBDs is ongoing, and my Web site is where I will regularly be updating the information in this book.

In closing, I thank you for reading this far. May the information I've shared guide you to a full and lasting recovery, and may your journey back to healing be filled with many blessings.

Resources

✴

www.lymedoctor.com—This site serves as an extension of *The Lyme Disease Solution* book and is intended to help you keep informed about the latest information related to Lyme and other tick-borne diseases. Be sure to sign up to receive free, ongoing email updates.

Lyme Disease Organizations
* Lyme Disease Association
  www.lymediseaseassociation.org
  P.O. Box 1438
  Jackson, NJ 08527
  (888) 366-6611

This is the Web site that I most commonly refer patients to, along with ILADS. It is a tremendous information resource about Lyme/TBDs, as well as current events related to Lyme, especially on the political front. I believe regular visitation to this site is essential for anyone interested in seeing the Lyme-awareness movement move in the right direction. An excellent doctor referral resource is located via this site.

* Lyme Net
www.lymenet.org
43 Winton Road
East Brunswick, NJ 08816

This Web site contains extremely good information and resources for the Lyme/TBD patient. It is very accurate and should be on the "regular read" list for all patients.

* Lyme Disease Foundation, Inc.
www.lyme.org
P.O. Box 332
Tolland, CT 06084
(860) 870-0070

The Lyme Disease Foundation (LDF) is a leading nonprofit organization dedicated to finding solutions for tick-borne disorders. The LDF Web site is another valuable online resource for people with Lyme and other TBDs.

* International Lyme and Associated Diseases Society (ILADS)
  www.ilads.org
  P.O. Box 341461
  Bethesda, MD 20827
  (301) 263-1080

ILADS is a nonprofit, international, multidisciplinary medical society, dedicated to the diagnosis and appropriate treatment of Lyme and its associated diseases. ILADS promotes understanding of Lyme and its associated diseases through research and education and strongly supports physicians and other health care professionals dedicated to advancing the standard of care for Lyme and its associated diseases.

Most of us doctors who have become Lyme-aware (or "Lyme-literate") became that way as a direct result of the educational efforts of ILADS. I am deeply grateful for this wonderful resource and urge you to support it in any way that you can (including financially). It is truly a voice crying in the wilderness.

Locating a Lyme-Aware Physician

* Lyme Disease Association (LDA)
  www.lymediseaseassociation.org
  888-366-6611

Lyme Disease Support Groups

To locate support groups across the United States, as well as in Canada, Europe, Australia, and on the Internet, visit www.lymenet.org/SupportGroups. There you will find an extensive listing of such groups.

Recommended General Lyme Information Resources

- www.openeyepictures.org This film company is producing the film "Under Our Skin" to be released in late 2007. Telling the story of Lyme patients themselves, I believe this powerful film will take Lyme awareness to a whole new level.

- www.publichealthalert.org This is a very informative Web site with a monthly newsletter that I highly recommend. More than most other Lyme information resources, it is open to the "integrative" approach to Lyme—conventional and alternative medical aspects.

- www.lymeinfo.net This is a wonderful source of useful Lyme-related Web links and other helpful information about Lyme and the co-infections. It is an excellent place to start when doing research about Lyme and the other tick-borne diseases.

- www.tickencounter.org This excellent Web site will teach you virtually everything you need to know about ticks, including identification and removal.

- *Coping with Lyme Disease*, Denise Lang with Kenneth B. Liegner, M.D. (Owl Books, 2004).

This book is an excellent resource for diagnosis and treatment principles from a practical standpoint. It deals with different age groups and with many commonly encountered problems and issues (such as insurance coverage) of Lyme patients seeking to cope with a difficult problem for which the medical community generally has no answers.

* *Everything You Need to Know About Lyme Disease*, Karen Vanderhoof-Forschner (Wiley Books 2003) and the Lyme Disease Foundation (www.lyme.org).

This classic book is arguably the most helpful printed resource since Lyme was recognized nearly three decades ago. It is must-reading for all students of Lyme disease. The non-profit organization that Ms. Vanderhoof-Forschner founded continues to be extremely helpful for education of the public, of our political leaders, and of the medical community in terms of Lyme and the other TBDs.

* *Healing Lyme*, Stephen Harrod Buhner (Raven Press 2005).

Written by master herbalist, Stephen Buhner, there is no better resource, in my opinion, available for understanding the biology of Lyme and the TBDs. It is thoroughly researched and highly useful for anyone who wants to understand the medical research available concerning these disorders. I refer to this book frequently for its wisdom in the use of natural products such as herbs.

Where to Send Ticks for Testing

* Local and State Health Departments. Check there first, as some do offer testing.

* Tick Testing Centers (from www.dig-itmag.com). Please note that pricing at each of these laboratories is subject to change, and therefore you should check with the lab for current prices.

Analytical Services, Inc.

Williston, VT

800-723-4432, www.analyticalservices.com

> (PCR test: $75, dead or alive. Ziplock bag, no tape, overnight it.
> Turnaround time: two weeks)

Connecticut Pathologies Laboratories, Inc.

Willimantic, CT

860-423-2775

> (PCR test: $49, dead or alive, Lyme disease only. Turnaround
> time: one week)

IgeneX, Inc.

Palo Alto, CA

800-832-3200, www.igenex.com

> (PCR test: $55, dead or alive. Can test for 5 organisms at $55/test.
> Turnaround time: ten to twelve business days; ziplock bag)

Imugen, Inc.

Norwood, MA

781-255-0770, www.imugen.com

> (Tests for Lyme and/or Babesia—$98 for both; tests only deer
> ticks, no alcohol allowed; see their Web site for instructions
> before sending ticks.)

Medical Diagnostic Laboratories

Mt. Laurel, NJ

877-269-0090, www.mdlab.com

> (Able to test ticks for the usual TBDs plus four different types
> of Bartonella and also Mycoplasma; Lyme PCR test: $155 plus
> doctor's prescription; dead or alive)

New Jersey Division of Health and Senior Services

Division of Public Health and Environmental Laboratories
Trenton, NJ
609-292-5819

> ($25 for Lyme disease test; $35 for both Lyme disease and Rocky
> Mountain spotted fever. Live ticks only. Send in film container
> or other hard container with moist cotton ball. No baggies.)

New Jersey Laboratories
New Brunswick, NJ
732-249-0148, 877-TICK-TEST

> ($60, if freshly dead or alive with no tick exposure to chemicals,
> alcohol, or antibiotics; if exposure to any of those agents has
> occurred, Lyme disease PCR is done at $175, dead or alive.)

Tick Repellent Information

* Avon Corporation
  800-FOR-AVON

They produce a very effective tick repellent, and it is the one
that I most often recommend to patients—Avon Skin-So-Soft
Mosquito, Flea, and Deer Tick Repellent Lotion. It is FDA
approved and is safe and non-toxic.

* Lewey's Eco-Blends
  www.BUZZOFF.us
  866-LEWEYS-1

This product is ecologically friendly and is made up of all
natural, deet-free, gmo (genetically modified organism)-free
ingredients. It works for up to four hours, and early feedback
from patients is very positive.

Reliable Labs for Lyme and Tick-Borne Disease Testing

* IGeneX Reference Laboratory
  www.igenex.com
  800-832-3200

This lab performs a very good battery of tests for Lyme (including the sensitive Western Blot) and tests for all the major co-infections. It is a reliable source of basic tick-disease testing and includes three important and useful tests: the Babesia PCR, Babesia flourescent in-situ hybridization (FISH) test, and the Lyme dot assay (LDA). *They report all bands on Lyme Western Blot.*

* Medical Diagnostics Laboratory
  www.mdlab.com
  877-269-0090

This lab performs comprehensive testing for Lyme, many co-infections, and viruses that may be confused with Lyme and offers many other valuable diagnostic tests. I find it especially useful when evaluating a patient for Bartonella/BLO. An advantage of this lab is that it works with many insurance companies, reducing the financial cost to the patient.

Other Labs Frequently Used in Lyme-Aware Practices

* Genova Labs
  www.genovalabs.com

This lab performs many useful unconventional tests used by practitioners of complementary and alternative medicine, such as tests of gastrointestinal function, heavy metal blood and urine analysis, and many others.

- Doctor's Data Lab
  www.doctorsdata.com

Similar to Genova Labs, this lab performs many useful tests for complementary and alternative practitioners.

- Metametrix Clinical Laboratory
  www.metametrix.com

Similar to Genova and Doctor's Data, Metametrix does salivary hormone testing, urinary porphyrin evaluation, and urinary organic acid analysis.

Other Useful Organizations

- American College for Advancement in Medicine (ACAM)
  www.acam.org
  24411 Ridge Route Suite 115
  Laguna Hills, CA 92653
  (949) 309-3520

This excellent organization trains medical professionals in the safe and effective use of alternative and complementary therapies, such as intravenous vitamin C and intravenous glutathione. If your Lyme-aware physician is also a member of ACAM, you are indeed in good hands. Contact ACAM for physician referrals.

- American Holistic Medical Association (AHMA)
  www.holisticmedicine.org
  P.O. Box 2016
  Edmonds, WA 98020
  (425) 967-0737

The AHMA is one of the oldest advocacy groups for the practice of holistic medicine, which it defines as an integration of all aspects of well-being, including physical, environmental, mental, emotional, spiritual, and social health. A number of AHMA members are also Lyme-Aware medical practioners (LAMPs).

Biological Dentist Information
* International Academy of Biological Dentistry and Medicine
  www.iabdm.org

* Mercury Free Dentists
  www.mercuryfreedentists.com

Pain Management Resources
* American Academy of Pain Management
  www.aapainmanage.org

* American Academy of Pain Medicine
  www.painmed.org

* American Board of Pain Medicine
  www.abpm.org

* American Pain Society
  www.ampainsoc.org

Homeopathy Resources
* National Center for Homeopathy

www.nationalcenterforhomeopathy.org

* British Institute of Homeopathy
  www.britinsthom.com

* North American Society of Homeopaths
  www.homeopathy.org

Herbal Medicine Resources

* United States Department of Agriculture (USDA)—Dr. James A. Duke's Phytochemical and Ethnobotanical Database
  www.ars-grin.gov/duke

Acupuncture Resources

* American Academy of Medical Acupuncture
  www.medicalacupuncture.org

* Tai Sophia Institute
  www.tai.edu

* American Association of Oriental Acupuncture
  www.aaoa.org

* National Acupuncture and Oriental Medicine Alliance
  www.acuall.org

Massage Therapy Resources

* American Massage Therapy Association
  www.amtamassage.org

Low Dose Naltrexone Information

www.lowdosenaltrexone.org

This novel therapy has been very useful in my practice. Although not effective for everyone, it is dramatically effective in those for whom it does work. The ideal candidates for this inexpensive and non-toxic treatment are those with autoimmune manifestations of chronic Lyme, such as chronic arthritis, multiple sclerosis, fibromyalgia, and other such disorders. Further research is needed, and I believe that research will validate the usefulness of this simple immune system "re-regulation" therapy.

Detoxification Resources

* American Academy of Environmental Medicine (AAEM)
  www.aaem.com

Sleep Medicine Resources

* American Academy of Sleep Medicine
  www.aasmnet.org

Nutritional Products for People with Lyme/TBDs

* Nutrition Essentials, Inc.
  www.nutritionessentialsinc.com
  8501 LaSalle Rd.
  Suite 310
  Towson, MD 21286
  (800) 816-2160

Co-founded by Dr. Singleton, Nutrition Essentials is a sup-

plier of top quality unique nutritional supplements and homeopathic products designed to address identified health needs of
targeted populations, including people with Lyme and other
TBDs. Nutrition Essentials is committed to a social mission
of supporting nonprofit organizations that benefit humanitar-
ian causes, world peace, and environmental responsibility. Ten
percent of all profits from the sale of their products are donated
to worthwhile charitable organizations. Among the Nutrition
Essential product line is Q-Nique, the excellent multiple vitamin supplement that contains co-enzyme Q10 (CoQ10)—a
vital co-enzyme involved in energy production that is often
deficient in people with Lyme/TBDs.

References

✱

Aberer E., et al. Why is chronic Lyme borreliosis chronic? *Clin Infect Dis.* 1997;25(Suppl 1):S64–S70.

Ackerman R., et al. Chronic neurological manifestations of erythema migrans borreliosis. *Annals of the New York Academy of Sciences.* 1987;539:16-23.

Adelson M., et al. Prevalence of *Borrelia burgdorferi, Bartonella spp., Babesia microti,* and *Anaplasma phagocytophilia* in Ixodes scapularis ticks collected in northern New Jersey. *J of Clinical Microbiology.* 2004;42:2799-2801.

Afonso V., et al. Reactive oxygen species and superoxide dismutases: Role in joint diseases. *Joint, Bone, Spine.* 2007.

Aguero-Rosenfeld M., et al. Evolution of the serologic response to *Borrelia burgdorferi* in treated patients with culture-confirmed erythema migrans. *J of Clinical Microbiology.* 1996;34:1-9.

Aktas O., et al. Green tea epigallocatechin-3-gallate mediates T cellular NF-kB inhibition and exerts neuroprotection in autoimmune encephalomyelitis. *J Immunol.* 2004;173:5794-5800.

Appel M., et al. Persistence of *Borrelia burgdorferi* in experimentally infected dogs after antibiotic treatment. *Clinical manifestations*, case series and treatment (Abstract D607).

Appleton N. *Stopping Inflammation.* Garden City Park, NJ: Square One Publishers; 2005.

Armstrong P., et al. A new *Borrelia* infecting lone star ticks. *Lancet.* 1996;347:66-67.

Bakken J., et al. Clinical diagnosis and treatment of human granulocytotropic anaplasmosis. *Annals of NY Acad of Sci.* 2006;1078:236-47.

Bakken J., et al. Ehrlichiosis and anaplasmosis. *Infect Med.* 2004;21(9):433-451.

Bassuk S., et al. High-sensitivity C-reactive protein: Clinical importance. *Curr Probl Cardiol.* 2004;29(8):439-493.

Belongia E. Epidemiology and impact of coinfections acquired from Ixodes ticks. *Vector Borne Zoonotic Dis.* 2002;2(4):265-273.

Berger A. Th1 and Th2 responses: What are they? *BMJ.* 2002;321:424.

Black P. Stress and the inflammatory response: A review of neurogenic inflammation. *Brain Behav Immun.* 2002;16(6):622-53.

Bock K. *The Road to Immunity.* New York: Pocket Books; 1997.

Breitschwerdt E., et al. *Bartonella* species in the blood of immunocompetent persons with animal and arthropod contact. *Emerging Infectious Diseases.* 2007;13(6):938-941.

Brorson O., Brorson S. Transformation of cystic forms of *Borrelia burgdorferii* to normal mobile spirochetes. *Infection.* 1997;25:240-246.

Brown S., Trivieri L. *The Acid-Alkaline Food Guide.* Garden City Park, NJ: Square One Publishers; 2006.

Buhner S.H. *Healing Lyme.* New York: Raven Press; 2005.

Bujack D., et al. Clinical and neurocognitive features of post-Lyme syndrome. *J Rheumatol.* 1996;23(8):1392-1397.

Burgdorfer W., et al. Lyme disease: A tick-borne spirochetosis? *Science.* 1982;216:1317-1319.

Burrascano J. M.D. Diagnostic Hints and Treatment Guidelines for Lyme and Other Tick Borne Illnesses. International Lyme and Associated Diseases Society. Available at: http://www.ilads.org/burrascano_0905.html.

Cambra K. Back to basics: Implicating insulin. *Brown Medicine.* 2006;11(2):10-11.

Cameron D., et al. Evidence-based guidelines for the management of Lyme disease. *Expert Rev Anti Infect Ther.* 2004;2(1 Suppl):S1-13.

Cantorna M., et al. Vitamin A deficiency exacerbates murine Lyme arthritis. *J Infect Dis.* Vol 1996;174(4):747-51.

Cantorna M., et al. Mounting evidence for vitamin D as an environmental factor affecting autoimmune disease prevalence. *Experimental Biology and Medicine*. 2004;229:1136-1142.

Centers for Disease Control and Prevention (CDC). Learn about Lyme disease. Available at: http://www.cdc.gov/ncidod/dvbid/lyme.

Lyme Disease (*Borrelia burgdorferi*), 1996 Case Definition. Case Definitions for Infectious Conditions Under Public Health Surveillance. Available at: http://www.cdc.gov/epo/dphsi/casedef/lyme_disease_current.htm.

Lyme Disease: Questions and Answers. Centers for Disease Control and Prevention. Available at: http://www.cdc.gov/ncidod/dvbid/lyme_QA.htm.

Reported Cases of Lyme Disease, United States, 2005. Centers for Disease Control and Prevention. Available at: http://www.cdc.gov/ncidod/dvbid/lyme/ld_statistics.htm.

Cole G., Morihara T., Lim G., et al. NSAID and antioxidant prevention of Alzheimer's disease: Lessons from in vitro and animal models. *Ann NY Acad Sci*. 2004;1035:68-84.

Cousins N. *Anatomy of an Illness*. New York: Norton; 1979.

Crook T., et al. Effects of phosphatidylserine in age-associated memory impairment. *Neurology*. 1991;41:644-449.

Coulter P., et al. Two-year evaluation of *Borrelia burgdorferi* culture and supplemental tests for definitive diagnosis of Lyme disease. *J Clin Microbiol*. 2005;43(10):5080-5084.

Deluca H., et al. Vitamin D: Its role and uses in immunology. *The FASEB Journal*. 2001;15:2579-2585.

Dempsey P., et al. The art of war: Innate and adaptive immune responses. *Cell Mol Life Sci*. 2003;60(12):2604-2621.

Dossey L. *Healing Words*. San Francisco, CA: Harper San Francisco, 1993.

Dossey L. *Prayer Is Good Medicine*. San Francisco, CA: Harper San Francisco, 1996.

Duvoix A., et al. Chemopreventive and therapeutic effects of curcumin. *Cancer Lett*. 2005;223(2):181-190.

Ebnet K., et al. *Borrelia burgdorferi* activates NF-kB and is a potent inducer of chemokines and adhesion molecule gene expression in endothelial cells and fibroblasts. *J of Immunology*. 1997;158:3285-3292.

Ergas D. N-3 fatty acids and the immune system in autoimmunity. *Isr Med Assoc J*. 2002;4(1):34-8.

Eskow E., et al. Concurrent infection of the central nervous system by *Borrelia burgdorferi* and *Bartonella henselae*: Evidence for a novel tick-borne disease complex. *Arch Neurol*. 2002;58(9):1357-1363.

Fallon B., et al. Neurology 2007, doi:10. 1212/01. WNL.0000284604.61160.2d. (abstract published online October 10, 2007).

Fallon B. Heavy metal: Matrix metalloproteinases in Lyme disease. *Medscape* [serial online]. 2005.

Fallon B., et al. Repeated antibiotic treatment in chronic Lyme disease. *J of Spiro Tick Dis*. 1999;6:94-102.

Fife W., et al. Preliminary clinical study on the use of hyperbaric oxygen therapy for the treatment of Lyme disease (in print). *Texas A&M University*. 1997.

French A., et al. Natural Killer Cells and Autoimmunity. *Arthritis Res Ther*. 2004;6:8-14.

Gao X. Immunomodulatory activity of resveratrol: Discrepant in vitro and in vivo immunological effects. *Biochem Pharmacol*. 2003;66(12):2427-2435.

Goldberg B., Trivieri L. *Chronic Fatigue, Fibromyalgia & Lyme Disease*. 2nd edition. Berkeley, Calif: Ten Speed/Celestial Arts; 2004.

Greenberg H., et al. Sleep quality in Lyme disease. *Sleep*. 1995;18(10):921-926.

Grimble R. Effect of antioxidative vitamins on immune function with clinical applications. *Int J Vitam Nutr Res*. 1997;67(5):312-320.

Grzanna R., et al. Ginger—an herbal medicinal product with broad anti-inflammatory actions. *J Med Food*. 2005;8(2):125-132.

Guerau-de-Arellano M., et al. Development of autoimmunity in Lyme arthritis. *Curr Opin Rheumatol*. 2002;14(4):388-393.

Haller J., et al. Vitamins for the elderly: Reducing disability and improving quality of life. *Aging Clinical and Experimental Research*. 1993;5 (supple 1):65-70.

Hamilton E. Lyme disease guidelines focus of antitrust probe. *Hartford Courant*. 2006.

Harris N., et al. *Borrelia burgdorferi* antigen levels in urine and other fluids during the course of treatment for Lyme disease: A case study presented at the VII International Congress of Lyme Borreliosis. San Francisco, CA: 16-21 June 1996.

Harvey W., et al. Lyme disease: Ancient engine of an unrecognized borreliosis pandemic? *Medical Hypotheses.* 2003;60(5):742-759.

Hendricks G. *Conscious Breathing.* New York: Bantam Books; 1995.

Position Paper on the CDC's Statement Regarding Lyme Diagnosis. ILADS (International Lyme and Associated Diseases Society). Available at: http://www.ilads.org/cdc_paper.html.

Johnson L., et al. Treatment of Lyme disease: A medicological assessment. Expert *Rev Anti Inf Ther.* 2004;2(4):533-557.

Kenefick K., et al. *B. burgdorferi* stimulates release of Interleukin-1 from bovine peripheral blood monocytes. *Infect Immun.* 1992;60(9):3630-3634.

Kiecolt-Glaser J., et al. Psychoneuro-immunology: Psychological influences on immune function and health. *J Consult Clin Psychol.* 2002;70(3):537-547.

Kosik-Bogacka, D. Detection of B. *burgdorferi* sensu lato in mosquitoes (Culicidae) in recreational areas of the city of Szczcin. *Ann Agri Environ Med.* 2002;9(1):55-7.

Krause P., et al. Concurrent Lyme disease and babesiosis: Evidence for increased severity and duration of illness. JAMA. 1996;275(21):1657-60.

Krupp, L.B., et al. Study and Treatment of Post Lyme Disease: A randomized double masked clinical trial. *Neurology.* 2003;60(12): 1923–1930.

Lac G. Saliva assays in clinical and research biology. *Pathol Biol* (Paris). 2001;49(8):660-7.

Landers S.J. Lyme disease debate provokes treatment divide, legal action (in what may be a first, the government has taken steps to investigate the drafting of medical guidelines). *AMNews*. 2006.

Lang D. *Coping with Lyme Disease*. 3rd edition. New York: Owl Books; 2004.

Lawrence C., et al. Seronegative chronic relapsing neuroborreliosis. *Eur Neurol*. 1995;35:113-117.

Lewis J. Controversies surround treatment of Lyme disease. *Infectious Disease News*. 2006.

Liegner K., et al. Recurrent erythema migrans despite extended antibiotic treatment with minocycline in a patient with persisting *Bb* infection. *M. Dermatology*. 1992.

Li Q., et al. NF-kappa B regulation in the immune system. *Nat Rev Immunol*. 2002;(10):725-734.

Luger S. Lyme disease transmitted by a biting fly. *New Eng J Med*. 1990;322(24):1752.

Magnarelli L., et al. The etiological agent of Lyme disease in deer flies, horse flies, and mosquitoes. *J Infect Dis*. 1986;154(2):355-8.

Marangon, K., et al. Comparison of the effect of alpha-lipoic acid and alpha-tocopherol supplementation on measures of oxidative stress. *Free Radical Biology & Medicine*. 1999;27(9,10):1114-1121.

Masaki K., et al. Association of vitamin E and C supplement use with cognitive function and dementia in elderly men. *Neurology.* 2000;54:1265-1272.

Masters E. Lone star vectored Lyme like disease. Available at: http://www.secebt.org/uploads/documents/Masters.pdf.

Masters E., et al. Physician-diagnosed erythema migrans and erythema mingrans-like rashes following Lone Star tick bites. *Archives of Dermatology.* 1998;134:955-960.

Nardelli D., et al. Association of CD4+CD25+ T cells with prevention of severe destructive arthritis in *B. burgdorferi*-vaccinated and challenged gamma interferon deficient mice treated with anti-Interleukin 17 antibody. *Clin Diag Lab Immunol.* 2004;11(6):1075-1084.

Let's Tackle Ticks. Gardens Alive. Available at: http://www.gardensalive. com/article.asp?ai=568.

Oksi, J., et al. Borrelia burgdorferi detected by culture and PCR in clinical relapse of disseminated Lyme borreliosis, *Ann Med.* 1999;31:225–232

Oleson C. Transverse myelitis secondary to coexistent Lyme disease and babesiosis. *J Spinal Cord Med.* 2003;26(2):168-171.

Owen D.C. Is Lyme disease always polymicrobial?—The jigsaw hypothesis. *Medical Hypotheses.* 2006;67(4):860-864.

Paparone P.W. Cardiovascular manifestations of Lyme disease. *JAOA.* 1997;97, issue 3:156-161.

Pavia C.S. Immune response to the Lyme spirochete *Borrelia burgdorferi* affected by ethanol consumption. *Immunopharmacology.* 1991;22(3):165-73.

Perlmutter D. *Brain Recovery*. Naples, FL: Perlmutter Health Center; 2001.

Peterson J.D., et al. Glutathione levels in antigen-presenting cells modulate Th1 vs Th2 response patterns. *Immunology*. 1998;95(6): 3071-3076.

Phillips S. Lyme disease: A public health crisis ignored. *Hartford Courant*. 2005.

Phillips S., et al. Evaluation of antibiotic treatment in patients with persistent symptoms of Lyme disease: An ILADS position paper. Available at: http://www.ILADS.org.

Plapp F.W. The role of vitamin A deficiency in autoimmune diseases: Gulf war syndrome, chronic fatigue syndrome, multiple chemical sensitivity, and fibromyalgia. Immune Support. Available at: http://www.immunesupport.com.

Preac-Mursic V., et al. Survival of *Borrelia burgdorferi* in antibiotically treated patients with Lyme borreliosis. *Infection*. 1989;17:355-359.

Riso P. Effect of a tomato-based drink on markers of inflammation, immunodulation and oxidative stress. *J Agric Food Chem*. 2006;54(7):2563-2566.

Salazar J., et al. Coevolution of markers of innate and adaptive immunity in skin and peripheral blood of patients with erythema migrans. *J Immonol*. 2003;171(5):2660-2670.

Schaible H.G., Ebersberger A., and Von Banchet G.S. Mechanisms of pain in arthritis. *Ann N Y Acad Sci*. 2002;966:343-54.

Seelig M.S. The requirement of magnesium by the normal adult. *American Journal of Clinical Nutrition*. 1964;14:342-390.

Seelig M.S. Review and hypothesis: Might patients with chronic fatigue syndrome have latent tetany of magnesium deficiency? *J of Chronic Fatigue Syndrome.* 1998; 4(2):77-108.

Shealy C.N., et al. Osteoarthritic pain: A comparison of homeopathy and acetaminophen. *American Journal of Pain Management.* 1998;8:89-91.

Sherr V. Two detailed case histories involving patients with co-infections— Babesiosis, Ehrlichiosis, and Lyme disease. Available at: http://www.ilads.org/sherr4.html.

Sherr V. Panic attacks may reveal previously unsuspected chronic disseminated Lyme disease. *Journal of Psychiatric Practice.* 2000; 6(6).

Simopoulas A.P. Omega-3 fatty acids in inflammation and autoimmune diseases. *J of Am Coll Nutr.* 2002;21(6):495-505.

Steere A.C., et al. Erythema chronicum migrans and Lyme arthritis: The enlarging clinical spectrum. *Ann Intern Med.* 1977;86(6):685-698.

Steere A.C., et al. Lyme arthritis: An epidemic of oligoarthritis in children and adults in three Connecticut communities. *Arthritis Rheum.* 1977;20:7-17.

Sternberg E.M. *The Balance Within.* New York: W.H. Freeman and Company, 2001.

Stricker R.B., et al. The Lyme wars: Time to listen. *Expert Opin Investig Drugs.* 2003;12:1609-1614.

Stricker R.B., et al. Decreased lymphocytes CD57 subset in patients with chronic Lyme disease. *Immunol Letter.* 2001;76(1):43-48.

Stricker R.B., et al. Medical revisionists threaten effective Lyme treatment. *Hartford Courant.* 2006.

Szalai A.J. C-reactive protein (CRP) and autoimmune disease: Facts and conjectures. *Clin Dev Immunol.* 2004;11(3-4):221-226.

Tan A. *The Opposite of Fate.* New York: Penguin Group; 2004.

Trivieri L. *Alternative Medicine: The Definitive Guide.* 2nd ed. Berkeley, Calif: Ten Speed/Celestial Arts; 2002.

Trivieri L. *The American Holistic Medical Association guide to holistic health.* Hoboken, NJ: John Wiley & Sons; 2001.

Vanderhoof-Forschner K. *Everything You Need to Know about Lyme Disease and Other Tick-Borne Disorders.* 2nd edition. Hoboken, NJ: John Wiley & Sons. 2003.

Vining R.F. The measurement of hormones in saliva: Possibilities and pitfalls. *J. Steroid Biochem.* 1987;27(1-3):81-94.

Virginia Department of Health. Tips for Avoiding Ticks.

Wormser G., et al. The clinical assessment, treatment, and prevention of Lyme disease, human granulocytic Anaplasmosis, and Babesiosis: Clinical practice guidelines by the Infectious Diseases Society of America. *Clin Infect Dis.* 2006;43:1089-1134. Available at:
http://www.journals.uchicago.edu/CID/journal/issues/v43n9/40897/40897.
text.html-fn1#fn
1http://www.journals.uchicago.edu/CID/journal/issues/v43n9/40897/40897.
text.html - fn2#fn2.

Zandi P. Reduced risk of Alzheimer's disease in users of antioxidant vitamin supplements. *Archives of Neurology.* 2004;61(1):82-8.

Appendix

Lyme Inflammation Diet Sample Recipes

Salmon Patties
Hash Brown Potatoes
Tofu Salad
Broccoli with Cheddar Cheese
Miso Soup
Split Pea Soup
Brown Rice Casserole
Flounder Almandine
Sweet Potato Souffle
Baked Chicken with Onions and Bell Pepper
Basil-Walnut Vinaigrette Dressing
Stir-Fry Vegetable Medley
Spicy Cilantro Sauce
Lentil Soup
Mango Sorbet
Potato Salad
French Toast
Venison Stew
Peach Cobbler

Salmon Patties

1	can (16 ounce) salmon
1	small onion, finely grated
2	tablespoons fresh parsley, minced
2	teaspoons dry mustard
2	tablespoons lemon juice
	ground black pepper, to taste
2	large eggs, well beaten
3/4	cup fine dry (whole wheat) bread crumbs
1	tablespoon butter

Heat oven to 350°.

Drain salmon and flake with a fork, removing or mashing any bones (they are edible). Mix in grated onion, parsley, mustard, lemon juice, and pepper. Mix eggs with salmon. Add enough bread crumbs, about 1/2 cup, to make mixture thick enough to shape into small patties. Roll patties to coat in bread crumbs. Melt 1 tablespoon butter in oven-safe pan, add patties, and bake for 20 minutes.

Hash Brown Potatoes

3	large potatoes, peeled or unpeeled and well washed
2	tablespoons olive oil
	sea salt to taste
	herb seasoning blend to taste
1/2	large onion, sliced
1/2	green bell pepper, chopped

Heat oven to 375°.

Slice potatoes (medium to thin slices) into a large bowl. Mix potatoes with olive oil, sea salt, and herb seasoning. (More or less seasoning mixture may be desired.) Coat the bottom of a baking dish with olive oil. Place potato mixture into the baking dish. Bake for approximately 25 minutes. Remove from oven. Turn potatoes with a spatula. Add onion and bell peppers, and bake for an additional 15 minutes or until potatoes are golden brown.

Tofu Salad

1	block firm tofu
	sea salt and pepper
1	teaspoon fresh dill (or ½ teaspoon dried)
1/4	teaspoon dry mustard
1/4	cup cider vinegar
1/2	cup Omega-3 mayonnaise
	juice of 1 lemon or lime (or combination)
	dash of dried basil
1/2	teaspoon turmeric
1/2	cup fresh parsley, chopped
1	scallion, sliced
1	red onion, finely chopped
1	bell pepper, diced
1	stalk of celery, chopped
1	tomato, chopped

Drain tofu and dice into small pieces. Mix tofu with sea salt and pepper to taste, dill, mustard, cider vinegar, mayonnaise, lemon or lime juice, dash of dried basil, tumeric, and chopped parsley. Allow to marinate about 1 hour. Mix together the scallion, red onion, bell pepper, and celery. Add vegetables to tofu, mix gently, and serve. Garnish with fresh chopped tomato.

Broccoli with Cheddar Cheese

2-3   cups broccoli florets

       sea salt, to taste

1   tablespoon organic butter or ghee

3/4   cups organic sharp cheddar cheese, grated

Steam the broccoli until crisp tender, about 3 to 4 minutes. Season to taste with sea salt and butter or ghee. Heat cheese until completely melted. Pour over the steamed broccoli and serve at once.

Miso Soup

1 1/2	tablespoons miso paste
3	cups diluted chicken stock, warmed
3	ounces shitake mushrooms
1	tablespoon ginger, finely grated
2	medium spring onions, sliced
4 1/4	ounces fresh soft tofu or long-life silken tofu
1/4	cup chives, chopped

Soften the miso in a small bowl by stirring in tablespoonfuls of warm chicken broth.

Mixture should be very smooth like a thick sauce. In a pot over moderate heat, gradually stir softened miso into remaining broth and bring to a simmer. Add the mushrooms, ginger, onions, and tofu, and simmer gently until mushrooms are just tender. Be careful not to boil soup. Add chives. Ladle into bowls and serve immediately. May be topped with roasted sesame seeds.

Split Pea Soup

1	tablespoon olive oil
1	large carrot, chopped
1	large celery stalk, chopped
1/2	medium onion, chopped
1	bay leaf
6	cups fat-free chicken broth
1	pound dried split peas
	sea salt and pepper to taste

In a large saucepan, heat oil over medium heat. Add carrot, celery, onion, and bay leaf and sauté about 3-4 minutes. Add broth and split peas. Bring to a boil over high heat. Lower the heat, and simmer until peas are tender, about 1 hour. Puree 2/3 cup of soup in a blender, and then stir back into pot. Season with sea salt and pepper. If the soup is too thick, add more broth, and bring to a boil for an additional 20 seconds.

Brown Rice Casserole

1	cup raw brown rice
1	cup canned tomatoes
1/4	cup chopped onions
1	small garlic clove, grated
1/4	cup olive oil
1/4	cup black olives, chopped
1/4	cup green peppers, chopped
4	ounces mushrooms
2	cups boiling water

Heat oven to 350°.

Mix all ingredients in oven-safe casserole dish. Bake covered for 1½ hours.

Flounder Almandine

4	flounder filets
	Old Bay seasoning
1/3	cup butter, melted
1	cup almonds, slivered
	juice of 1 lemon
	fresh parsley sprig

Heat oven to 350°.

Place 4 flounder fillets in a well-greased, shallow baking dish. Baste the fillets with a mixture of Old Bay seasoning, melted butter, almonds, and lemon juice. Bake for 8 to 10 minutes. Top with sprig of fresh parsley.

Sweet Potato Souffle

2	cups mashed, cooked sweet potatoes
1/4	stick butter, melted
2	eggs
1/2	cup almond milk
1	teaspoon vanilla
1/3	cup apple juice
1/4	teaspoon nutmeg
1/2	teaspoon cinnamon
1/4	teaspoon allspice
1/2	teaspoon vanilla
1/3	cup of crushed pineapple, drained

Heat oven to 350°.

Mix all ingredients and place into a buttered baking dish. Bake for approximately 45 minutes or until mixture becomes firm and top is slightly browned.

Baked Chicken with Onions and Bell Pepper

2   tablespoons olive oil

1   clove garlic, minced

1/4   cup lemon juice

1   teaspoon dried basil leaves

1/2   teaspoon Old Bay seasoning

1/4   teaspoon ground black pepper

1/4   teaspoon sea salt

6   skinless, boneless chicken breast halves

1   small onion, sliced

1/2   bell pepper, sliced

Preheat oven to 350°.

Lightly oil a 9x13 baking dish. In a bowl, blend the olive oil, garlic, lemon juice, basil, Old Bay seasoning, pepper, and salt. Dip each chicken breast into the oil mixture. Arrange the chicken breasts in the baking dish. Top with slices of onion.

Bake approximately 25 minutes. Add slices of bell pepper, return to oven to cook for approximately an additional 5 minutes or until chicken is no longer pink and juices run clear.

Basil-Walnut Vinaigrette Dressing

1   tablespoon Dijon mustard

1/3   cup red wine vinegar

3/4   cup fresh basil leaves, coarsely chopped

       salt and black pepper, to taste

1   cup extra-virgin, cold pressed olive oil

1/2   cup walnuts (optional)

Combine mustard, vinegar, and basil in a food processor and season with salt and pepper. Blend for 1 minute. Stop and scrape down sides of processing bowl, and then blend for an additional 30 seconds. While blending, dribble olive oil into mixture, until completely blended. If walnuts are desired, add walnuts slowly, and blend until desired consistency is achieved. Cover and refrigerate until ready for use.

Stir-Fry Vegetable Medley

2	tablespoons olive oil
1	cup carrots, sliced
1	clove garlic, crushed
1	cup onion, sliced
1	cup green beans or broccoli
1	cup cauliflower or cabbage
2	tablespoons soy sauce
2	tablespoons lemon juice
1/4	cup vegetable or organic chicken broth
1/2	teaspoon sea salt (optional)
	dash pepper
2	tablespoons parsley, chopped

In wok or large heavy skillet, heat the oil. Add carrots, garlic, and onion; stir-fry 3-4 minutes. Stir in other vegetables, soy sauce, lemon juice, broth, salt, and pepper, and stir-fry 2 minutes, or cook until vegetables are just fork tender. Sprinkle chopped parsley over vegetable mixture.

Spicy Cilantro Sauce

1/2	cup fresh cilantro leaves
1/2	cup fresh parsley
1/4	cup water
1	teaspoon extra virgin olive oil
2	shallots, finely chopped
1	large garlic clove, minced
2	teaspoons fresh gingerroot, peeled and grated
1/4	teaspoon cumin
1	jalapeño pepper, seeded and chopped
2	tablespoons reduced sodium soy sauce
2	tablespoons fresh lime juice
	salt to taste
	ground pepper to taste

In a small saucepan of boiling water, blanch cilantro and parsley for 10 seconds and drain in a sieve. Refresh herbs in ice water for a few seconds, and drain in sieve again. Heat oil and 1 tablespoon of water in a small nonstick skillet. Add shallots, garlic, gingerroot, cumin, and jalapeño, and cook over moderately low heat, stirring, until shallots are softened. In a blender purée shallot mixture, blanched cilantro and parsley, the rest of the water, and the soy sauce until smooth, about 1 minute, and season with salt and pepper. Sauce may be made 1 day ahead and chilled, covered. Bring sauce to room temperature before serving. Just before serving, stir in lemon juice.

Lentil Soup

2	tablespoons olive oil
1	medium onion, chopped
2	carrots, diced
2	stalks celery, chopped
2	cloves garlic, minced
1	teaspoon dried oregano
1	bay leaf
1	teaspoon dried basil
2	cups dry lentils
8	cups water
1	(14.5 ounce) can crushed tomatoes
1/2	cup spinach, rinsed and thinly sliced
1	tablespoon vinegar
	sea salt to taste
	ground black pepper to taste

In a large soup pot, heat oil over medium heat. Add onions, carrots, and celery; cook and stir until onion is tender. Stir in garlic, bay leaf, oregano, and basil; cook for 2 minutes. Stir in lentils, and add water and tomatoes. Bring to a boil. Reduce heat, and simmer for at least 1 hour. When ready to serve stir in spinach, and cook until it wilts. Stir in vinegar, and season to taste with salt and pepper. Add more vinegar if desired.

Mango Sorbet

1/3	cup honey
1	cup water
2	tablespoons lemon or lime juice
4	medium-size ripe mangoes, peeled and coarsely chopped
2	egg whites, beaten until soft peaks form

Combine honey with water in a saucepan, and stir over medium heat until blended (do not allow to boil). Add juice, and simmer uncovered for about 3 minutes. Remove from heat and allow to cool. Blend or process mango until a smooth puree is achieved. Add lemon syrup and continue blending until well combined. Stir in egg whites, mixing thoroughly.

Pour mixture into a freezer-proof container and place in the freezer until it reaches a soft freeze. Remove mixture; chop and blend until smooth. Return to container and freeze until firm.

Potato Salad

2	pounds small red potatoes, unpeeled and well washed
2	large celery stalks, chopped
1/4	bell pepper
2	tablespoons minced purple onion or sweet onion
3/4	cup Omega-3 mayonnaise, or to taste
2	tablespoons cider vinegar
1	teaspoon tumeric
1	tablespoon mustard
1	teaspoon raw honey
1	teaspoon salt (add more if needed)
	several sprigs of fresh dill

Place whole unpeeled potatoes in a large saucepan or Dutch oven. Cover with water. Cover pan and bring to a boil. Simmer for 25 to 30 minutes, or until potatoes can be pierced easily with a fork. Drain and let cool until easy to handle, and then dice potatoes.

In a large bowl, combine potatoes with celery, bell pepper, and onion. Mix remaining ingredients in a small bowl. Add to potatoes and toss to blend. Place fresh dill over top of mixture. Cover and refrigerate until serving time.

French Toast

1	egg
1	cup almond milk
1	tablespoon honey
	dash of cinnamon
3	slices sprouted-grain bread
2	tablespoons ghee
1/4	cup blueberries (fresh or frozen)

In a bowl, beat the egg. Add almond milk, honey, and cinnamon. Beat mixture with a wire whisk. Dip sprouted-grain bread into mixture to coat both sides of bread. Melt ghee in pan. Place bread into pan. On low to medium heat, allow bread to slightly brown on both sides. Serve with maple syrup or top with blueberries.

Venison Stew

2	pounds venison, in one-inch cubes
2	tablespoons olive oil
1 1/2	quarts water
1	tablespoon salt
	beef bouillon or organic beef stock
4	large potatoes, peeled and cubed
4-5	large carrots, diced
2	large onions, cut into medium-size pieces
1/2	cup celery, chopped
1/3	cup bell pepper, chopped
1/2	tablespoon pepper
3	whole bay leaves
1/2	teaspoon of sage
1/4	teaspoon thyme
2	tablespoons parsley, chopped
	garlic clove, chopped

Brown venison with olive oil in Dutch oven. Add approximately 1 1/2 quarts of water. Add salt, bouillon (or beef stock). Add remaining spices and vegetables. Bring to a boil. Cover and reduce heat to low. Allow to cook slowly until meat is tender, about 2 1/2 hours.

Peach Cobbler

6-8	fresh firm peaches (or frozen)
1 1/2	cup peach nectar
1/2	teaspoon nutmeg
1/2	teaspoon cinnamon
1/4	teaspoon cloves
1	teaspoon lemon
1	tablespoon honey
1	teaspoon cornstarch (for thickening)

Topping Mix

1 1/2	cup almonds
3/4	cup instant oats
1	teaspoon vanilla
1	teaspoon cinnamon
2	tablespoons honey

Heat oven to 375°.

Heat all ingredients in a saucepan until peaches are just fork tender (not soft). For thickening, mix cornstarch with 3 tablespoons water. Stir until smooth. Pour into heated peach mixture. Continue to stir until mixture becomes slightly thickened. Place mixture in baking dish. Place topping mixture in food processor. Process until almonds are chopped and all ingredients are fully blended. Place topping mixture over peaches. Bake until cobbler turns golden brown. Remove from oven and allow cobbler to cool for about 20 minutes before serving.

Index

5-hydroxytryptophan (5-HTP), 224

A

acemannan, 153–154
acetaminophen, 155, 157, 293, 294, 376
Acid-Alkaline Food Guide, The (Brown & Trivieri), 226
Actos (pioglitazone), 386
acupuncture
    anxiety, 364
    general, 283–284
    immune system, 150, 156
    pain, 296–297, 299–301
    resources, 463
    sleep problems, 407
acute Lyme disease. *See* Lyme disease: stages
Adams, Patch, 437
adrenal glands
    anxiety, 364
    general, 147–149, 161–162, 165–166, 318, 323–327
    sleep, 186
    testing, 122, 340
    See also endocrine (hormonal) disruption
advanced glycation end products (AGEs), 182–183, 198
Afzelius, Arvid, 14
air quality, 393
alcohol, 66, 155, 157, 163, 223, 402
allergies and sensitivities
    depression, 367
    diet, 185, 198, 350–351
    inflammation, 179–180
    Continued

STARI, 40, 79–80
testing, 112–118, 121–124, 126
tick paralysis, 82
tularemia, 81, 85
West Nile virus, 81, 117
Colorado tick fever, 82, 118
complete blood count test (CBC), 119
comprehensive metabolic chemistry profile, 119
concentration problems. *See* brain fog
conjugated linoleic acid (CLA), 385
Conscious Breathing (Hendricks), 434
coordination problems, 54, 84
cortisol, 147–149, 323–324, 326–327. *See also* adrenal glands; endocrine
  (hormonal) disruption
cough, 65, 69, 81
counseling, 281, 364, 365–366, 443, 444–445. *See also* psychological health
countries more at risk for Lyme disease, 10–13, 41
Cousins, Norman, 437
C-reactive protein (CRP) test, 120, 191
culture tests, 106–107
curcumin, 157, 306–307, 375, 385
cyclical nature of Lyme disease, 54, 84, 252–253
Cymbalta (duloxetine), 295, 370
cystic fibrosis, 189
cytokines, 141–142, 143–144, 160, 181
cytomegalovirus (CMV), 117. *See also* viral diseases

D
dairy products, 204, 215, 218, 222
DEET, 32–33. *See also* insect repellents
dementia. *See* psychological health
dental health, 118, 391, 398–399, 462
depression
  causes, 263, 267, 292, 350, 366–367, 415
  general, 58, 84, 365–366, 411
  sleep problems, 405
  treatment, 270, 279, 336, 368–371 (see also antidepressants)
  See also psychological health
detoxification, 180, 332, 391–400, 412–413, 464. *See also* Lyme Inflammation
  Diet (LID):phase 1
devil's claw, 309

About the Author

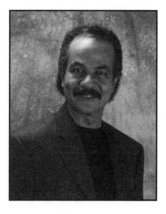

Kenneth B. Singleton, M.D., M.P.H., is a board-certified physician specializing in internal medicine. One of the most trusted voices in the medical field of Lyme disease today, Dr. Singleton earned his master's degree of public health from Johns Hopkins University and received training in acupuncture from UCLA. He completed his training in internal medicine at Wright State University in Dayton, Ohio, and has been practicing medicine since 1981. His medical practice is located in Towson, Maryland.

www.lymedoctor.com